LEGAL ASPECTS OF PHYSIOTHERAPY

LEGAL ASPECTS OF PHYSIOTHERAPY

BRIDGIT C. DIMOND

MA, LLB, DSA, AHSM, Barrister-at-law,
Emeritus Professor of the University of Glamorgan

Blackwell
Science

© 1999 Bridgit C. Dimond

Blackwell Science Ltd
Editorial Offices:
Osney Mead, Oxford OX2 0EL
25 John Street, London WC1N 2BL
23 Ainslie Place, Edinburgh EH3 6AJ
350 Main Street, Malden
  MA 02148 5018, USA
54 University Street, Carlton
  Victoria 3053, Australia
10, rue Casimir Delavigne
  75006 Paris, France

Other Editorial Offices:

Blackwell Wissenschafts-Verlag GmbH
Kurfürstendamm 57
10707 Berlin, Germany

Blackwell Science KK
MG Kodenmacho Building
7–10 Kodenmacho Nihombashi
Chuo-ku, Tokyo 104, Japan

First published 1999

Set in 10/12 pt Century
by DP Photosetting, Aylesbury, Bucks
Printed and bound in Great Britain at
the Alden Press, Oxford

The Blackwell Science logo is a trade mark of
Blackwell Science Ltd, registered at the United
Kingdom Trade Marks Registry

DISTRIBUTORS

Marston Book Services Ltd
PO Box 269
Abingdon
Oxon OX14 4YN
(*Orders:* Tel: 01235 465500
          Fax: 01235 465555)

USA
  Blackwell Science, Inc.
  Commerce Place
  350 Main Street
  Malden, MA 02148 5018
  (*Orders:* Tel: 800 759 6102
            781 388 8250
          Fax: 781 388 8255)

Canada
  Login Brothers Book Company
  324 Saulteaux Crescent
  Winnipeg, Manitoba R3J 3T2
  (*Orders:* Tel: 204 837-2987
          Fax: 204 837-3116)

Australia
  Blackwell Science Pty Ltd
  54 University Street
  Carlton, Victoria 3053
  (*Orders:* Tel: 03 9347 0300
          Fax: 03 9347 5001)

A catalogue record for this title is available
from the British Library

ISBN 0-632-05108-6

Library of Congress
Cataloging-in-Publication Data
is available

For further information on
Blackwell Science, visit our website
www.blackwell-science.com

TO CARMEL

Contents

Foreword

The impact of the law and the legal process continues to confuse and worry physiotherapists. The Society is continually contacted by members who may have been contacted by a solicitor, have heard that there may be a complaint made against them, or have had to deal with a patient who is threatening to sue. These members are naturally worried and often extremely fearful. This fear and worry is usually based on a lack of knowledge and understanding.

This book is a vital tool in supplying physiotherapists with knowledge of the law and its relevance to their practice, helping them to understand what the possible implications are of the solicitor's letter, or of the patient who decides to sue.

The profession of physiotherapy has expanded its boundaries: the physiotherapist can be found working in a wide range of environments; often as a lone practitioner or part of a multi-professional team. As the range of modalities, philosophies of care and approaches expand to encompass complementary therapies (including the application of prescription only drugs), as the demand for clinically effective interventions increase, and as handling patients for therapeutic purposes continues to be central to practice, the risk of physiotherapists being sued or subjected to complaints can only increase.

Professor Dimond gives physiotherapists the knowledge and understanding of the law to put practice into perspective and enable therapists to continue to evaluate, explore and expand their practice in the best interest of patient care. Taking real situations that therapists encounter on a day to day basis, she teases out the ethical and legal dilemas that may arise from these and sets out what the law says about these situations. The legal system is clearly explained and each chapter includes practical exercises that will appeal to the problem-solving approach adopted by therapists when caring for patients.

I first met Bridget Dimond many years ago on a University of Wales Masters course in the Philosophy of Health Care. A reasonable course of study for a therapist, but perhaps a slightly less obvious one for a lawyer. However, to my mind, it is this width and depth of perception that makes Bridgit's writing and advice so applicable to everyday practice. She understands that therapists are dealing with real people in real life, and assists therapists with practical information and advice to enable them to practise professionally with the added understanding of the legal and ethical context.

I know I will be using this book on a regular basis to give information and advice to members to reassure and inform.

Penelope Robinson
Director of Professional Affairs
Chartered Society of Physiotherapy

Preface

The legal issues which can arise in the practice of physiotherapy are vast and cover many areas of specialist law. It has been my task to provide physiotherapy practitioners, students, managers and those in related professions and posts with an introduction to the law which relates to the practice of physiotherapy. There is also a chapter for those in independent practice, covering the law and regulations which apply to a business. It is assumed that the reader will have no previous legal knowledge and a glossary has been provided to explain some of the technical legal language. This is essentially a book which is concerned with the practical aspects of the law as it applies to physiotherapy and examples of the specific legal concerns are derived to a considerable extent from the many questions raised with me by physiotherapists across the country. The anticipation is that this introduction to the law will enable the physiotherapist to develop the knowledge and awareness of the legal implications of her practice so that she can protect both her client and herself.

Terminology in relation to gender always causes concern and I have recognised the fact that the profession is mainly female and thus referred to the physiotherapist as 'she' or 'her'. This should be interpreted as including 'he' and 'him'. Persons cared for by physiotherapists are variously called 'patients, clients, residents, customers and consumers' and I have in the main used the term 'client', but where the context makes other terms more appropriate I have used these. I use the word 'physiotherapist', but it must be understood that by this I mean a Chartered Physiotherapist registered under the Council for Professions Supplementary to Medicine.

The statutory changes which took place in 1990 with the introduction of the internal market into health care and the developments within community care are due to be changed under proposals in the White Paper *The New NHS: Modern Dependable*, which will have major implications for the work of the physiotherapist. A National Institute for Clinical Excellence, a Commission for Health Improvements, National Standards of Clinical Practice, and Clinical Governance will all have a great impact on the practice of physiotherapy. Further major changes are to come with a comprehensive reorganisation of the regulation of the professions supplementary to medicine currently before the Government. It is hoped that the knowledge obtained from this book on the law applying to physiotherapy will enable the reader to meet these challenges and continue to develop a comprehensive and high quality service to her clients.

Section A describes the basic principles which apply to professional issues. Section B looks at the rights of the client: the right to care, to refuse treatment, to confidentiality and to have access to records. Section C considers the account-ability of the physiotherapist in the civil and criminal courts, looking at negligence, health and safety, record keeping, giving evidence in court and handling complaints. It also looks at the specific issues which arise in relation to equipment and transport. Section D looks at management in the employment and statutory organisation of the NHS, the community and in private practice. Section E covers specialist client groups and other areas not considered appropriate for the earlier sections. I had considered including chapters on all the different areas of work in which physiotherapists practise (respiratory, neurology, orthopaedics etc.), but I soon discovered that I could write a different book on each specialty. I therefore decided to concentrate on the general legal areas with separate chapters for the different client groups but to use examples from the different specialties across all chapters. Questions and exercises are included at the end of each chapter to enable the book to be used as a teaching aid.

Inevitably, even before the laptop is switched off, the law has changed as new statutes are passed and new cases decided. However, this book should provide the framework on which the physiotherapist can continue to build her knowledge of law in order to protect her patient/client, her colleagues and herself.

Acknowledgements

I am considerably indebted to the numerous chartered physiotherapists who have assisted me with topics which should be included and which were relevant to their practice. I should like in particular to thank Pen Robinson who is professional adviser of the Chartered Society for her encouragement, invaluable assistance and professional knowledge.

Many of the chairmen and members of the physiotherapy special interest groups have also given me considerable help in suggesting topics which I should include and I would therefore like to thank Ruth Hawkes, Olwen Finlay, Liz Holey, Liz Hardy, Susie Durrell, Susan Edwards, Nicola Ford, Patricia Shelley, Maggie Campbell, Jane Sclater and Judy Mead of the CSP; also Anna Sewerniak, Senior Information Officer of the CSP, who was extremely helpful in enabling me to access information held by them. Thanks are also due to Caroline Gordan, a physiotherapist and now trainee solicitor, Sue Smith, Allen Mason, Sybil Williams and her colleagues in the ACPPLD; also Eleri Cross and Ann Hughes at Whitchurch Hospital.

I would also pay tribute to Tamsin Bacchus, my exacting copy editor whose advice is gratefully received, and once again I acknowledge with thanks the encouragement and forbearance of my family, particularly Bette who read the typescript and prepared the index.

My special thanks are due to Carmel Richards for her support and encouragement and to whom this book is dedicated.

Abbreviations

ACAS	Advisory, Conciliation and Arbitration Service
ACPAT	Association of Chartered Physiotherapists in Animal Therapy
ACPC	Area Child Protection Committee
ADL	Activities of Daily Living
ADR	Alternative Dispute Resolution
ASW	Approved Social Worker
BAOT	British Association of Occupational Therapists
BCMA	British Complementary Medicine Association
BMA	British Medical Association
CA	Court of Appeal
CCAM	Council for Complementary and Alternative Therapies
CCP	Collaborative Clinical Care Profiles
CDI	Community Dependency Index
CHC	Community Health Council
CHP	Council for Health Professions
CIG	Clinical Interest Group
COSHH	Control of Substances Hazardous to Health [Regulations]
CPA	Care Programme Approach
CPA	Consumer Protection Act 1987
CPAUIA	Commissioner for Protection Against Unlawful Industrial Action
CPD	Continuing Professional Development
CPN	Community Psychiatric Nurse
CPS	Crown Prosecution Service
CPSM	Council for Professions Supplementary to Medicine
CRE	Commission on Racial Equality
CRTUM	Commissioner for the Rights of Trade Union Members
CSP	Chartered Society of Physiotherapy
DFG	Disabled Facilities Grants
DHA	District Health Authority
DISC	Disability Information and Study Centre
DSS	Department of Social Security
EC	European Community
EEA	European Economic Area
EL	Executive Letter
EOC	Equal Opportunities Commission
ESP	Extended Scope Practitioners
FHSA	Family Health Services Authority

GMC	General Medical Council
GP	General Practitioner
GPFH	GP Fundholder
HASAW	Health and Safety at Work etc. Act 1974
HC	Health Circular (from Department of Health)
HCHS	Hospital and Community Health Services
HIV	Human Immunodeficiency Virus
HL	House of Lords
HMSO	Her Majesty's Stationery Office
HRSW	Health Related Social Worker
HSC	Health Services Commissioner (Ombudsman)
HSE	Health and Safety Executive
HSG	Health Service Guidance
ICM	Institute of Complementary Medicine
ICP	Integrated Care Pathway
IV	Intravenous
JCC	Joint Consultative Committee
JP	Justice of the Peace
LA	Local Authority
LAC	Local Authority Circular
LEA	Local Education Authority
LREC	Local Research Ethics Committee
MDA	Medical Devices Agency
MHAC	Mental Health Act Commission
MHRT	Mental Health Review Tribunal
MND	Motor Neurone Disease
NAA	National Assistance Act
NAESC	National Association for the Education of Sick Children
NAHAT	National Association of Health Authorities and Trusts
NDC	National Disability Council
NHSME	National Health Service Management Executive
NFR	Not For Resuscitation
NFR	Neurophysiological Facilitation of Respiration
NSPCC	National Society for the Prevention of Cruelty to Children
NVQ	National Vocational Qualification
OOS	Occupational Overuse Syndrome
OPD	Out-patient Department
OT	Occupational therapist
PACE	Physiotherapy Access to Continuing Education
PC	Privy Council
PCC	Professional Conduct Committee
PPA	Prescription Pricing Authority
PPC	Preliminary Proceedings Committee
PPC	Professional Practice Committee
PRN	As Required (of medicines)
PSM	Profession Supplementary to Medicine
QBD	Queens Bench Division (of the High Court)
RCN	Royal College of Nursing

RMO	Responsible Medical Officer
RPSGB	Royal Pharmaceutical Society of Great Britain
RSC	Rules of the Supreme Court
RSI	Repetitive Strain Injury
SENT	Special Educational Needs Tribunal
SOAD	Second Opinion Appointed Doctor
SRV	Social Role Valorisation
SSD	Social Services Department
SSI	Social Services Inspectorate
SWD	Short Wave Diathermy
TENS	Transcutaneous Electrical Nerve Stimulation
TU	Trade Union
UKCC	United Kingdom Central Council for Nursing, Midwifery and Health Visiting
UKCP	United Kingdom Council for Psychotherapy
WHC	Welsh Health Circular
WRULD	Work Related Upper Limb Disorder

Clinical interest and occupational groups of the Chartered Society of Physiotherapy

Acupuncture Association of Chartered Physiotherapists (AACP)

British Association of Chartered Physiotherapists in **Amputee Rehabilitation** (BACPAR)

Association of Chartered Physiotherapists in **Animal Therapy** (ACPAT)

Association of **Blind** Physiotherapists (ABCP)

British Association of **Bobath Trained Therapists** (BABTT)

Association of Chartered Physiotherapists in **Cardiac Rehabilitation** (ACPICR)

Association of Chartered Physiotherapists in the **Community** (ACPC)

Chartered Physiotherapists in **Education** (CPE)

Association of Chartered Physiotherapists interested in **Electrotherapy** (ACPIE)

British Association of **Hand Therapists** (BAHT)

Hydrotherapy Association of Chartered Physiotherapists (HACP)

Association of Chartered Physiotherapists in **Independent Hospitals** (ACPIH)

Association of Chartered Physiotherapists for People with **Learning Disabilities** (ACPPLD)

Manipulation Association of Chartered Physiotherapists (MACP)

Association of Chartered Physiotherapists in **Management** (ACPM)

Association of Chartered Physiotherapists interested in **Massage** (ACPIM)

Chartered Physiotherapists in **Mental Health** (ACPMH)

Association of Chartered Physiotherapists in **Neurology** (ACPIN)

Association of Chartered Physiotherapists in **Occupational Health** (ACPOH)

Chartered Physiotherapists working with **Older People** (AGILE, formerly ACPSIEP)

Association of Chartered Physiotherapists in **Oncology & Palliative Care** (ACPOPC)

Association of **Orthopaedic** Chartered Physiotherapists (AOCP)

Association of Chartered Physiotherapists in **Orthopaedic Medicine** (ACPOM)
Association of **Paediatric** Chartered Physiotherapists (APCP)
Physiotherapy **Pain** Association (PPA)
Organisation of Chartered Physiotherapists in **Private Practice** (OCPPP)
Association of Chartered Physiotherapists in **Reflex Therapy** (ACPIRT)
Association of Chartered Physiotherapists in **Respiratory Care** (ACPRC)
Rheumatic Care Association of Chartered Physiotherapists (RCACP)
Association of Chartered Physiotherapists in **Therapeutic Riding** (ACPTR)
Association of Chartered Physiotherapists in **Sports Medicine** (ACPSM)
Association of Chartered Physiotherapists in **Women's Health** (ACPWH)

Chapter 1
Introduction

Why does a physiotherapist need to know the law?

A twenty year old girl, Sandra, was injured in a road accident when a lorry went out of control and crashed into her as she was walking along the pavement. She survived with severe brain damage and was transferred to a neurosurgical unit. The consultant neurologist warned the parents that she might never recover fully and in fact might stay in a persistent vegetative state. The nurses however encouraged the parents to be more optimistic and gave them contact addresses for voluntary organisations. Her father thought it might be best if she was taken off the ventilator, but her mother wanted all possible treatment and care to continue. Sandra remained in a coma for several months, during which time she had intensive physiotherapy. She developed a severe pressure sore as a result of a splint which was badly applied at the time of the accident. She slowly recovered consciousness and had suffered a severe left sided hemiplegia. She moved to a specialist rehabilitation unit, returning home for the weekends. Her parents paid for her to have private physiotherapy at the weekends. The occupational therapist recommended that she should have a bed downstairs and should use a hoist for bathing. Sandra refused since she was determined to be independent. She was however concerned that her compensation following the road accident might be reduced the more she persevered in her exercises. She was also hoping to be able to drive a specially adapted car but, since she suffered epileptic fits following the brain injury, was advised to wait till these were clearly under control. Later she ended in-patient treatment, returning to the centre for check ups and relying upon local physiotherapists for her care. They liaised with the centre.

Legal issues which arise

The facts describe a situation well known to many physiotherapists and repeated in various guises across the country every day. On examination however it gives rise to numerous legal issues. Some of them are shown in Figure 1.1.

Figure 1.1 **Legal issues arising from Sandra's situation.**

(1) Consent issues in treating a mentally incapacitated adult. Do parents have the right to give and withhold consent?

(2) Standard of care in caring for a comatose patient. At what point and on the basis of what circumstances can active treatment be withdrawn? What rights do the relatives have?

(3) Giving information to relatives about prognosis and about voluntary groups.

(4) Liability for causing pressure sores and for treating them.

(5) Manual handling implications when a client refuses to use a hoist.

(6) Duty of carers when a patient with uncontrolled epilepsy wishes to drive a car.

(7) Duty of staff if patients are incapable of driving because of conditions such as epilepsy but refuse to accept their advice.

(8) Entitlements to NHS and Social Services care.

(9) Financial support for disabled.

(10) Rights to have specially adapted wheelchairs and cars.

(11) Compensation following a road traffic accident. How it is calculated and the extent to which it will be reduced if a patient puts more effort into recovery.

(12) Who would have administered the finances if she had remained in a comatose state but had been awarded substantial compensation.

Physiotherapists and the law

Figure 1.1 shows only a few of the legal issues which can confront the physiotherapist in one particular case. It provides the justification for this book which aims to explain within the context of physiotherapy the law which applies to physiotherapists' practice. Physiotherapists need to have sufficient familiarity with the basic principles of law, so that when they are in a difficult situation they know immediately the laws which apply and the point at which they need to seek expert advice.

Research was undertaken by Herman Triezenberg[1] to identify present and future ethical issues arising in physical therapy practice. Sixteen issues were raised: six involving patients' rights and welfare, five professional issues and five business and economic factors. Of these, 13 had never been discussed in previous physical therapy literature. The list is shown in Figure 1.2. It will be noted that each ethical issue also raises legal questions. The fact that the respondents to his questionnaires were US citizens is reflected in the number of topics relating to the financial relationship between therapist and patient and the dangers of exploitation and fraud. Legal issues arising from private practice are considered in Chapter 19. In a commentary on the research Ruth Purtilo[2], Director of the Center for Health Policy and Ethics, Creighton University, Omaha states:

'The more physical therapists can do to create a broad base of understanding about the ethical issues facing the profession, the more likely we are to enter the new millennium prepared to make a meaningful contribution.'

Exactly the same point could be made about a legal understanding.

Figure 1.2 **Ethical issues in physical therapy practice.**

(1) Overutilisation of services.
(2) Identification of the factors that constitute informed consent.
(3) Confidentiality of patient.
(4) Justification of fees charged.
(5) Maintenance of truth in advertising.
(6) Identification and prevention of sexual misconduct by therapists.
(7) Maintenance of clinical competence.
(8) Adherence to ethical guidelines in research.
(9) Endorsement of equipment and products in which the therapist has a financial interest.
(10) Determination of appropriate level of resourcing.
(11) Involvement of therapists in business relationships which could have potential for patient exploitation.
(12) Identification and elimination of fraud in billing.
(13) Duty to provide treatment according to needs of patient irrespective of patient's personal or social characteristics.
(14) Responsibility of therapists to respond to the environment.
(15) Duty of physical therapists to report misconduct in colleagues.
(16) Need for therapists to define the limits of personal relationships within the professional setting.

Taken from Figure 5 of Herman L. Triezenberg's 'The Identification of Ethical Issues in Physical Therapy Practice'. *Physical Therapy*, October 1996 Vol. 76, no. 10

Definition of physiotherapy

A Royal Charter was granted in 1920 to the body which later became the Chartered Society of Physiotherapy and established as the only recognised examining and professional body for physiotherapists in the UK. It was authorised to

> 'promote a curriculum and standard of qualification for persons engaged in the practice of massage, medical gymnastics, electrotherapeutics and kindred methods for treatment [and] to make and maintain lists of persons considered to be qualified to practise in such methods of treatment.'

The new Curriculum Framework drafted by the CSP in 1996 defines physiotherapy as:

> 'a health care profession which emphasises the use of physical approaches in the promotion, maintenance and restoration of an individual's physical, psychological and social well-being, encompassing variations in health status.'[3]

It then identifies eight outcomes – qualities which a graduate physiotherapist would be expected to possess.

Anne Parry points out the dangers of researchers defining physiotherapy in a minimalist way, i.e. by limiting it to exercise therapy, massage and physical applications, and then concluding that it is ineffective[4]. She urges 'Complain vociferously when "physiotherapy" is misused. If you don't care, no one else will.'

Once need for a physiotherapist has been determined, the physiotherapist will:

- Agree long and short term goals with the patient, carer and team.
- Determine the cost-effective type, frequency, duration, progression and mix of skills needed.
- Give a degree of priority to the case.
- Take the case onto the case load when a full care régime can be undertaken.
- Continue to re-assess and review the treatment plan.
- Discharge the patient when goals are met or progress is optimal.
- Take full legal responsibility for his/her care.[5]

All these stages have legal implications which will be covered in this book.

History of physiotherapy

Physiotherapy has ancient origins. In a review of the use of physiotherapy in health and lung conditions Diana Innocenti[6] discusses how massage and gymnastics were practised in the ancient world and were documented in China by Kong-Fu at around 3000 BC. There is also evidence of the use of massage and gymnastics for the improvement of health in Greece at around 700 BC. John Hutchinson presented his research on lung volumes and spirometry to the Royal Medical and Chirurgical Society on 28 April 1846. Allen Mason's many articles on the history of individual aspects of physiotherapy practice provide an amusing insight into its ancient past and into the different forms of treatment.

The modern development of the profession which led to state registration of physiotherapy practice probably begins with the establishment of the Society of Masseurs in 1894. Jane Wicksteed has researched the history of the Chartered Society of Physiotherapy from 1894–1945[7] and describes how the original founders, nurses or midwives by training but all practising as masseuses, were anxious to establish their credibility as masseuses in the eyes of the public. They therefore set up a Council and Society, establishing examinations and membership rules and sought support from doctors as patrons and external examiners.

The development of the Society in the 20th century illustrates the way in which new groups and new practices were assimilated within the main structure. In 1900 the Society became incorporated and linked in with Swedish physical exercises or gymnastics. New training schools were established and popularity increased. In 1916 Queen Mary became patron of the Society. In 1920 a Royal Charter was awarded and the Chartered Society of Massage and Medical Gymnastics (CSMMG) was formed with the amalgamation of the Incorporated Society of Trained Masseurs and the Institute of Massage and Remedial Gymnasts, the chairman being a member of the medical profession. Light and electrotherapy and hydrotherapy were added to the syllabus and examinations. In 1942 the name of the Chartered Society of Physiotherapy was adopted when the CSMMG and the Incorporation of Physiotherapists amalgamated. In 1986 the Chartered Society merged with the Society of Remedial Gymnastics and Recreational Therapy and 726 remedial gymnasts became members of the CSP[8].

In 1960 physiotherapists obtained state registration under the Professions Supplementary to Medicine Act 1960.

The future

The Heathrow debate was a meeting in 1995 of the Chief Nursing Officers of England, Scotland, Wales and Northern Ireland to consider the future development of nursing. Following this Jean Potts[9], in the Founders' Lecture (established in honour of the Founders in 1914), looked at:

- the changing context of physiotherapy practice
- the nature of that practice
- regulation
- implications for education and training and
- future challenges, including the number and diversity of health care professions involved in the primary care of patients.

She identified a core area of practice, knowledge and skills common to a variety of professions, with each profession building on this with their own particular and unique skills. Similarly distinct branches of care lead from common foundation studies: namely, care of the elderly, children and adolescents, women, those with learning disabilities, those with musculoskeletal or neurological disorders and the mentally ill. In summarising the impact of this in terms of education and regulation Jean Potts says:

'From the education point of view, it would be relatively easy to design multi-competency professional health care routes, and would be extremely cost-effective in terms of staff resources.'

Clinical interest groups of the CSP

The breadth of physiotherapy practice is supported by clinical interest groups and special interest groups within the CSP. They have been described by Ruth Dubbey[10] as serving

'as a forum for physiotherapists to encourage, promote and facilitate interchange of thoughts and ideas as well as providing expertise with education, practice and research in their specialty.'

There are 22 recognised CIGs and many more non-recognised groups representing the diverse interests and specialties of physiotherapists. Criteria for a CIG to be recognised by the CSP were developed by the Professional Practice Committee in 1992 and are shown in Figure 1.3.

***Figure 1.3* Criteria for recognition of a Clinical Interest Group (CIG).**

- That the proposed group has a minimum number of 50 subscribers who are chartered physiotherapists, and that it has been in existence for at least 2 years.
- That the group provides for a distinct clinical area or client group for physiotherapy.
- That the group demonstrates a clear and valid relationship between its area of expertise/specialism and the core of physiotherapy as described in the Charter.
- That the group demonstrates a commitment to developing areas of expertise through education, practice and research, and will be of benefit to the current and future needs of both the general public and the profession.

There exists a Clinical Interest Group Liaison Committee which meets four times a year at the CSP headquarters.

Recent developments in terms of training etc. and Continuing Professional Development (CPD) are considered in Chapter 5.

The diversity and range of treatments provided by the physiotherapist means that the laws covered in this book will be extensive and many specialist areas will be discussed. First however it is necessary to understand the basic structure, language and sources of law and it is this to which we turn in the next chapter.

 Questions and exercises

1 How would you define the core work of the physiotherapist?
2 To what extent do you consider it is appropriate to describe a physiotherapist as 'supplementary to medicine'?
3 Do you consider the personal beliefs and philosophies of the physiotherapist are relevant to her work? To what extent, if any, should they be taken into account by a prospective employer?

References

1 Triezenberg, H.L. (1996) The Identification of Ethical Issues in Physical Therapy Practice, *Physical Therapy* **76** 10, 1097–1108.
2 Purtilo, R. (1996) Invited Commentary, *Physical Therapy* **76** 10, 1107–8.
3 Thornton, E. (1996) Framework for Flexibility: A new Physiotherapy curriculum, *Physiotherapist* **82** 7, 387–8.
4 Parry, A. (1997) Choice Treatment for Physiotherapy, *Physiotherapy* **83** 6, 277.
5 Squires, A. & Hastings, M. (1997) Physiotherapy with Older People: Calculating Staffing Need, *Physiotherapy* **83** 2, 58–64.
6 Innocenti, D. (1996) An Overview of the Development of Breathing Exercises into the Specialty of Physiotherapy for Heart and Lung Conditions, *Physiotherapy* **82** 12, 681–93.
7 Wicksteed, J.H. (1948) *The Growth of a Profession*, Edward Arnold, London (reprinted by the CSP in 1994 to celebrate the centenary).

8   Barclay, J. (1994) *In Good Hands: the History of the Chartered Society of Physio-therapists 1894–1994*, Butterworth Heinemann, Oxford.

9   Potts, J. (1996) Physiotherapy in the Next Century: Opportunities and Challenges, *Physiotherapy* **82** 3, 150–5.

10 Dubbey, R. (1996) Clinical Interest Groups, *Physiotherapy* **82** 5, 283–4.

Chapter 2
The Legal System

Law can be perplexing to those who have never studied it. The jargon, the complexity of a lawyer's answer to the simplest question, can place a significant barrier between the ordinary health professional and the law practitioner. However any health professional or health service manager has to work within the context of the law, and therefore has to know the basic legal principles which constrain or empower her. She also needs to have a clear understanding of the point at which it is essential to bring in legal advice and support. This chapter is aimed at providing an introduction to the basic terms which are used and a description of the framework within which the law is implemented. A glossary at the end of this book provides an explanation of some of the technical terms which are used. The following topics will be covered:

- Sources of law
- Civil and criminal law
- Civil and criminal courts
- Types of civil action
- Public and private law
- Legal personnel

- Procedure in civil courts
- Procedure in criminal courts
- Accusatorial system
- Law and ethics
- Guidance on conduct and procedures

Sources of law

Law derives from two main sources: statute law and the common law. These are illustrated in Figure 2.1.

Figure 2.1 **Derivation and sources of law.**

Statute Law	Common Law
EC Regulations	**EC Court rulings**
Acts of Parliament/Statutes	**House of Lords** – cases on
made by House of Commons	important points of law
House of Lords	**Court of Appeal**
Royal Assent	**High Court/Crown Court**
Statutory Instruments	Decisions binding on basis of rules of
made by relevant Ministry	precedent and hierarchy
laid before Parliament	

Statutes and statutory instruments as well as previous cases are interpreted by judges and the decisions become part of the common law

Statute law

Statute law is based on legislation passed through the agreed constitutional process. Legislation of the European Community now takes precedence over the Acts of Parliament of the United Kingdom Government. This country must observe the Treaties of the European Community, and is bound by Regulations made by the European Council and the European Commission. These have direct application to Member States. This is in contrast to the European Directives, which must be incorporated into UK law to be effective (although they do apply directly to state authorities).

A bill is introduced into either the House of Lords or House of Commons, sometimes by the Government and sometimes by a private member, and follows through a recognised procedure by way of hearings, committee stages and the report stage. Eventually, following agreement by both Houses and the signature of the Queen, it becomes an Act of Parliament. The actual date it comes into force will either be set out in the Act itself or will be determined at a later date by Statutory Instrument. The Act of Parliament may provide for powers to be delegated to Ministers and others to enact detailed supplementary rules. These are known as Statutory Instruments. They must be formally placed before Parliament before coming into effect but there is no provision for debate and discussion.

Common law

Decisions by judges in courts create what is known as the common law. A recognised hierarchy of the courts determines which previous decisions are binding on courts hearing similar cases. The European Court of Justice based in Luxembourg can hear cases between member states on European law, such as quota disputes or applications by domestic courts for a ruling on a particular point of law.

Figure 2.2 shows the civil court system and Figure 2.3 shows the criminal court system.

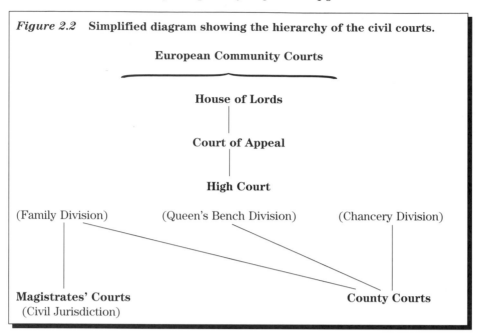

Figure 2.2   **Simplified diagram showing the hierarchy of the civil courts.**

European Community Courts

House of Lords

Court of Appeal

High Court

(Family Division)   (Queen's Bench Division)   (Chancery Division)

Magistrates' Courts   **County Courts**
(Civil Jurisdiction)

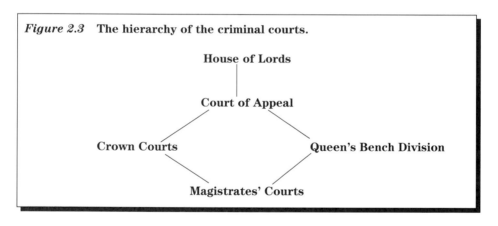

Figure 2.3   **The hierarchy of the criminal courts.**

House of Lords

Court of Appeal

Crown Courts   **Queen's Bench Division**

Magistrates' Courts

A recognised system of reporting of judges' decisions ensures certainty over what was stated and the facts of the cases. The main principles which are set out in a case are known as the *ratio decidendi* (reasons for the decision). Other parts of a judge's speech which are not considered to be part of the *ratio decidendi* are known as *obiter dicta* (things said by the way). Only the *ratio decidendi* is directly binding on lower courts, but the *obiter dicta* may influence the decision of judges in later court cases. It may be possible for judges to 'distinguish' previous cases and not follow them on the grounds that the facts are significantly different. For example before the Occupier's Liability Act 1984 was passed which defined the liability of an occupier of premises towards trespassers, the liability was based on decisions made by judges on particular facts. Cases which involved harm to children (where the occupier had been held liable) were held not to be binding on judges hearing cases involving adults, so that occupiers were not liable to an adult trespasser. The earlier cases relating to children were 'distinguished'.

Judges are however bound by statute and if case law results in an unsatisfactory situation, then this may be remedied by new amending legislation. Statutes nevertheless have to be interpreted by judges in court cases if disputes arise in relation to what the statute means. Thus law develops through a mix of statutory promulgation and common law decision making.

Procedure for judicial review

The decisions of judicial and administrative bodies can be challenged by an application to the Queen's Bench Division for the decision or adjudication to be reviewed. Thus if a person detained under the Mental Health Act 1983 were to appeal unsuccessfully to a Mental Health Review Tribunal (MHRT) and considered that the decision not to discharge him was based upon a failure to apply the correct law or because the principles of natural justice were infringed (e.g. the chairman was prejudiced against him personally), he could apply to the High Court, Queen's Bench Division for the decision of the MHRT to be reviewed[1]. However this procedure is not recommended where an Act of Parliament lays down a specific procedure for challenging the decision of a statutory body. For example in the case of *Gossington* v. *Ealing Borough Council*[2], Mr Gossington applied for judicial review of the decision of London Borough of Ealing to provide him with only five hours of home help per week instead of the original ten hours. The judge held that, since the Act provided for an application to the Secretary of State if a local authority fails to carry out its statutory functions, the applicant had not exhausted the other available routes open to him to remedy the wrong he felt that he had suffered, and therefore the application for judicial review was refused.

The Human Rights Act 1998

The European Convention on Human Rights (1950) provides protection for the fundamental rights and freedoms of all people[3]. The UK is a signatory as are many European countries which are not members of the European Community. Thus Norway is a signatory to the European Convention on Human Rights but not a member of the European Community. It is enforced through the European Commission and the European Court of Human Rights, which meets in Strasbourg. However following the passing of the Human Rights Act 1998 most of the Articles will be directly enforceable in the UK courts in relation to alleged infringement by a public authority or an organisation which performs a public function. The Articles included in the Human Rights Act 1998 are shown in Appendix 1.

Other international charters relating to health

This country is also a signatory to, or has recognised, many other International Charters which recognise rights in a variety of fields. These include: UN

Convention on the Rights of the Child, the UN Convention on the Elimination of All Forms of Discrimination against Women, the Universal Declaration of Human Rights, the Declaration of Helsinki developed by the World Health Organisation in 1964 (relating to research practice). These Charters are not directly enforced in this country, though their principles may be contained in statutory or common law, and reflected in guidance provided by the Department of Health and professional bodies and organisations.

Civil and criminal law

The civil law covers the law which governs disputes between citizens (including corporate bodies) or between citizens and the state. Thus contract law and the law of torts (civil wrongs excluding breach of contract), rights over property, marital disputes and the wrongful exercise of power by a statutory authority all come under the civil law.

Criminal law relates to actions which can be followed by criminal proceedings in which an accused is prosecuted. The sources of criminal law are both statutory and the common law: thus the definition of murder derives from a decision of the courts in the seventeenth century whereas theft is defined by a 1968 Act of Parliament as amended by subsequent legislation.

An illustration of some of the principal differences between a civil case and a criminal case are shown in Figure 2.4.

Figure 2.4 **Differences between civil and criminal hearings.**

	Criminal hearings	**Civil hearings**
basis of action	a charge of a criminal offence	an alleged wrong by one person against another
action brought by	Crown Prosecution Service (CPS) – occasionally a private prosecution	the person wronged (the Plaintiff or Claimant) or if a child, a person on his/her behalf
standard of proof	beyond reasonable doubt	balance of probabilities
facts decided by	Magistrates Courts – the magistrate(s) Crown Court – the jury	the judge
law applied by	Magistrates Courts – the magistrate(s) (lay magistrates advised by legally qualified clerk) Crown Court – the judge	the judge(s)

There is an overlap between civil and criminal wrongs: thus touching a person without his consent may be a civil wrong, known as trespass to the person. It may also be a crime i.e. a criminal assault or battery. Similarly driving a car carelessly may lead to criminal proceedings for driving without due care and attention but if someone was injured as a result would also lead to civil proceedings for negligence as it is almost certain that the driver would have been in breach of a duty of care owed to that person. In one case where a patient alleged that an unregistered physiotherapist had raped and indecently assaulted her, the police decided not to prosecute. However the patient brought a civil action for assault and obtained compensation of over £25 000, including an amount representing aggravated damages because the defendant put her through the harrowing ordeal of having to appear in court[4].

In another case an anaesthetist failed to realise that during an operation a tube had become disconnected as a result of which the patient died. He was prosecuted in the criminal courts and convicted of manslaughter[5]. There would also be liability on him and his employers in the civil courts for his negligence in causing the death of the patient (see Chapter 10). The Law Commission[6] has recommended that the law should be changed to enable it to be made easier for corporations and statutory bodies to be prosecuted for manslaughter and this may lead to more charges being brought in connection with deaths which arise from gross negligence. Punishment and possibly imprisonment can therefore be meted out to the perpetrators of grossly negligent or reckless practice rather than just payment of compensation awarded by the civil courts which would in any event be covered by insurance.

Both criminal proceedings and civil proceedings could thus arise from the same set of facts or incidents.

Types of civil action

Figure 2.5 illustrates some of the kinds of civil action which may be brought. In this book we are principally concerned with the law relating to negligence, breach of statutory duty and trespass to the person, but the physiotherapist should also be aware of the civil law relating to defamation and nuisance.

Figure 2.5 **Civil actions.**

- Negligence
- Nuisance
- Defamation
- Breach of statutory duty
- Trespass (to the person, goods or land)
- Breach of contract

Public and private law

Another distinction in the classification of laws is that of public and private law. Figure 2.6 illustrates the difference between the two.

Figure 2.6 **Differences between public and private law.**

Public Law	Private Law
Matter of public concern e.g.	*Matter arising between individuals (people or organisations) e.g.*
● protection of children	● purchasing a house
● public nuisance	● suing for personal injury
● how statutory duties are carried out	● suing for breach of contract

---

Public law deals with those areas of law where society intervenes in the actions of individuals. In contrast private law is concerned with the behaviour of individuals or corporate bodies to each other. The Children Act 1989 covers both private law and public law relating to children: care proceedings, protection orders, child assessment orders are part of the public law; orders in relation to children made following divorce or nullity, such as with whom the child is to live, are part of the private law. Thus the Cleveland Report was concerned with the public law: the duty of Social Services Departments to take action to protect children. In contrast a dispute over whether consent has been given for a child to have treatment would be part of private law.

Scotland and Northern Ireland

This book describes the law which applies to England and Wales. This for the most part also applies to Scotland and Northern Ireland, but there are some differences since there are specific statutory provisions for these countries and Scots common law has different roots.

Legal personnel

If patients believe that they have a claim for compensation because of the actions or omissions of health professionals, after possibly seeking advice from the Community Health Council, they could ask a solicitor to take the case. A solicitor is a professionally qualified person (usually a law degree followed by completion of the Law Society's professional examinations and completion of a set time in supervised practice) who tends to have direct contact with the client. The solicitor may seek the opinion of a barrister (known as counsel) on liability and the amount of compensation. A barrister will usually have a law degree and must complete the examinations set by the Council for Legal Education. The barrister must be a member of an Inn of Court and complete a term of apprenticeship known as pupillage. Traditionally the barrister has had the role of conducting the case in court and preparing the documents which are exchanged between the parties in the run up to the court hearing (known as the pleadings). However increasingly the right of solicitors to represent the client in court has been extended until it is now possible for solicitors with special training and recognition to undertake the work of advocacy formerly undertaken by barristers alone. Many would see the final result of this development to be a single legal profession.

Procedure in civil courts

Figure 2.7 sets out a summary of the stages which take place in civil litigation in the High Courts. Lord Woolf[7] has conducted an inquiry to determine how access to justice could be simplified and speeded up, and the main changes are discussed in Chapter 10. Major reforms in civil proceedings came into force in April 1999.

For personal injury claims under £1000 and other civil claims under £3000 the claim would normally be heard in the small claims court through a process of arbitration. Above these amounts and for claims up to £50 000 the claim could be heard in the County Court. Above £50 000 the claim would usually be heard in the High Court.

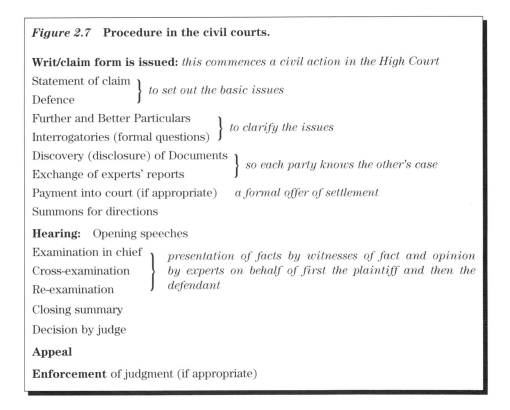

Figure 2.7   Procedure in the civil courts.

Writ/claim form is issued: *this commences a civil action in the High Court*

Statement of claim
Defence
} *to set out the basic issues*

Further and Better Particulars
Interrogatories (formal questions)
} *to clarify the issues*

Discovery (disclosure) of Documents
Exchange of experts' reports
} *so each party knows the other's case*

Payment into court (if appropriate)   *a formal offer of settlement*

Summons for directions

Hearing: Opening speeches

Examination in chief
Cross-examination
Re-examination
} *presentation of facts by witnesses of fact and opinion by experts on behalf of first the plaintiff and then the defendant*

Closing summary

Decision by judge

Appeal

Enforcement of judgment (if appropriate)

Procedure in criminal courts

Figure 2.8 sets out the stages which would be followed in a criminal prosecution of an offence triable only on indictment. The magistrates, who are either lay people known as justices of the peace (JPs) sitting in threes (the bench) or legally qualified persons known as stipendiary magistrates (who sit alone), can only hear charges which relate to offences known as summary offences or offences such as theft which can be heard either as summary offences or on indictment (i.e. which are triable either way). Only the crown court (with judge and jury) can hear charges of offences which can only be made on indictment (indictable only offences). Such offences are the most serious e.g. murder, rape, grievous bodily harm, and other offences against the person. The magistrates however have a gate-keeping role in relation to these offences and oversee committal proceedings where they decide whether there is a case to answer and if the case should therefore be committed to the crown court for the trial to take place. In criminal cases, the Crown Prosecution Service (CPS) has the responsibility for preparing the case, including statements, witnesses, etc. for the prosecution in criminal cases.

Figure 2.8 **Procedure in a criminal case.**

Committal proceedings: *in Magistrates Court*
Crown Court trial:
Arraignment of jury
Plea is taken
Prosecution opening address
Prosecution witnesses   *examination in chief*
                            cross-examination
                            re-examination
Defence witnesses   *examination in chief*
                            cross-examination
                            re-examination
Final speeches – *prosecution and defence summarise the case*
Judge address to the jury – *explaining the law*
Jury retire and consider verdict – *to decide on the facts*
Finding of guilt or innocence – *by jury*
Sentencing if guilty verdict – *by judge*

Accusatorial system

A feature of the legal system in this country is that it consists of one side tasked with the responsibility of proving that the other side is guilty, liable or at fault of the wrong or crime alleged. This is known as an 'accusatorial' system (or sometimes 'adversarial') and applies to both civil and criminal proceedings as can be seen from the stages illustrated in Figures 2.7 and 2.8. In criminal cases the prosecution attempts to show beyond all reasonable doubt that the accused is guilty of the offence with which he is charged. The magistrates, or the jury in the crown court, determine whether the prosecution has succeeded in establishing the guilt of the accused, who is presumed innocent until proved guilty. In civil proceedings the plaintiff, i.e. the person bringing the action, has to establish on a balance of probability that there has been negligence, trespass, nuisance or whatever civil wrong is alleged. In civil cases (apart from defamation) there is no jury and the judge has the responsibility of making a decision on disputed facts and determining whether the plaintiff has succeeded in establishing the civil wrong.

In this accusatorial system of law one party to a case confronts the other party and the role of the judge is to chair the proceedings, intervening where necessary in the interests of justice and clarifying points of law and procedure. It contrasts with the system of law which is known as 'inquisitorial' where the judge plays a far more active role in determining the outcome. An example of an inquisitorial system in the UK is the coroner's court. Here the coroner is responsible for deciding which witnesses would be relevant to the answers to the questions which are placed before him by statute (i.e. the identity of the deceased and how, when and where he came to die). The coroner asks the witnesses questions in court and decides who else can ask questions and what they can ask. As a result of this 'inquisition' he, or a jury if one is used, determines the cause of death.

Some may feel that an inquisitorial system of justice is fairer since the outcome of the accusatorial system may depend heavily upon the ability of the barristers representing the party in court. However the strengths of the accusatorial system probably outweigh the weaknesses; there are after all many challenges to the decisions of the coroners. The proposals put forward by Lord Woolf envisage a case management approach to civil claims in order to speed their progress and reduce the costs. The adversarial system would be kept, but in certain cases it is envisaged that expert witnesses would be agreed or appointed by the court. These proposals are considered in Chapters 10 (Negligence) and 13 (Giving Evidence in Court). They were implemented in April 1999.

Law and ethics

Law is both wider and narrower than the field of ethics. On the one hand the law covers areas of practice which may not be considered to give rise to any ethical issue, other than the one as to whether the law should be obeyed, for example, to park in a no parking area would not appear to raise many ethical issues other than the decision to obey or to ignore the law. On the other hand there are major areas of health care which raise significant ethical questions where there appears to be little law. For example elective ventilation of a corpse in order to keep the organs alive for transplant purposes, raises considerable ethical issues for health professionals and relatives, but provided the requirements of the Human Tissue Act and the Transplant Acts are satisfied there is no legal issue. At any time, of course, a practice which is considered to be contrary to ethical principles can be challenged in court and, on the basis of any existing statute law or decided cases, the judge will determine the legal position.

Situations may arise where a health professional considers the law to be wrong and contrary to her own ethical principles. In such a case she has to decide personally what action to take, in full awareness that she could face the effects of the criminal law, a civil action, disciplinary procedure by her employer and professional proceedings by her registration body. In certain cases the law itself provides for conscientious objection. Thus no one can be compelled to partici-pate in an abortion unless it is an emergency situation to save the life of the mother. (Abortion Act 1967). Similar provisions apply to activities in relation to human fertilisation and embryology where the Human Fertilisation and Embry-ology Act 1990 provides a statutory protection clause.

The Law Commission in its report on Mental Incapacity[8] drafted legislation to cover advance refusals of treatment but considered it would be inappropriate to have a conscientious objection clause for a health professional to ignore the existence of the previously declared wishes of the patient. A health professional may have strong ethical views about the need to save the life of a mentally incompetent adult who made an advance directive refusing treatment in the specified circumstances that now exist (e.g. naso-gastric feeding), but, if the Law Commission's proposals are enacted the law would not permit the refusal to be overruled, provided that it was expressed when the adult was mentally competent.

It is inevitable that any discussion of the function of physiotherapy should be concerned with the ethical or philosophical beliefs of the therapist who is providing the treatment and it is essential that the physiotherapist understands the extent to which the law is in harmony with her ethical beliefs and values.

Guidance on conduct and procedures

Rules of Professional Conduct

The Chartered Society of Physiotherapy has issued Rules governing professional practice[9]. These are not in themselves directly enforceable in a court of law, but could be used as evidence in civil or criminal proceedings that their reasonable professional standards of practice have not been followed. An allegation of a breach of the Rules could also be used as a basis for professional conduct proceedings, for which the ultimate sanction is removal from the Register. This is discussed in Chapter 4.

Charters and their enforcement

Recent years have seen an increase in the publication of Charters across both the public and private sector. In July 1992 the Citizen's Charter was published and it was followed by a Patient's Charter, with different editions being published by the different parts of the UK. Since then health authorities and NHS Trusts have prepared their own charters for their patients. Shortly after the Labour Government came into office in May 1997 a working party was set up to review the Patient's Charter which was to take into account patients' responsibilities as well. At the time of writing the results of this initiative are still awaited, but a revised charter of patients' rights and responsibilities is expected in the Spring of 1999.

These charters are not legally enforceable in themselves, except insofar as they recognise existing legal rights. Thus every patient is entitled to have a reasonable standard of care and this is enforceable whether or not it is included in a charter (see Chapter 10). They do however provide to the public a measure of the quality of service which it can expect and a failure could always lead to a complaint being made (see Chapter 14). The implementation of the standards set out in charters is monitored by the individual hospitals and health authorities and by the government.

Other guidance

Many other organisations and public bodies issue guidance for professional conduct and procedures for the provision of health care. The National Health Service Executive and Department of Health issue circulars and executive letters providing advice for health and social services organisations and staff. These do not have the direct force of law but it is expected that they are to be followed. Thus in 1997 the High Court ruled against the North Derbyshire Health Authority, which had refused to fund the purchase of beta-interferon for the treatment of multiple sclerosis[10]. The judge found that the health authority had knowingly failed to apply national guidance in an NHS circular. It cannot be assumed however that the guidance is always correct in law, and in *R* v. *Wandsworth Borough Council*[11] the court held that ministerial guidance was contrary to the law as stated in statute.

Directions issued by the Secretary of State under statutory powers, e.g. under the National Health Service and Community Care Act 1990, are directly enforceable against health authorities through the default mechanisms provided for in the legislation.

Conclusions

The variety of the sources of law and perplexity as to what a law is can be very confusing, but it is helpful for professionals when confronted with a statement that 'the law says...', to seek an explanation as to whether the basis for the assertion is a statute or decision of a court or whether it is derived from a charter or professional code of practice or, as often may be the case, a pronouncement which has no proper foundation in law at all.

 Questions and exercises _____

1   A client has consulted you about the possibility of bringing a claim for compensation. What advice would you give her on the procedure which would be followed and the steps which she should take?
2   Draw up a diagram which illustrates the difference between civil and criminal procedure.
3   Turn to the glossary and study the definitions of legal terms included there.
4   In what ways do you consider that conflict between ethical beliefs and the law should be resolved?

References

1   *R* v. *Hallstrom, ex parte W; R* v. *Gardener, ex parte L* [1986] 2 All ER 306.
2   *Gossington* v. *Ealing Borough Council* (CA) 18 November 1985, Lexis transcript.
3   *See* briefing note prepared by the Children's Legal Centre (address given in appendix)
4   *Miles* v. *Cain* 25 November 1988, Lexis transcript.
5   *R* v. *Adomako* (H of L) The Times Law Report, 4 July 1994.
6   Law Commission (1996) *Report on Criminal Prosecutions.*
7   Lord Woolf (January 1996) *Access to Civil Justice Inquiry Consultation Paper* HMSO, London; Lord Woolf (July 1996) *Access to Justice Final Report* HMSO, London.
8   Law Commission Report (1995) No. 231 *Mental Incapacity* HMSO, London.
9   Chartered Society of Physiotherapy (1995) *Rules of Professional Conduct* CSP, London.

10   Michael Horsnell (1997) 'Refusal to give MS victim new drug was illegal' *The Times* 12 July 1997.
11   *R* v. *Wandsworth Borough Council, ex parte Beckwith* [1996] 1 All ER 129 (discussed in Dimond, B. (1997) *Legal Aspects of Care in the Community* pp 465–6. Macmillan, Basingstoke).

Section A
Professional Issues

Chapter 3
Registration and the Role of the Statutory Bodies

In this chapter we consider the statutory basis of physiotherapy in the UK and the provisions for registration. We also discuss the role of the Council for Professions Supplementary to Medicine (CPSM) and the Physiotherapy Board. The following topics will be covered:

- Statutory basis of the CPSM
- Physiotherapy Board
- Registration machinery
- Private practitioners
- Non-registered professionals
- Projected changes

Statutory basis of the CPSM

The Council for the Professions Supplementary to Medicine was established under the Professions Supplementary to Medicine Act 1960. It is an independent, self-regulating, statutory body. At present it covers the professions shown in Figure 3.1.

Figure 3.1 **Professions covered by the CPSM.**

- chiropody
- dietetics
- medical laboratory science
- occupational therapy
- orthoptics

- physiotherapy
- radiography
- art therapy (added 1997)
- prosthetics and orthotics (added 1997)

There is a Board for each of the nine professions under its aegis.

The PSM reports to the Privy Council (PC) but there is also direct access from the professional Boards to the PC. The PSM appoints a Registrar who runs a secretariat for the PSM and the Boards, administering the registration scheme and providing support services. The Chairman of the PSM is appointed by the Privy Council.

Activities of the CPSM

Under section 1 of the Act the CPSM has the general function of co-ordinating and supervising the activities of the Boards established under the Act and the additional functions assigned to it. These functions are set out in Figure 3.2.

Figure 3.2 **Functions of the CPSM.**

- General function of co-ordinating and supervising the activities of the Boards –
  - by making to each Board, or inviting the Boards to make to Council, proposals as to the activities to be carried on by the Board;
  - by recommending a Board to carry on such activities, or to limit its activities, in such manner as the Council considers appropriate after consultation with the Board on the proposals;
  - by concerning itself with matters appearing to it to be of special interest to any two or more of the Boards, and by giving the Boards such advice and assistance as it thinks fit with respect to such matters;
  - by exercising its powers under the following provisions of this Act in such manner as the Council considers most conducive to the satisfactory performance by each Boards of the Board's function under this Act.
- Keeping the registers from each Board and lists deposited open at all reasonable times for inspection by members of the public.

The CPSM acts as the mediator between the Boards and the Privy Council. In its explanatory booklet published in March 1995, it describes itself as having eight primary areas of activity shown in Figure 3.3.

Figure 3.3 **Primary areas of activity of the CPSM.**

(1)   NHS purchasers and providers, current changes, private practice and insurance cover
(2)   Educational changes and relationships
(3)   Department of Employment, Occupational Standards Council, National Vocational Qualifications (NVQs)
(4)   Issues relating to regulation, relationships with educational providers and government departments, disciplinary functions, and statements of conduct
(5)   Professional bodies
(6)   European and international dimension
(7)   Reviewing possible changes to the 1960 Act and the framework for regulations and registration set up under it
(8)   Internal efficiency of the CPSM

Composition of the Council

The Council is constituted in accordance with Part I of the First Schedule to the Act. There are 25 members of whom:

- **Four** are appointed by the PC (one of these must be resident in Scotland and one in Wales) and **one** is appointed by the Secretary of State (none of these can be a registered medical practitioner or a member of the stated professions)

- **Four** are jointly appointed by the Secretary of State for Social Services, the Secretary of State for Wales, the Secretary of State for Scotland and the Minister of Health and Local Government (two of these only shall be registered medical practitioners and none shall be a member of the stated professions)
- **Nine** shall be representative members of the Council appointed by each Board
- **Three** are registered medical practitioners (one appointed by each of English colleges)
- **Three** are registered medical practitioners appointed jointly by the Scottish Corporation
- **One** is a registered medical practitioner appointed by the General Medical Council.

Each Board is entitled to appoint an alternate member for each representative member. In addition each Board may appoint two persons to act as additional members of the Council (without right to vote) at any meeting at which the Council is considering a matter appearing to the Council to be of special interest to registered members of the profession for which the Board is established.

The Physiotherapy Board

The Physiotherapy Board is constituted in accordance with the provisions of Part II of the first Schedule. There are 17 members of whom:

- **Nine** are representative members
- **Four** from the English colleges jointly
- **One** from the Scottish Corporations
- **One** from the British Medical Association
- **One** from experts in professional education
- with **one** other member who shall be a physicist. (Before making the appointment of this member the CPSM shall consult such other bodies or persons as appear to it to be appropriate in relation to that appointment.)

The members of the Board, other than the representative members, are appointed by CPSM. For each representative member, an alternate can be elected or appointed.

The Board has the functions shown in Figure 3.4.

Figure 3.4 **Functions of the Physiotherapy Board.**

(1) To promote the high standards of professional education and professional conduct.

(2) To prepare and maintain a register of the names, addresses and qualifications, and such other particulars as may be prescribed, of all persons who are entitled in accordance with the provisions of the Act to be registered by the Board and who apply in the prescribed manner to be so registered.

(3) To cause the register to be printed, published and put on sale to members of the public.

(4) To publish corrections to the register.

(5) To cause a print of each edition of the register and of each list of corrections to be deposited at the offices of the CPSM.

(6) To approve
    (a) any course of training
    (b) any qualification
    (c) any institution
with a view to registered status being conferred and also to refuse its approval or withdraw such an approval previously given.

(7) To keep itself informed (under a duty) of the nature of:
    (a) the instruction given at approved institutions to persons attending approved courses of training and
    (b) the examinations as the result of which approved qualifications are granted.

(8) To appoint persons to visit approved institutions or attend examinations for the purposes under (6) above. Visitors appointed have the duty to report to the Board:

- as to the sufficiency of the instruction given to persons attending approved courses of training at the institutions;
- the sufficiency of the examinations; and
- as to any other matters relating to the institutions or examinations.

However no such visitor shall interfere with the giving of any instruction or the holding of any examination.

When it approves a course of training or a qualification, the Board sends its recommendations to the CPSM and the CPSM shall send the application and the recommendations together with its own recommendations to the PC and the PC shall determine whether the approval is to be given or refused. Before approval is refused the PC must give an opportunity to the applicant to make representations to it.

When the Board approves an institution as being properly organised and equipped for conducting the whole or any part of a course of training approved by the Board, the approval does not have to go before the CPSM or the PC.

The Board also has a duty to publish statements of 'infamous conduct' and enforce professional discipline (see below). Ultimately it can strike a practitioner from the register (see Chapter 4).

The Board appoints its own Chairman, usually from amongst the profession that the Board represents. Each Board elects a practising member of the profession to the CPSM.

Registration machinery

Each Board under the CPSM maintains a register. The NHS requires professions supplementary to medicine to have registered status to work in the NHS. The CPSM describes state registration as guaranteeing a threshold of competence, an acceptance of professional discipline, and duties of care to cover 'omission' as well as 'commission'. It acts as a gateway into the NHS and to the wider 'family' of medical professions[1].

In the annual report for 1993–4[2] the CPSM set out a statement about state registration defining more fully what benefits state registration gives to registrants. This statement is set out in Figure 3.5.

Figure 3.5   **Statement about State Registration.**

The unique qualities of State Registration
Only relevant practitioners able to demonstrate current 'State Registration' (as opposed to just 'registration')

- are intentionally defined in a range of statutes as 'health professionals';
- have attended courses and gained qualifications under a system of quality control approved by the Privy Council;
- accept the discipline of the judicial sanction of being 'struck off' for 'infamous conduct';
- are automatically accepted on that basis alone by the General Medical Council and the British Medical Association as being persons to whom it is proper for medical practitioners to delegate treatment;
- have their qualifications statutorily recognised in other European countries under the EC directive on mutual recognition of higher education diplomas;
- are automatically deemed in statutes governing local authorities to be of such probity as not to require (medical) inspection of their professional activities;
- are recognised by the great majority of private health care and medical insurance providers as meeting the highest standards in their profession (and state registration is a requirement for all but a handful of these providers), and
- if Chiropodists, are legally able to administer local anaesthetics (and perform surgery on the foot) and to be exempted from relevant prescription-only drugs regulations.

State registration is a universal standard and a kitemark of excellence. Such importance was attached to it by Parliament that it is a specific offence to make a false claim to State Registration.

Private practitioners

The only difference between private practitioners and others is that the former are not employees. They may in fact be employers in their own right. No difference is made in the registration procedure between those who are employed and those who are in private practice. Chapter 19 is concerned with the legal aspects of private practice.

Non-registered physiotherapists

Only physiotherapists who have registered status can be employed within the NHS. It is the duty of the employer to check the registered status of its employees. Under the NHS and Community Care Act 1990 from 1 April 1991 the Secretary of State issued directions requiring local authorities to employ only practitioners registered with Council for Professions Supplementary to Medicine when using those professionals who come under its jurisdiction. The direction is shown in Figure 3.6.

Figure 3.6 **Directions on professions supplementary to medicine employed by local authorities and their agents.**

The Secretary of State for Health in exercise of powers conferred on him by section 7(A) of the Local Authority Social Services Act 1970 as inserted by Section 50 of the National Health Service and Community Care Act 1990 has issued the following direction:

(1) Subject to paragraph 2, no local authority shall in exercise of its social services functions under the 1970 Act employ any person as an officer of the authority in a capacity specified in column 1 of the Schedule unless the name of that person is included in a register maintained under section 2(1) of the Professions Supplementary to Medicine Act 1960.

[Nor is the local authority permitted to make arrangements with an agent to do so.]

This direction raises some interesting points since it prohibits the employment of unregistered professionals in the capacity covered by the 1960 Act. It does not seem to cover the case where a registered physiotherapist acquires skills normally undertaken by a registered occupational therapist. Nor does it appear to cover the situation where a care assistant is employed as a care assistant but undertakes work which would normally be undertaken by one of the listed professions. In other words the directions ensure that non-registered physiotherapists cannot be employed to do physiotherapy work, but they do not prevent the functions normally provided by registered physiotherapists from being undertaken by non-registered practitioners employed in another capacity.

Many chartered physiotherapists would like to have the actual word 'physiotherapist' restricted to the use of those who are registered under the 1960 Act. They argue that the general public does not appreciate the difference between those who are registered and those who are not.

Confirmation of this lack of understanding is shown by the words of a judge in a case where an unregistered physiotherapist was charged with assault on a patient[3]. The judge said:

'Although the Defendant is not a physiotherapist of the Chartered Institute [sic.] and he does not hold himself out as such, he has considerable experience and has had some training in physiotherapy principally through the Football Association. Soccer has been his great love and remains so. He is not a trickster in physiotherapy. Eamonn Martin, the international athlete and Olympic competitor, was one of his regular patients.'

The judge did not refer to the lack of the professional code of practice and assessed level of training and competence which all registered practitioners and Chartered Society members must have.

Evidence of the confusion in the public mind over the significance and value of registration is apparent from the CPSM annual report for 1997/8 which states that:

'It has come to light that the number of members of the professions under the aegis of the Professions Supplementary to Medicine Act 1960 who are working for the NHS and for local authorities without state registration is far higher than had been thought. This is caused by employers not complying with the Government directives and failing to check annual registration certificates.'

Of great concern to registered professionals is the use of professional titles by those who might well be excluded by the registration process. The police now report convictions and cautions to the CPSM and it is significant that, of the 45 convictions reported to the CPSM at the time of writing, only 14 were registered practitioners who were reported to the appropriate Board. Twenty five of the others had never been registered but used the common title of one of the professions when charged.

The situation will only be remedied if the use of the title physiotherapist without being registered becomes an offence under a new health bill (see recommendations of the Review Committee below).

The registered practitioner is increasingly expected to work with support from non-registered practitioners known variously as health support workers, care assistants, physiotherapy assistants and other titles. The legal aspects relating to the supervision of the activities of non-registered practitioners and delegation to them are considered in Chapter 10 on negligence.

Projected changes

There has been much concern that the framework established in 1960 for the regulations and registration of professions supplementary to medicine no longer meets the changing circumstances for the delivery and purchase of health care, the growing diversity of health professions and the relationship between these professions and the medical profession.

The review of the 1960 Act

A review of the Professions Supplementary to Medicine Act 1960 was undertaken by JM Consulting Ltd under a steering group chaired by Professor Sheila McLean. Following a consultation document issued in October 1995, a report[4] was published in July 1996.

The report describes the present weaknesses of the Professions Supplementary to Medicine Act, identifying two broad areas:

- the weaknesses in the powers provided by the 1960 Act; and
- the weaknesses in the statutory bodies and working arrangements.

It explores the developments which have taken place since 1960 including:

- the development of primary care;
- the introduction of the internal market;
- the use of multi-disciplinary teams and the possibility of non state registered professionals being employed in the NHS by GPs;
- the growth of private sector provision; and
- the changes which have taken place within the professions including strong professional associations with regulations for discipline.

Other changes include:

- the new professions which have sought state registered status;
- developments within higher education with degree status for many professions and education provision being made outside the NHS; and
- changing attitudes in society and higher public expectations.

The inappropriateness of the term 'Professions Supplementary to Medicine' was also considered.

The recommendations of the report

The report's recommendations cover the following areas:

- basic recommendations (see Figure 3.7);
- the establishment of the Council for Health Professions (CHP) (see Figure 3.8);
- the establishment of Statutory Committees and a Panel of Professional Advisers (see Figure 3.9); and
- protection of title.

Figure 3.7   Basic recommendations of the review body on the 1960 Act.

(1)   A new statutory body should be established with new powers.
(2)   Legislation should allow for the growth in the number of professions.
(3)   The purpose of the new legislation should be the protection of the public.
(4)   Professions to be covered should be based on the potential for harm arising from either invasive procedures or the application of unsupervised judgment by the professional which can substantially impact on patient/client health or welfare.
(5)   All the professions under the CPSM should be included.
(6)   Other professional groups may be eligible.
(7)   Protection of common title for all of the regulated professions should be established.
(8)   The new statutory body should have more effective and flexible powers.
(9)   The government, through the Secretary of State or Privy Council, should continue to provide oversight and the ultimate court of appeal, but with reduced involvement in policy and administrative matters.
(10) The normal costs of the regulatory body should be funded from registration fees.

Figure 3.8   Recommendations of the review body on the Council.

(1) A new enlarged Council for Health Professions (CHP) should be established, with stronger powers to decide on matters currently referred to the Privy Council and with broader membership.

(2) The overall function of the CHP should be 'to provide protection to the public by specifying and monitoring standards of education, training and conduct for health professions'.

(3) The CHP would be a policy-making and supervisory body rather than an executive one.

(4) There would be three main types of duty for the CHP:
    (a) matters which it could determine itself;
    (b) matters needing government approval;
    (c) major matters which would eventually require placing before Parliament for affirmative resolution.

(5) Membership of the Council:
    (a) One third not registered professionals;
    (b) each professional group to be represented equally;
    (c) professional representatives to be elected by registrants;
    (d) other interests to be represented – medicine, other health professions, consumer groups;
    (e) nominations by Secretary of State or Privy Council.

(6) The Government should appoint the initial CHP, following these principles, but in future the Council should be allowed to recommend changes to adapt to future circumstances.

Figure 3.9   Recommendations of the review body on Statutory Committees.

The Council should delegate much of its work to Statutory Committees:

(1) **Preliminary Proceedings Committee** – to investigate and deal with all initial complaints or other professional performance matters (see Chapter 4).

(2) **Professional Conduct Committee** – to define and enforce standards of conduct, acting in a judicial capacity when cases are heard (see Chapter 4).

(3) **Health Committee** – to deal with matters of conduct possibly originating from health causes (see Chapter 4).

(4) **Education Committee** – dealing with pre-registration qualifications, continuing professional development (CPD), and registration criteria including those for overseas and European Economic Area (EEA) applicants.

(5) **Panel of Professional Advisers** – appointed by CHP to provide the resources and the expertise to carry out much of the detailed work in education and other areas. Members of the Panel would be nominated by professional bodies and would provide:

- members of working parties;
- members of Committees;
- members of course validation panels;
- members of the Education Committee's working committees; and
- a source of consultation on specific issues.

The CHP could also set up other non-statutory committees.

The role of the government
The Government's role would be:

- to establish the initial CHP
- to appoint specific members to the CHP on a continuing basis
- to approve minor matters such as the rules and procedures of the CHP
- to receive and consider applications for major changes such as the admission of the new professions and to submit these to Parliament
- to act as a final court of appeal when appropriate.

Protection of title
The report recommends that all professions regulated under CHP would have a protected title. This would be agreed by affirmative resolution of Parliament. The CHP would promote and publicise the titles and their significance to the public and employers and would have powers to monitor compliance with the protected title requirements and to request court action against non-state registered practitioners using protected titles or otherwise holding themselves out to be state registered.

Comment on the recommendations

Perhaps the most controversial of the recommendations is the recommendation that the existing statutory boards should cease to exist and the CHP should be the umbrella organisation, emphasising the shared approach of all the professions. The report looks at the opposition to this proposal which is based on a perceived loss of professional autonomy and which emphasises the lack of commonality across the professions. The report concludes:

'It is illogical to welcome the thought of 15 or twenty autonomous professional boards, each with its own sub-structure of education, discipline, investigation and liaison committees. This cannot be efficient or effective.'

Legislation is now awaited following this report but the CPSM Annual Report for 1997/8 states that with

'the increasing legislative load it is not known whether the time will be made available in the 1998/9 [Parliamentary] session.'

The CPSM is giving its full support to the new legislation.

Implications for physiotherapists

In its annual report for 1997 the Chartered Society of Physiotherapy states that it and other professions ancillary to medicine (PAMs) have agreed a common position paper on the proposed Health Professions Bill. It would support protection of title and education with joint validation arrangements. However on disciplinary procedures the annual report states:

'The Health Departments advocate the creation of a multi-professional committee for hearing disciplinary complaints. The assumption is that most misconduct issues centre on "generic" problems such as sexual misconduct. However experience has shown that most cases have a strong profession specific component. Potentially a large proportion of committee members may not be qualified to assess these cases. A suitable solution to this problem must be found.'[5]

The CSP will obviously continue to have a significant role in the maintenance and development of high standards of professional practice and conduct. Its work will be underpinned by the CHP (or whatever the new body is called) which will ensure common standards for state registration and practice across all those health professions under its aegis. The protection of a title for state registered physiotherapists, together with the education of the general public which must accompany this, should ensure that registered physiotherapists receive the public recognition which they deserve. However to be effective this must be accompanied by greater marketing skills on the value that registered physiotherapists can bring to the patient/client.

 Questions and exercises _____

1 What changes do you consider should be made to the present system for the registration of the profession of physiotherapy?
2 Draw up a table illustrating the relationship between the Council for Professions Supplementary to Medicine, the Physiotherapy Board, the

Chartered Society of Physiotherapy and the universities providing education for student physiotherapists.

3 Do you consider that the functions of the registered physiotherapist should be protected rather than just the title?

References

1 Council for Professions Supplementary to Medicine (1995) *Who we are and what we do*, CPSM, London.
2 Council for Professions Supplementary to Medicine (1994) *Annual Report 1993–4* page 14 CPSM, London.
3 *Miles* v. *Cain* 25 November 1988, Lexis transcript.
4 JM Consulting Ltd (1996) *The Regulation of Health Professions: Report of a review of the Professions Supplementary to Medicine Act 1960 with recommendations for new legislation* JM Consulting Ltd, Bristol.
5 Chartered Society of Physiotherapy *Annual report 1997* CSP, London.

Chapter 4
Professional Conduct Proceedings

In the last chapter we considered the law relating to the statutory bodies set up to control the entry onto the register and the functions and constitutions of the machinery for professional regulation set up under the Council for the Professions Supplementary to Medicine (CPSM). In this chapter we consider the regulation of professional discipline. The following areas will be discussed:

- Disciplinary machinery
- Role of the Chartered Society of Physiotherapists (CSP)
- Code of ethics and professional practice
- Scope of professional practice
- Post-registration control and supervision
- Insurance and indemnity
- The future

Disciplinary machinery

The committees

Sections 8 and 9 of the Professions Supplementary to Medicine Act 1960 make provision for the disciplinary function of the Council for Professions Supplementary to Medicine and the relevant Boards.

Section 8 requires each Board to set up two committees, to be known respectively as the investigating committee and the disciplinary committee.

The investigating committee has the duty of conducting a preliminary investigation into any case where it is alleged that a person registered by the Board is liable to have his or her name removed from the register, and of deciding whether the case should be referred to the disciplinary committee.

The disciplinary committee has the duty of considering and determining any case referred to it by the investigating committee and any other case of which the disciplinary committee has cognisance under section 9(1) of the 1960 Act. Provisions are laid down in the second schedule of the 1960 Act covering the constitution of the investigating and disciplinary committees and the procedures to be followed by the disciplinary committee.

Reasons for and effect of removal

The disciplinary committee (by section 9(1) of the Act) may if it thinks fit direct that a person's name should be removed from the register:

- where a registered person is convicted of a criminal offence which, in the opinion of the disciplinary committee set up by the Board, renders him unfit to be registered; or
- a registered person is judged by the disciplinary committee to be guilty of infamous conduct in any professional respect; or
- the disciplinary committee is satisfied that the name of a registered person has been fraudulently entered on the register maintained by the Board.

When the disciplinary committee directs that a person's name shall be removed from the register, the committee shall cause notice of the direction to be served on that person. Within 28 days of service of this notice, the person can 'appeal to Her Majesty in Council'. In practice this will lead to a hearing of the Judicial Committee of the Privy Council to which appeals to Her Majesty in Council are referred. The Board concerned may appear as the respondent on any such appeal (section 9(3)).

The direction for the removal of a name from the register shall take effect:

- where no appeal is brought, on the expiration of the 28 days;
- where an appeal is brought and is withdrawn or struck out for want of prosecution, on the withdrawal or striking out;
- where an appeal is brought and is dismissed, on the dismissal (section 9(4)).

Once a person's name is removed from the register, the person is not entitled to be registered on that register again except following a direction given by the committee as a result of an application by that person. The committee can, in its direction for removal, specify a time limit within which the person cannot apply for registration.

Infamous conduct

Under section 9(6) each disciplinary committee has a duty to prepare and from time to time revise, in consultation with its Board and the Council, a statement as to the kind of conduct which the committee considers to be infamous conduct in a professional respect. The Board has the duty to send by post to each registered member, a copy of the statement being revised. However it is specifically stated that

> 'the fact that any matters are not mentioned in such a statement shall not preclude the disciplinary committee from judging a person to be guilty of infamous conduct in a professional respect by reference to such matters.'

Constitution of the committees

Part 1 of Schedule 2 sets out the constitution of the investigating and disciplinary committees. The Board can in consultation with the Council, make rules regulating the following:

- the membership of each of the committees,
- the times and places of the meetings,
- quorum, and
- the mode of summoning members.

A person is not eligible for membership of a committee unless he is a member of the Board. (Special provisions apply to Northern Ireland.)

No person who acted as a member of the investigating committee with respect to any case shall act as a member of the disciplinary committee with respect to that case.

Rules made by the Boards do not come into force until they have been approved by the Privy Council (PC).

Procedure for the disciplinary committee

Part 2 of Schedule 2 sets out the procedure for disciplinary committees and covers the following matters:

- administration of oaths and issuing writs of *subpoena ad testificandum* (requiring a person to give oral evidence) and *duces tecum* (requiring a person to bring documentary evidence);
- rules:
  - relating to the securing of notice of proceedings,
  - as to who is to be a party to the proceedings,
  - relating to representations,
  - requiring proceedings to be in public (except as provided by the rules),
  - for records relating to findings that a person is not guilty of infamous conduct; and
- rules relating to the registration situation of a person whose name has been removed.

The committee is required to consult the relevant Board before making or amending rules under this provision and the Board must consult relevant persons and organisations. Rules and amendments do not have to be approved by the PC before they come into force.

The CPSM is required to appoint, after consultation with the Board, an assessor to advise the disciplinary committee on legal matters.

Cases and annual reports

The Physiotherapy Board reports to the CPSM on disciplinary proceedings undertaken in the event of any allegation of infamous conduct. In the CPS report for 1997/98, the Chairman of the Physiotherapy Board, Professor Brook, stated

'Both the Board's Investigating and Disciplinary Committees, unfortunately have been working very hard this year as we continue to see an increase in complaints of improper behaviour. In addition to the usual sources of complaint, notifications of criminal convictions and cautions are now being received by the Board. The need to follow correct procedures, particularly with regard to patient/client informed consent, cannot be emphasised and we urge practitioners to be alert to the importance of delivering best practice at all times.'

The CPSM in its annual report for 1997/8 stated that a serious anomaly had been found in that professions under the aegis of the Professions Supplementary to Medicine Act 1960 did not appear on the Home Office Circular which requires the Police to report to the Statutory Body any convictions or cautions. This has now been rectified. However, as mentioned in the previous chapter less than one third of those reported were registered practitioners and the information was passed to the appropriate Board. Most of the others just used the common title of one of the professions when charged.

Role of the Chartered Society of Physiotherapy (CSP)

Most registered physiotherapists join the CSP, although there are a few who do not become chartered even though they are registered. The CSP has its own regulations for membership and there could well be parallel proceedings in the case of infamous conduct with the disciplinary committee under the Council for Professions Supplementary to Medicine deciding whether there are grounds for removing the person from the register and the CSP determining on the basis of the misconduct whether the physiotherapist should remain a member of the Chartered Society.

The CSP plays an important part in the setting and maintenance of educational standards which is discussed in Chapter 5 and also has a significant role in the preparation of standards on professional conduct. The *Rules* are considered below. It has also issued other guidance and free information sheets on a variety of topics, many of which are referred to in the relevant chapters of this book.

Code of ethics and professional practice

The Rules of Professional Conduct[1]

The Rules are not law in the sense that a breach of their provisions would not lead directly to criminal or civil proceedings, but such a breach could be used in evidence in professional conduct or other proceedings where the activities of a physiotherapist were in question. The Rules cover the topics shown in Figure 4.1.

Figure 4.1 **Rules of Professional Conduct.**

(1)   Scope of practice
(2)   Relationships with patients
(3)   Confidentiality
(4)   Relationships with professional staff and carers
(5)   Duty to report
(6)   Advertising
(7)   Sale of services and goods
(8)   Personal and professional standards.

The principles on which the Rules are based are reflected in the Society's *Standards of Physiotherapy Practice*[2], which also include criteria to provide measures of how these principles and standards are being adhered to.

A Code of Conduct has also been prepared for physiotherapist assistants[3], which is discussed in Chapter 10.

The CSP has also issued guidance on standards of business conduct[4]. This applies to physiotherapists wherever they practice (see Chapter 19 for the physiotherapist in private practice) and covers the topics of:

- conflict of interests,
- conflict of stance/position,
- changes in employment status,
- restrictive clauses,
- incentives,
- favouritism, and
- gifts and hospitality.

Receipts of gifts from clients

This is one area of professional practice which frequently concerns health professionals. Clients/patients are often grateful for the help they have received and wish to make a small gesture in recognition of this. Most Trusts have policies prohibiting the receipt of gifts except under strict procedures. These might include accepting a gift to a department or unit rather than to an individual and ensuring that any gift is notified to a senior manager and a record is made. It is, of course, axiomatic that the gift should not have any influence on the standard of care provided or lead to any priority for that patient which is not justified on clinical grounds. Any large gift should be dealt with through the unit manager's office since it may become part of the charitable funds held in trust by the Health Authority or Trust. Similarly, if a patient indicates that they wish to make a bequest in a will, the solicitors of the trust should be involved to ensure that there is no question of undue influence and that the patient receives independent advice.

Scope of professional practice

There is increasing pressure on physiotherapists to expand their field of activities. On the one hand many are attracted by the uses of complementary therapies as an adjunct to their practice. They are therefore acquiring training in such therapies as acupuncture, reflexology, aromatherapy and similar fields. The legal implications of this are considered in Chapter 27.

On the other hand, some physiotherapists are being asked by their employers and managers to undertake activities not usually associated with the core physiotherapy role. The guidance issued by the CSP[5] cites such tasks as injections, phlebotomy, electrocardiography, suturing and acting as a clinical assistant in filtering patients for orthopaedic, rheumatology and neurological clinics. The guidance suggests that such activities could be undertaken by physiotherapists provided that they are properly trained to carry out the new procedures, and have appropriate professional liability insurance. It is the personal responsibility of each physiotherapist to determine her competence to perform these activities.

Where the employee has been asked by the employer to undertake these extended role activities then in the event of a successful claim for compensation being made the employer will be vicariously liable (see Chapter 10). If, however, the physiotherapist is a self-employed practitioner she must seek additional insurance cover to include these activities (see below). The CSP has made it clear that even when the physiotherapist is working outside the scope of physiotherapy practice, she will still be subject to the Rules of Professional Conduct:

> 'Chartered Physiotherapists shall adhere at all times to personal and professional standards which reflect credit on the profession.' (Rule 8)

Specific guidance has been given by the CSP for chartered physiotherapists working as Extended Scope Practitioners[6] (known as ESPs). ESPs are clinical physiotherapy specialists with an extended scope of practice. They see patients referred for assessment, clinical diagnosis and management of neuro-musculoskeletal disorders. Some of the extended role activities they can undertake include:

- requesting investigations (X-rays, scans, blood tests, etc.);
- using the results of investigations to assist clinical diagnosis and appropriate management of patients;
- listing for surgery and referring to other medical and health care professionals.

The CSP guidance lists the considerations which should be taken into account when setting up an ESP post. It also stresses the importance of clear protocols for the role of the ESP and the importance of evaluation and audit of the ESP post. The use of expanding the scope of practice in orthopaedics is considered below and in Chapter 20.

The personal and professional responsibility of the advanced practitioner is recognised by Mel Stewart[7] who points out the necessity to rethink professional development and links with other professions.

One of the greatest difficulties for practitioners in entering into a new area of expertise is knowing when they are competent to practise in this field. Unless there is a system of accreditation for individual training courses the practitioner does not know the strengths and limitations of any training course they follow. Since the individual is personally accountable it is suggested that developments in the scope of professional practice should be through a mix of education/training and supervised practice.

Orthopaedics (an example of extended role practice)

An interesting example of the extended role of the physiotherapist in specialist clinics is given by Durrell[8]. She shows how an appropriately trained physiotherapist can act in selecting referrals from a general case mix and request and interpret investigations (such as blood tests, X-rays, and scans), forming a working diagnosis and planning patient management. The issues which arise from this extended activity include:

- consent from the patient that the referral is to a physiotherapist and not a doctor;
- responsibility for the patient being with the physiotherapist once an appointment is booked;
- the importance of good communication with the consultant and GP;
- open access to medical advice, including an immediate opinion if necessary, and cross referral;
- adequate training for the physiotherapist to undertake these activities;
- agreement on the scope of professional practice between doctors and physiotherapists;
- appropriate professional liability cover;
- the employer's agreement over the expansion to ensure their vicarious liability (see Chapter 10) for these activities;
- guidelines and protocols need to be developed to cover the increasing number of extended role activities.

Sue Thomas describes how the use of skilled chartered physiotherapists as the first line assessment of orthopaedic patients has speeded up the referral process in orthopaedics[9].

The employer's responsibility

In a discussion of the history, present situation and future developments of the ESP, Hourigan and Weatherley[10] make the following point.

'The medico-legal position of the physiotherapist has not always been clearly defined. In most units the employing Trust has assumed vicarious liability for the actions of the physiotherapists which are beyond the normal scope but advisably the role expansion needs to be stated in the job description. The potential lack of knowledge of physiotherapists, in particular with regards to more general medical conditions, may be of concern.'

The concept of vicarious liability is discussed in Chapter 10 where it is pointed out that the activities of the negligent employee must be in the course of employment in order for the employer to be held vicariously liable. If there is written evidence of the employer's agreement to these extended roles, then the argument that the employee was not acting in the course of employment whilst undertaking these extended role activities is unlikely to succeed.

Collaborative practice

Physiotherapists, unlike many other professions supplementary to medicine, have for some years seen themselves as able to take direct referrals (i.e. other than through a doctor) and the CSP has been concerned to protect this power. Thus in a collaboration[11] with occupational therapists and speech and language therapists there was a reassurance from the then Secretary of State for Health, Virginia Bottomley (Appendix D to the paper), that the NHS reforms of 1990 were not intended to restrict referral to physiotherapists, so that physiotherapists could continue to accept referrals from sources other than consultants and general practitioners.

It should be borne in mind when the expansion of the scope of professional practice of the physiotherapist is being considered that there may well be many overlaps with the professional ambitions of other health professions including nurses and occupational therapists. Collaboration with these groups therefore becomes extremely important. The document referred to covers collaborative practice in the following areas:

- professional organisations
- education and
- undergraduate education
- research, clinical research and evaluation
- manpower planning and support workers
- staff retention and job satisfaction.

Post-registration control and supervision

Once physiotherapists are qualified and registered they are professionally accountable for their actions and are not subject to any system of professional supervision comparable to the statutory supervision of the midwife. They are expected to provide the reasonable standard of care the patient is entitled to have (see Chapter 10) and it would be no defence for them to argue that they were only recently qualified and that was why negligence occurred. In practice, however, senior colleagues provide support for junior staff and would ensure that some form of supervision and training was in place. It is, of course, more difficult in those work areas where a physiotherapist would be working on her own. Schemes for continuing education and training are considered in Chapter 5.

Insurance and indemnity

It is essential that any physiotherapist should ensure that she is covered in relation to the possibility of claims for compensation. If she is employed, she will be covered by the vicarious liability of the employer, provided that the situation giving rise to the claim occurs whilst she is working in the course of her employment. However, if she does work outside the course of her employment or as a self-employed physiotherapist she would be personally responsible for the payment of any compensation (see further Chapter 10 on negligence and Chapter 19 on private practice).

The CSP has prepared guidance on the chartered physiotherapist and insurance[12]. It explains the circumstances in which insurance might be needed, explains what is covered by the annual subscription and how additional cover can be obtained. Excluded from the CSP insurance cover are the categories of work shown in Figure 4.2.

Figure 4.2 **Categories of work excluded from the CSP insurance scheme.**

- Treatment of animals (unless a member of the Association of Chartered Physiotherapists in Animal Therapy (ACPAT))
- Provision of any treatment that is not deemed by the CSP to be part of the normal work of a physiotherapist
- Acting as a clinical assistant in an orthopaedic or other medical clinic
- Liability of those who are not permitted to practise in the country in which they are working
- Liability of student members unless working under the direct supervision of a chartered physiotherapist or person of equal status in the profession of physiotherapy
- Liability arising out of work in the USA/Canada (with exceptions)

Where the physiotherapist is involved in treating sports injuries additional 'top-up' insurance is available beyond the usual cover of £1.5 million. The guidance also covers insurance for students, assistants and research.

The insurance scheme does not cover for personal injuries incurred by the physiotherapist herself and those who wish to have compensation beyond the scale of benefit provided by the NHS Injury Benefit Scheme would need to have their own personal cover for situations where they cannot hold another person or organisation liable.

The industrial relations department of the CSP has given details of its legal advice and assistance scheme[13]. This is distinct from the Society's professional liability insurance scheme and covers the defence costs in criminal cases, and legal advice and representation for some civil matters such as industrial injury claims, industrial tribunal cases and employment contract disputes. It does **not** cover business matters such as partnership disputes or the collection of debts and does not cover fines or compensation awards in criminal or civil cases. The scheme applies to assistants, students and chartered physiotherapists. CSP reserves the right to decide in each individual case the extent to which support will be provided and to amend the scheme as the CSP Council decides.

For details on education reference should be made to Chapter 5, and for the law relating to teaching and research, Chapter 25.

The future

The following recommendations were made by the Review on the Professions Supplementary to Medicine and the 1960 Act[14] relating to the conduct of professional conduct proceedings:

(1) Criminal conviction, continued incompetence (proven), misconduct (proven) would all be grounds for suspension or removal of registration.
(2) Adhering to CPD should be a requirement once Council-approved schemes are in place. Applicants applying for continued registration would be required periodically to certify that they are conforming with the requirement.
(3) Statutory committees should be set up as detailed below.

Preliminary Proceedings Committee (PPC)

The main function of this committee would be to consider whether cases involving allegations or information about a regulated professional should be referred to the Professional Conduct or Health Committees for inquiry. Complaints should be considered initially by the Registrar or Chairman and then come to the PPC. They could cover any situation where professional competence is being challenged in the public interest. The Council should propose procedures drawing upon best practice in other regulatory bodies.

The PPC should be chaired by a person with a judicial/legal background (e.g. a JP or retired judge) nominated by the Government who would then become a Council member *ex officio*. This would be both to ensure familiarity with Council policies and procedures and to provide feed-back to the Council on issues arising in investigations. Membership of the PPC should have a strong representation of non-registrants (the Review suggested at least 33%) and include a registered medical practitioner (to advise on health problems as they affect professionals).

Professional Conduct Committee (PCC)

The main role of the PCC would be:

- to consider issues of discipline and ethics, referring (if appropriate but not as a requirement) to its own statements of conduct or those issued by professional bodies
- to sit in public where a registrant has been the subject of an allegation using a procedure akin to that of court in order to decide
  - first whether the facts are proved and if so
  - whether these constitute misconduct
- to determine whether a registrant guilty of a criminal offence is also guilty of misconduct
- to refer cases at its discretion to the Health Committee.

The definition of misdemeanour would be 'misconduct' rather than 'infamous conduct'.

The PCC would have powers:

- to expel from the register
- to endorse or reprimand
- to make a 'condition of practice' order
- to suspend registration and
- to apply financial penalties and
- to suspend any such judgment

The Health Committee

The role of the Health Committee would be to consider the action to be taken in cases where a registered professional's fitness to practise may be seriously impaired by reason of ill health. Referrals could be made by the PPC. It was recommended that the GMC model should be followed. The Health Committee's powers would include suspension of registrants, or imposition of conditions on their continued registration, but not to strike them off the register.

All three committees should have the power to suspend from registration pending the hearing of a case where the need to protect the public overrides the practitioner's right to continue to practise. The Chairmen should have legal expertise.

At the time of writing the Government's response to this review is awaited.

Conclusions

Standards of professional practice are constantly increasing and the onus is on the professional personally to ensure that her competence is maintained and that she upholds the reasonable standards of professional practice. She therefore has the responsibility of ensuring that she obtains the necessary training and instruction to remain competent and to develop safely in new areas of practice. Registered nurses have now a statutory duty to undertake at least 5 days of study or professional development every three years in order to remain on the register. There is at present no such stipulation for physiotherapists but it is likely that any revised legislation following the review undertaken by JM Consultants of the Professions Supplementary to Medicine (see Chapter 3) may impose similar requirements.

 Questions and exercises _____

1   A colleague tells you that she has been reported to the Council for Professions Supplementary to Medicine for infamous conduct. Advise her on the procedure which will be followed and how she could defend herself. What changes are recommended?

2   Do you consider that the following conduct by a registered physiotherapist should be the subject of professional conduct proceedings:
    (a) A parking fine
    (b) An offence of shop-lifting
    (c) Being cited in a divorce as an adulterer
    (d) Being found guilty of a breach of the peace following a New Year's Eve party?

3   Explain the legal situation in relation to insurance cover for an employed and a self-employed physiotherapist.

References

1   Chartered Society of Physiotherapy (1995) *Rules of Professional Conduct*, CSP, London.
2   CSP Professional Affairs Department (1993) *Standards of Physiotherapy Practice.* CSP, London.
3   Chartered Society of Physiotherapy (1995) *Rules of Professional Conduct.* pp 45–8 CSP, London.
4   CSP Professional Affairs Department (1995) No. PA 26 (May 1995) *Standards of Business Conduct*, CSP, London.
5   CSP Professional Affairs Department (1994) No. PA 21 (November 1994) *Physiotherapists Working Outside the Scope of Physiotherapy Practice.* CSP, London.

6   CSP Professional Affairs Department No. PA 29 *Chartered Physiotherapists working as extended scope practitioners*, CSP, London.
7   Stewart, M. (1998) Advanced Practice in Physiotherapy. *Physiotherapy* **84** 4, 184–6.
8   Durrell, S. (1996) Expanding the scope of physiotherapy: clinical physiotherapy specialists in consultants clinics. *Manual Therapy* **4** 210–13.
9   Thomas, S. (1994) Speeding up the referral process in orthopaedics. NHS Executive VFM Update No. 11, June 1994.
10 Hourigan, P.G. & Weatherley, C.R. (1998) Developments in Physiotherapy: The extended scope practitioner. *ACPM Journal*, Spring 1998, 3–5.
11 Chartered Society of Physiotherapy, the College of Occupational Therapists and the College of Speech and Language Therapists (no date) *Promoting collaborative practice*, CSP, COT, CSLT, London.
12 CSP Professional Affairs Department (1998) No. PA 32 (Revised May 1998) *Physiotherapists & Insurance*. CSP, London.
13 CSP Industrial Relations Department (no date) *Legal Advice and assistance*. CSP, London.
14 JM Consulting Ltd. (1996) *The Regulation of Health Professions: Report of a review of the Professions Supplementary to Medicine Act 1960 with recommendations for new legislation*. JM Consulting Ltd., Bristol.

Chapter 5
Education and the Physiotherapist

This chapter is concerned with the statutory provisions for controlling the education of the physiotherapist both pre- and post-registration. The following issues will be considered:

- Council for Professions Supplementary to Medicine (CPSM)
- Role of Chartered Society of Physiotherapists (CSP)
- Accreditation and generic skills
- External placement for clinical training
- Post registration education
- Supervision and mentoring
- The future

(Reference should be made to Chapter 26 on the legal aspects of teaching and research.)

Council for Professions Supplementary to Medicine

As has been seen in Chapter 3 the regulations for the registration of physiotherapists are designed by the Physiotherapy Board under the aegis of the CPSM. The Physiotherapy Board is the statutory body which, in conjunction with the CPSM, lays down the requirements for registration and can approve courses, successful completion of which can lead to registration. The Board also gives institutional approval to those colleges and universities which provide the training which leads to registered status. The recommendations of the Board on approval of courses, examinations, qualifications and institutions are forwarded to the CPSM, which in turn sends them with any comments it wishes to make to the Privy Council for final approval.

In its annual report for 1997/98 the CPSM noted that it was brought to the notice of the CPSM that not all Higher Education Institutes were requiring evidence as to good conduct from potential students applying for places on approved courses leading to state registration. This led to wastage, when checks prior to clinical placements or by potential employers resulted in the refusal of a placement or a contract because of a serious offence or offences in the person's past. The Boards are now requiring clearance of students prior to the start of a programme as a condition of validation or revalidation of courses. The current method is by the potential student obtaining a Police Certificate under the Data Protection Act 1984 (Subject Access) or the Data Protection Act 1998 (when implemented).

Role of Chartered Society of Physiotherapy (CSP)

The CSP supports the work of the Physiotherapy Board in developing the criteria for the recognition of courses for registration.

A new framework with a new approach to undergraduate physiotherapy studies was adopted by the CSP Council in 1996[1]. The new curriculum is designed to reflect the developments in education and practice since the last review in 1991. Physiotherapy in the UK and the Republic of Ireland is an all-graduate profession. Each educational institution sets its own admission requirements in addition to those required by the registration body and the CSP. A study by Ann Green and Jackie Waterfield looked at admission and progression trends in physiotherapy undergraduate education[2] and concluded that the mode of pre-entry academic study is not the best predictor of academic performance in terms of degree classification. It suggested that further work was required to explore whether different pre-entry qualifications influence students' performance on different elements within the programmes.

Accreditation and generic skills

The accreditation of courses for physiotherapists and of the colleges is carried out jointly by the Physiotherapists Board of the Council for Professions Supplementary to Medicine, the CSP and the educational representatives. This work is essential in maintaining the standards of education and clinical practice required by students before registration can take place.

A review article by Adrienne Hunt *et al.*[3] sought to look at current teaching in physiotherapy and determine the extent to which curriculum and teaching strategies could be used to ensure that new graduates meet the needs of the community. The researchers drew on experience at the University of Sydney which set out the generic skills and attributes which are expected of all graduates. The main areas are:

(1)   Knowledge skills
(2)   Thinking skills
(3)   Personal skills
(4)   Personal attributes
(5)   Practical skills (where appropriate)

They conclude that in order to function better within a changing health care environment, professional education curricula should extend beyond the learning of discipline-specific skills to encompass broader learning goals, in particular the acquisition of 'generic' university skills.

External placement for clinical training

Whilst the theoretical content of the training and education will take place largely within universities or colleges of higher education, it is necessary for the colleges to agree placements for clinical training and instruction with NHS Trusts and Social Services Departments (SSDs). Trusts and departments used for clinical placements will be subject to approval of the Physiotherapy Board.

A memorandum of agreement is drawn up between college and Trust or SSD, to set down the basic principles behind the placement. It should cover:

- the number of students to be taken by the Trust/SSD,
- the liability for any harm caused *by* the student,
- the liability for any harm caused *to* the student,

and should also clarify the duties of the clinical instructor. Some agreements may now include payment for the clinical placements from the college to the Trust/SSD or even from the Trust to the college – third year students may be valuable members of the multi-disciplinary team.

Post registration education

As in pre-registration training and education, the colleges and the Board are both concerned to maintain standards of competence in the profession.

Since Chartered Physiotherapists are directed that they should only 'practise to the extent that they have established and maintained their ability to work safely and competently' (first rule of the CSP *Professional Conduct Rules*), continuing professional development is a professional obligation.

The CSP is therefore concerned with post-registration professional development and in 1996 undertook a review of its existing post-qualifying education, known as physiotherapy access to continuing education (PACE). The principal recommendations were that CPD (continuing professional development) should replace PACE as the umbrella term for the Society's initiatives on post-qualifying learning. In addition it recommended that physiotherapists providing post-qualifying education should make links with higher education institutions to develop, deliver and gain recognition for their programmes and the CSP should explore the feasibility of accrediting its members' professional development[4]. From July 1996 to September 1997 the CSP commissioned a feasibility study on developing a framework for CPD, funded jointly by the CSP Charitable Trust and the NHS Executive[5]. At the time of writing the development of such a framework is on-going.

It is the responsibility of the individual practitioner to maintain his or her post registration competence, experience and knowledge. The CSP has assisted members in preparing standards for continuing professional development covering the following areas[6]:

- Assessment of current skills and knowledge
- Recording CPD
- Identifying the need for CPD
- Planning CPD
- Selecting an activity for CPD
- Evaluating CPD
- Sharing knowledge and skills
- Self-audit tools.

If the Trust or SSD is unwilling to fund post-registration courses or study leave, individual practitioners may have to be prepared to meet the cost themselves. Registered nurses and midwives have a responsibility to complete a personal profile of their professional development to be reregistered and such a record can also be extremely useful for physiotherapists, as well as occupational therapists[7].

Supervision and mentoring

It cannot be assumed that only full time clinical teachers have responsibilities in education and training. Increasingly, the colleges are looking for practitioners to provide not only clinical supervision for pre-registration students, but also a mentoring role for students and newly qualified registered staff. The responsibilities of the senior practitioner in relation to supervision and delegation cannot be underestimated and reference should be made to Chapter 10 on this topic.

 Questions and exercises _____

1   Define a development plan to ensure your continued professional competence.
2   What improvements do you consider could be made in ensuring the integration of theoretical and clinical training for the pre-registration student?
3   Design a protocol which could be used for those physiotherapists who act as mentors for junior colleagues.

References

1   Thornton, E. (1996) Framework for Flexibility: A new Physiotherapy curriculum. *Physiotherapist*, **82** 7, 387–8.
2   Green, A. & Waterfield, J. (1997) Admission and Progression Trends in Physiotherapy Undergraduate Education. *Physiotherapy*, **83** 9, 472–9.
3   Hunt, A., Adamson, B., Higgs, J. & Harris, L. (1998) University Education and the Physiotherapy Professional. *Physiotherapy*, **84** 6, 264–73.
4   Gosling, S. (1996) From PACE to CPD. *Physiotherapy*, **82** 9, 499–501.
5   Gosling, S. (1997) Continuing Professional Development. *Physiotherapy*, **83** 11, 563–5.
6   CSP Professional Affairs Department (1995) *Standards for Continuing Professional Development (CPD) CPD Guidelines for Physiotherapists, Managers & Educators*. CSP, London.
7   Alsop, A. (1995) The Professional Portfolio – Purpose, Process and Practice. *British Journal of Occupational Therapy*, **58** 7, 299–302.

Section B
Client-Centred Care

Chapter 6
Rights of Clients

In this Section we consider the rights of the client. First we take an overview of the basic statutory and common law rights. The next chapter looks at consent to treatment and information to be given to the client and the remaining chapters consider confidentiality and the right of access to health records.

In this chapter the following topics are considered:

- Statutory basis of the client's rights
- The right to care and treatment
- The Charter movement
- Questionable claims

Statutory basis of the client's rights

When the Human Rights Act 1998 is implemented there will be a statutory duty on public authorities to recognise the Articles of the European Convention on Human Rights. These are shown in Appendix One but it will be noted that there is no specific right to access health care that is free at the point of delivery.

Rights to health care and social care derive from the legislation shown in Figure 6.1. and from the common law (see Chapter 2 and the glossary for an explanation of these terms).

Figure 6.1 **Statutes giving rights to health care and social care.**

- National Health Service Act 1977 (based on the National Health Service Act 1946)
- National Assistance Act 1948
- Health Service and Public Health Act 1968
- Chronically Sick and Disabled Persons Act 1970
- Disabled Persons (Service, Consultation and Representation Act 1986
- Health and Social Services and Social Security Adjudications Act 1983
- Mental Health Act 1983 (as amended)
- National Health Service and Community Care Act 1990

Some of these Acts are considered in more detail in the chapters covering specific client groups.

Absolute or discretionary rights

It should be noted that very few statutes bestow absolute rights on clients or patients. The National Health Service Act 1977 re-enacted the duty of the Secretary of State to continue to promote in England and Wales a comprehensive health service designed to secure improvement:

- in the physical and mental health of the people of those countries, and
- in the prevention, diagnosis, and treatment of illness.

The duty however left much to his discretion as can be seen from Figure 6.2.

Figure 6.2 **Discretionary duties of the Secretary of State – section 3(1).**

It is the Secretary of State's duty to provide ... *to such extent as he considers necessary* to meet *all reasonable* requirements:

(a) hospital accommodation;
(b) other accommodation for the purpose of any service provided under this Act;
(c) medical, dental, nursing and ambulance services;
(d) such other facilities for the care of expectant and nursing mothers and young children *as he considers are appropriate* as part of the health service;
(e) such facilities for the prevention of illness, the care of persons suffering from illness and the after-care of persons who have suffered from illness *as he considers are appropriate* as part of the health service;
(f) such other services as are required for the diagnosis and treatment of illness.

(author's emphasis)

The rights recognised by the statutes and common law are summarised in Figure 6.3.

Figure 6.3 **Summary of client rights in the NHS and under social services.**

- To receive care and treatment (not absolute)
- To receive a reasonable standard of care and treatment
- To give or withhold consent to treatment and/or care
- To confidentiality
- To access health and personal social services records
- To complain
- To receive rights recognised in the Human Rights Act 1998

These are covered in the chapters which follow.

Enforcement of rights

These rights can be enforced by the individual patient in many ways through administrative and judicial machinery.

Administrative machinery includes the following:

- Complaint through the set procedure (see Chapter 14)
- Inquiry by Secretary of State
- Independent inquiry.

Judicial remedies include the following:

- An action for negligence – when harm has occurred (see Chapter 10)
- An action for trespass to the person – where treatment has been given without consent (see Chapter 7)
- An action for breach of statutory duty – where it is alleged that a statutory authority has not fulfilled its duties.
- An action for judicial review of the decisions of a statutory authority or other administrative body.

The right to care and treatment

Unenforceable rights

As can be seen from Figure 6.2 there is not an absolute right to obtain treatment under the NHS. In the inevitable situation where resources are finite and demand outmatches supply providers and purchasers have to weigh priorities. Where individual patients have sought to enforce the statutory duty to provide services, the courts have refused to intervene unless there is evidence that there has been a failure to make a reasonable decision about the allocation of resources[1]. Thus patients who brought an action for breach of statutory duty against the Secretary of State for Health and the Regional and Area Health Authorities on the grounds that they had waited too long for hip operations failed in their claim.

More recently Jamie Bowen, a child suffering from leukaemia, was refused a course of chemotherapy and a second bone marrow transplant on the grounds that there was only a very small chance of the treatment succeeding and therefore it would not be in her best interests for the treatment to proceed. The Court of Appeal upheld the decision of the health authority[2] as they were unable to fault its process of reasoning and allowed the appeal.

The Master of the Rolls (Sir Thomas Bingham) stated:

> 'While I have every sympathy with B, I feel bound to regard this as an attempt – wholly understandable, but nevertheless misguided – to involve the court in a field of activity where it is not fitted to make any decision favourable to the patient.'

The inability to provide all the services the patient requires is a major concern of physiotherapists. This mismatching between needs and supply of services may never reach court, but physiotherapists are aware when they do not have the resources to provide as intensive or extensive treatment as the patient would appear to require. For example an audit of elderly care in-patient physiotherapy services revealed that patients received around half of the treatment that staff felt was necessary[3]. This issue is discussed further in Chapter 10 in the context of rationing and prioritising services.

Since the patient has no absolute right to receive treatment, the patient cannot insist that the care is provided by a specific member of staff (though the patient could probably require a member of staff of the same gender); nor could the patient insist on the provision of clinical treatment which was clinically contra-indicated or not supported by professional opinion; nor, if the physiotherapist was of the view that continued treatment in a chronic condition was no longer effective, could the patient insist on receiving it. The patient could however refuse to accept treatment from a student (but probably not from a physiotherapy assistant if the activity is within her sphere of competence) and normally the patient's consent would be requested in advance to the presence of and care by students.

Enforceable rights

Some rights to care are however enforceable. These arise in circumstances of:

- a failure to provide a general practitioner; and
- a failure to provide appropriate emergency services in an accident and emergency department.

Here the claim would be based upon the duty to ensure that a reasonable standard of care was provided (see Chapter 10 on negligence).

Duty to follow DoH guidelines

In July 1997 the High Court ruled against North Derbyshire Health Authority which had refused to fund the purchase of beta-interferon in the treatment of multiple sclerosis[4]. In its press announcement following the decision a spokeswoman for the authority stated that the drug had not yet been supported by clear research findings on its effectiveness. It lost the case because the health authority had failed to follow DoH guidelines in the supply of the drug to MS patients. On the other hand even following ministerial guidelines to the letter would not render an authority immune from a successful claim being made against it. In *R* v. *Wandsworth Borough Council*[5] the Court found that the guidance itself was incorrect.

The Charter movement

Effect of the charters

There are now national Charters for patients in both secondary and primary care; and many hospitals, community health services and GP practices have prepared their own charters. These give certain assurances to clients and patients that services will be provided within set times and to a specific quality.

However these charters do not bestow legal rights and the client or patient cannot enforce them unless the services they offer are already part of the law. For example the client might be advised that full information will be given to him or her about the range of services available and about any contra-indications or side effects. Should a health professional fail to give the appropriate information and the client suffers harm of which she had not been warned, then the client would have a legal right of action. However this would not be on the basis of the charter, but because of an existing common law right to be given appropriate information as part of the duty of care owed by the health professional to the client (see Chapter 7). In contrast, a charter may declare that a patient has the right to receive in-patient admission within eighteen months. Nevertheless if a patient waits for over two years for in-patient admission he would have little hope of success in a court action.

He may however be able to bring a complaint to the NHS Trust and this could reach the Health Service Commissioner. He could also complain to the health authority or primary health group/trust (PCG) because of the Trust's failure to comply with patient charter standards and therefore with the NHS agreement it has with the health authority or PCG.

Where the client is receiving private health care under a contract agreed with a physiotherapist in private practice, then a charter might be seen as part of the agreement and the client may then be able to sue for breach of contract (see Chapter 19).

The CSP has given advice on the existing Patient's Charter[6].

Enforcement of charters

Complaints can be made about failure to fulfil charter terms through the recognised complaints procedures (see Chapter 14). Otherwise the enforcement of the charters lies not in the right of the individual patient to enforce them but through the monitoring carried out by the health authorities and GP fundholders (or in the future primary health or local health groups as purchasers on behalf of the Department of Health and the Welsh Office). NHS agreements contain stipulations about meeting charter requirements and these are reviewed through the quality assurance mechanisms. At the time of writing a new charter which covers the responsibilities of the patient as well as the rights of the patient is being drafted with the intention that it should be published in the spring of 1999.

Questionable claims

Physiotherapists may be confronted by clients who, in contrast to those who are ignorant of their rights, are anxious to exploit the system for any benefits which are obtainable. This can be seen from a letter to the *British Journal of Occupational Therapy* by Rosemary Barnitt[7]. Her point is that in undertaking research into ethical dilemmas experienced by several hundred occupational therapists and physiotherapists, she is 'surprised by the number who have found themselves being referred "patients" with apparently substantial physical disabilities, but who turn out to have insignificant or no health problems'. She gave an example of a referral to a social services occupational therapist of a man in a wheelchair who had requested home adaptations. On assessment, the therapist felt that the man could walk and function normally but had chosen to take on a disabled role. She asked for information about this phenomenon and followed up with a letter five months later in the same journal[8] saying that she had over 40 letters and telephone calls on this subject.

The requirement for the physiotherapist to follow the professional standards of assessment (and not be biased in favour of the claimant or defendant) in making reports to be used in court action is considered in Chapter 13.

Situation: unjustified claims

A physiotherapist has been providing home treatment to a patient following a stroke. She is anxious that the treatment should be continued in the OPD, but the patient says that he is not able to attend because of his disability which prevents him leaving the house. She subsequently hears from a colleague that the patient was seen in a super-market. Can the physiotherapist refuse to provide physiotherapy services at home?

There are of course limited resources for health care which must be used justly and wisely. Abuse or unjustified expenditure in one area limits resources for use elsewhere and may mean that justifiable claims are not met. In this situation, the patient should be advised that he must attend the clinic in order to receive his treatment and that transport will be made available. If the patient is mentally competent and decides that he is not prepared to attend then that is his decision (see Chapter 18 on care in the community).

Conclusions

This is a complex area of law, partly because there has been no attempt to codify the rights to which a patient/client is entitled nor has there been any attempt to ensure that such a code is enforceable through the legal system. Any potential litigant therefore has first to ascertain if the wrong which he claims to have suffered is one recognised by the common law or statute law and then to take advice on the means of enforcement. The following chapters cover patient/client separate rights which are currently recognised in law and enforceable in the courts. Chapter 14 covers the procedures relating to complaints and to the enforcement mechanism for standards within NHS care.

Questions and exercises _____

1 What client rights do you consider that the law should recognise?
2 There will never be the resources to meet all demands upon health and social services. What criteria would you draw up to determine priorities for patients to receive physiotherapy services?
3 What do you consider are the advantages of the Human Rights Act 1998? (see Appendix One)

References

1 *R* v. *Secretary of State for Social Services, ex parte Hincks and others.* Solicitors Journal, 29 June 1979, page 436.

2 *R* v. *Cambridge and Huntingdon Health Authority, ex parte B* [1995] 2 All ER 129.

3 David, C., Noon, J. & Abdulla, A. (1998) An audit of elderly care in-patient physio-therapy services. *Agility* January 1998, 13–16.

4 *R* v. *North Derbyshire Health Authority, ex parte Fisher* [1997] 8 Med LR 327.

5 *R* v. *Wandsworth Borough Council, ex parte Beckwith* [1996] 1 All ER 129 (discussed in Dimond, B. (1997) *Legal Aspects of Care in the Community* pp 465–6, Macmillan, Basingstoke).

6 CSP Professional Affairs Department (1997) No. PA 17 (August 1997) *The Patient's Charter*. CPS, London.

7 Barnitt, R. (1995) Letter to the editor on 'Ethical dilemmas'. *British Journal of Occupational Therapy*, **58** 2, 78.

8 Barnitt, R. (1995) Letter to the editor. *British Journal of Occupational Therapy*, **58** 7, 308.

Chapter 7
Consent and Information Giving

This chapter covers the legal issues relating to consent to treatment. It will be concerned with those issues which arise in relation to the mentally competent adult. The laws relating to consent in the case of children, mentally ill, elderly and those with learning disabilities are covered in the chapters in Section E dealing with those specialist client groups. The topic of disclosure is considered in the Chapter 8 on confidentiality. The following topics are considered in this chapter.

- Basic principles
- Trespass to the person
- Duty to inform
- Conclusion

Basic principles

There are two distinct aspects of the law relating to consent to treatment. One is the actual giving of consent and the possibility that a trespass to the person has occurred because the patient did not give consent to the treatment. The other is the duty to give information to the patient prior to the giving of consent. The absence of consent could result in the patient suing for trespass to the person. The failure to provide sufficient relevant information could result in an action for negligence. These two different legal actions will be considered separately.

Trespass to the person

A trespass to the person occurs when an individual either apprehends a touching of her person (an assault) or the individual is actually touched (a battery) and has not given consent. The person who has suffered the trespass can sue for compensation in the civil courts (and a prosecution could also be brought in criminal cases).

In the civil cases, the victim has to prove:

- the touching or the apprehension of the touching; and
- that it was a (potentially) direct interference with her person.

The victim does not have to show that harm has occurred. This is in contrast to an action for negligence in which the victim must show that harm has resulted from the breach of duty of care (see Chapter 10).

Defences to an action for trespass to the person

The main defence to an action for trespass to the person is that consent was given by a mentally competent person. In addition there are two other defences in law which are:

- statutory authorisation e.g. Mental Health Act 1983 (discussed in Chapter 21)
- the common law power to act out of necessity.

Consent

For consent to treatment to be valid, the person giving it must be mentally competent (a child of 16 and 17 has a statutory right to give consent, as may a child below 16 if 'Gillick competent' (see Chapter 23)) and the consent must be given without any duress or force or deceit.

Competence and capacity

It will be seen below that in the case of *Re T*[1] the Court of Appeal emphasised the duty of the health professional to ensure that a person who was refusing a necessary treatment had the capacity to do so. Of relevance here is the work of Jennifer Fleming and Jenny Strong[2] in the research of self-awareness of deficits following acquired brain injury and what must be taken into account in rehabilitation. Where there is any doubt about the competence of an individual to give a valid consent there are considerable advantages if the capacity to give a valid consent could be checked by a person who is not involved in the treatment which is being recommended. This person should record her actions and observations.

Different ways of giving consent

Consent can be given by word of mouth, in writing or can be implied i.e. the non-verbal conduct of the person may indicate that she is giving consent. All these forms of giving consent are valid, but where procedures entail risk and/or where there is likely to be a dispute over whether consent was given it is advisable to obtain consent in writing. It is then easier to establish in a court of law that consent was given.

Although consent can be given by word of mouth or by non-verbal communication, there are a few situations where consent must be recorded in writing by law and Chapter 21 covers the provision of the Mental Health Act 1983 and consent by detained patients.

Application to physiotherapy

In practice there are many physiotherapy activities and treatments which cannot proceed without the co-operation of the patient and consent to the involvement is often implied from the patient's non-verbal communication. In such cases, therefore, trespass to the person actions are unlikely. The focus is more likely to be on the nature of the information which is made available before the consent is given (see below).

Care should however always be taken if it is necessary to examine patients or have physical contact with them to ensure that the patient consents to this contact and continues to consent.

Consent for intimate examinations

Physiotherapists are particularly concerned when they are required to carry out intimate examinations on their patients. Often in even basic care the physio- therapist might have to ask a patient to undress completely. In such circum- stances it is advisable for the patient to be warned about this possibility before they attend, so that they can be prepared and bring with them a friend or chaperon. If such examination is necessary and it is a male physiotherapist who is working in the department, a female patient should be given a choice over whether she is to be attended by a male physiotherapist or not. If she agrees, the male physiotherapist should ensure that he is chaperoned and watch carefully for any signs which would suggest that a female colleague should take over. It must be remembered that this is also to protect the male physiotherapist from any allegations in such circumstances.

In some conditions it may be necessary for the physiotherapist to carry out a pelvic floor examination which would require vaginal examination and occa- sionally rectal examination. The patient should be clearly informed about what this examination would entail and specific consent to this should be obtained, preferably in writing. Although consent by word of mouth would be valid in law, it would be more difficult to establish in court where it may be one person's word against another. Rule 2 of the CSP *Rules of Professional Conduct*[3] suggests that written consent may not usually be necessary but continues:

> 'Procedures that may however require such a form [i.e. of consent] are movements of force to the cervical spine, vaginal and rectal examinations and exercise tolerance tests from cardiac patients. If consent forms are used some indication of the information given, the options offered and how consent was received should be included to ensure that the form has some legal credibility.'

There are clear advantages for the physiotherapist in obtaining consent in writing from the patient at the beginning of any treatment plan. At this time the physiotherapist can explain to the patient the nature and extent of the treatment, its likely effects and any side effects or inherent risks. If it is the intention to use electrotherapy or manipulation, the physiotherapist could explain any risks of the treatment and also obtain the consent of the patient in writing. If at any time, the treatment plan is significantly changed, this may be reflected in a new written consent by the patient.

Consent forms

It will be noted that many physiotherapy treatments will be given without any written evidence of consent. Where however, it is feared that there may be sig- nificant risks of substantial harm or there is likely to be any dispute as to whether consent was given, it is advisable for consent to be obtained in writing. The NHS Management Executive has issued guidance[4] and gives in the appendix a form which can be used for the consent for treatments given by professions other than a doctor and dentist. This should act as a reminder that the relevant information should be given to patients for them to give valid consent and ensure that all the requisite details are recorded.

The NHSME also recommends that a form could be completed when an adult who lacks mental capacity to give consent to treatment is provided with care in the absence of consent (see below). This form could be adapted for completion by the physiotherapist.

Withdrawal of consent

■ What if someone wishes to leave hospital?

It is a principle of consent that a person who has given consent can withdraw it at any time, unless there is a contractual reason why this is not so. This means that if people wish to leave hospital contrary to their best interests then, unless they lack the capacity to make a valid decision, they are free to go. Clearly there are advantages in obtaining the signature of such patients that the self-discharge or refusal to accept treatment is contrary to clinical advice, but if they refuse to sign a form that they are taking discharge contrary to clinical advice, that refusal must be accepted. It would in such a case be advisable to ensure that there is another professional as a witness to this and that a careful record is made by both professionals.

Refusal to consent

The Court of Appeal set out the basic principles of self-determination of the mentally competent adult in the case of *Re T*[1]. However it also emphasised the importance of the health professional ensuring that any refusal to give consent to life saving treatment and care was valid.

Case: *Re T*

A woman suffering from complications after childbirth had made it clear that she would not wish to have a blood transfusion. She was very much under the influence of her mother, a Jehovah's Witness. When it became evident that she would need blood to stay alive, the Court allowed the application of the cohabitee and father for blood to be given. This was on the grounds that her refusal was not valid. This decision was confirmed by the Court of Appeal.

The Court of Appeal laid down the following propositions.

(1) *Prima facie* every adult has the right and capacity to decide whether or not he will accept medical treatment, even if a refusal may risk permanent injury to his health or even lead to premature death. It matters not whether the reasons for the refusal are rational or irrational, unknown or even non-existent. However this presumption of capacity is rebuttable.
(2) An adult may be deprived of his capacity to decide either by long-term mental incapacity or retarded development, or by temporary factors such as unconsciousness or confusion or the effects of fatigue, shock, pain or drugs.
(3) If an adult patient did not have the capacity to decide at the time of purported

refusal and still does not have that capacity, it is the duty of the doctors to treat him in whatever way they consider (in the exercise of their clinical judgment) to be in his best interests.

(4) Doctors faced with a refusal of consent have to give very careful and detailed consideration to what was the patient's capacity to decide at the time when the decision was made.

(5) Doctors must also consider if the refusal has been vitiated because of the will of others who have sought to persuade the patient to refuse. If his will has been overborne, the refusal will not represent the true decision.

(6) In all cases doctors will need to consider what is the true scope and basis of the refusal.

(7) Forms of refusal should be redesigned to bring the consequences of a refusal forcibly to the attention of patients.

(8) In cases of doubt as to the effect of a purported refusal of treatment, where failure to treat threatens the patient's life, doctors and health authorities should not hesitate to apply to the courts for assistance.

The right of the adult mentally competent person to refuse food was upheld in the case of a prisoner who had gone on hunger strike. Although the prisoner was diagnosed as suffering from a personality disorder he was held to be of sound mind so that the law required the Home Office, prison officers and doctors to accept his refusal to take food or drink[5]. This case overruled a case where suffragettes who went on hunger strike were force fed[6] and the defence of acting out of necessity was applied. It is now clear that this defence is only available when the adult is mentally in competent (see below).

The principle of the right of self-determination if the adult is mentally competent has subsequently been considered and extended by the Court of Appeal in two cases where a compulsory caesarean had been carried out. In the first case[8], where the pregnant woman suffered from needle phobia and would not agree to an injection preceding the caesarean, the court held the needle phobia to be so acute as to render her mentally incapable and therefore it was declared that doctors performing a caesarean, acting in her best interests, would not be acting illegally. (For the common law power to act in the best interests out of necessity see below.)

The Court of Appeal laid down principles to assist clinicians in treating a pregnant woman.

- In cases where the competence of the mother to make a decision is in doubt, the doctors are advised to seek a ruling from the High Court on the issue of competence.
- Those involved with the pregnancy should identify a potential problem as early as possible so that both hospital and patient can seek legal advice.
- The need for an emergency application to court should be avoided as far as is possible.
- Both parties should be represented, unless the mother refuses. An unconscious mother should be represented by the guardian ad litem.
- The Official Solicitor should be notified of all applications.
- There should be some evidence of the lack of competence of the patient (not necessarily from a psychiatrist).

The facts of the second case[8] are shown below:

Case: *St George's Healthcare National Health Service Trust* v. *S*

S was diagnosed with pre-eclampsia and advised that she needed urgent attention, bedrest and admission to hospital for an induced delivery. Without that treatment the health and life of both herself and the unborn child were in real danger. She fully understood the potential risks but rejected the advice. She wanted her baby to be born naturally.

She was then seen by an approved social worker and two doctors in relation to compulsory admission to hospital under section 2 of the Mental Health Act 1983 for assessment. They repeated the advice which she had been given and she refused to accept it. On the basis of the written medical recommendations of the two doctors the approved social worker applied for her admission to hospital for assessment under section 2 of the Mental Health Act 1983. Later that day, again against her will, she was transferred to St George's Hospital. In view of her continuing adamant refusal to consent to treatment an application was made *ex parte* on behalf of the hospital authority to Mrs Justice Hogg who made a declaration that the caesarean section could proceed, dispensing with S's consent to treatment. The operation was carried out and a baby girl delivered. S was then returned to Springfield Hospital and two days later her detention under section 2 of the Mental Health Act was ended.

She then sought judicial review of her detention, the High Court judgment and the caesarean operation.

The Court of Appeal held that the Mental Health Act 1983 could not be deployed to achieve the detention of an individual against her will merely because her thinking process was unusual, or even apparently bizarre and irrational, and contrary to the view of the overwhelming majority of the community at large. A woman detained under the Act for mental disorder could not be forced into medical procedures unconnected with her mental condition unless her capacity to consent to such treatment was diminished. The Court of Appeal was not satisfied that S was lawfully detained under section 2 of the Mental Health Act 1983 because she was not suffering from mental disorder of a nature or degree which warranted her detention in hospital for assessment. Although on the face of the documents her admission would appear to have been legal, her transfer to St George's Hospital was unlawful and at any time she would have been justified in applying for a writ of *habeas corpus* which would have led to her immediate release. The declaration made by the High Court judge should not have been made on an *ex parte* basis (i.e. without representation of the woman) and was unlawful.

The difference between the two cases is that in the first case the woman was held, as a result of the extreme needle phobia, to be mentally incompetent, and therefore the caesarean could be carried out in her best interests without her consent; whereas in the second case S was not to be held mentally incompetent, and therefore the compulsory caesarean was a trespass to her person. In neither case did the Court consider the rights of the foetus to influence the decision making. The foetus is not regarded in law as a legal personality until birth. Until then the wishes of a mentally competent pregnant woman will prevail whatever the effect on the unborn child.

The existence of a mental illness will not automatically mean that people are incapable of giving a valid refusal of consent to treatment in their best interests, as in the case of *Re C*[9], where a patient in Broadmoor was considered to have the capacity to refuse a leg amputation which doctors had advised him was indicated as a life saving measure. An injunction (see glossary) was ordered against any doctors carrying out an amputation on him without his consent.

The principles established by the Court for consent to be seen as competent were:

- comprehending and retaining treatment information;
- believing it; and
- weighing it in the balance to arrive at a choice.

In applying this test to C the judge was completely satisfied that the presumption that C had the right of self-determination had not been replaced. Although his general capacity had been impaired by schizophrenia, he had understood and retained the treatment information, and believed it and had arrived at a clear choice. (See Chapter 21 for further details of the law of consent and the mentally ill.)

Common law power to act out of necessity

Where, but only where, the patient lacks the capacity to give consent to treatment, treatment can proceed on the basis that it is in the best interests of that individual and is given according to the reasonable standard of the profession. This is known as the right at common law (i.e. judge-made law) to act out of necessity in the best interests of the mentally incompetent person. In such circumstances, the health professional would not be committing a trespass to the person. This was the ruling in the House of Lords in the case of *Re F*[10]. In that case the House of Lords declared that it was lawful for doctors to sterilise a mentally handicapped person who lacked the capacity to give a valid consent provided that they acted in her best interests. The court did, however, require a reference to the court to be made in future cases, and a Practice Direction[11] was issued. Under the principle established in *Re F* many health professionals provide care to persons who are unable to give consent to treatment. (This is further discussed in Chapter 21.).

The House of Lords, in the case of *R* v. *Bournewood Community and Mental Health NHS Trust*[12], held that the common law power to act out of necessity in the best interests of the patient also included the right to admit adult mentally incapacitated patients to psychiatric hospital. It overruled a decision of the Court of Appeal that such patients had to be detained under the Mental Health Act 1983 where this applied.

Consent on another's behalf

At present there is a vacuum in the law. If a mentally incapacitated adult is unable to make their own decisions no relative can give or withhold consent on their behalf. The Law Commission has made recommendations on how this vacuum should be filled[13] and this was followed by a Consultation paper issued by the

Lord Chancellor's Office in 1997[14]. At the time of writing the Government's proposals are awaited (see Chapter 21).

Situation: Who decides?

> An elderly man had a stroke and decisions had to be made about his on-going treatment. The Consultant asked his daughter if she would give consent for him to have an operation.

In this situation, the daughter does not have a legal right to give or withhold consent on behalf of her father. Clearly her views on the operation are relevant, but, in the absence of any person with the legal right to make decisions on behalf of the mentally incapacitated adult, doctors must decide in the light of the prognosis and the views of the multi-disciplinary team and of the relatives what is in the best interests of the patient. They can then act on the basis of the common law power described above. The NHS Executive has recommended specific forms to be used when treatment is given to a mentally incapacitated adult[15].

Duty to inform

As part of the duty of care owed in the law of negligence the professional has a duty to inform the patient about the significant risks of substantial harm which could occur if treatment were to proceed.

If the harm has not been explained to the patient and the harm then occurs, the patient can claim that, had she known of this possibility, she would not have agreed to undergo the treatment. She could then bring an action in negligence. To succeed the patient would have to show:

- that there was a duty of care to give specific information;
- the defendant failed to give this information and in so doing was therefore in breach of the reasonable standard of care which should have been provided;
- as a result of this failure to inform, the patient agreed to the treatment; and
- subsequently suffered the harm.

The leading case is that of *Sidaway*[16] where the House of Lords stated that the professional was required in law to provide information to the patient according to the Bolam test i.e. the standard of the reasonable practitioner following the accepted approved standard of care (see Chapter 10).

To ensure that the patient understands the information which is given, there are considerable advantages in a written hand out being provided (checking of course that the patient is literate). This would also assist if there were any dispute over the information having been given.

In Chapter 9 the duty of a doctor to give full information as a requirement by the GMC is considered.

Application to physiotherapy

The duty placed upon the physiotherapist is that she should ensure that the patient is given information about the significant risks of substantial harm which could arise from treatment. She would be judged by the standard of the reasonable practitioner in that situation with that specific patient. (This is further discussed in Chapter 10 on negligence.) This requires the physiotherapist to ensure that she maintains her competence and knowledge about current issues and research. It also requires the physiotherapist to make an assessment of the competence of clients to understand what they are being told, and to use language which conveys the necessary information accurately and effectively. In difficult situations it would be advisable for a physiotherapist to ask a colleague, possibly a psychologist, to provide an independent assessment of the mental competence of the patient.

Kim Jones discusses the problems involved in explaining rehabilitation theory to neurologically impaired patients and their families[17], in particular explaining the concept of neural plasticity. She uses the analogy of a path between a house and a grain store through a corn field to communicate to patients how rehabilitation can take place.

Debate arose over the information, including pictorial information, which should be given to patients about lymphoedema following publication of the book written by Michael Mason[18], *Living with Lymphoedema*. He argues that

> 'most patients . . . request as much information as possible about their medical problems. Lymphoedema patients are no different. They want to know, among other things, the prognosis, the treatment and how bad their condition can become if left untreated. Once they have all of this information, patients are then in the position to make an informed decision about their treatment.'

This therefore justifies the use of before and after pictures. Most physiotherapists would probably accept that this is sound practice, providing the information is given sensitively.

Written information provided in a department should be reviewed critically to assess its readability by patients. Judith Chapman and John Langridge assessed the physiotherapy health education literature distributed by a physiotherapy service[19] and concluded that many leaflets were written at a level too high for the average comprehension of their patients. The authors recommend the use of an uncomplicated method for assessing reading levels of written materials.

Communication should of course be a two-way process and in a stimulating paper Barbara Martlew describes a study in a day hospice to examine patients' perceptions of the problems caused by their terminal illness, the relevance and benefit of physiotherapy and the factors contributing to quality of life[20]. Recommendations are made on the benefits of listening sensitively, of being aware of the underlying fear that symptoms indicate disease progression, and on utilising the quality of life indicators when setting goals for physiotherapy intervention.

Analysing the reasons why patients fail to attend for out-patient treatment can also provide an important way of improving communication with patients. Jane Armistead studied initial non-attendance rates for physiotherapy[21]. Rates of attendance were better if made by telephone than by post and referrals from GPs were more likely to lead to non-attendance than referrals from consultants. The author concludes that there is a need to 'provide a flexible, responsive service and stimulate the moral responsibility of the consumers.'

Conclusion

The physiotherapist must accept that the law recognises the autonomy of the mentally competent patient to decide whether or not to participate in treatment activities. The onus is on the health professional to inform the patient fully about the benefits and risks of the treatment.

 Questions and exercises

1   Analyse your practice in relation to obtaining consent from the patient and decide if it could be improved.
2   Draw up a form for consent to physiotherapy.
3   Prepare a hand out for the client/patient giving information about the nature of any specific treatment which you provide, setting out any inherent risks.

References

1   *Re T (Adult: Refusal of Medical Treatment* [1992] 4 All ER 649.
2   Fleming, J. & Strong, J. (1995) Self-awareness of deficits following acquired brain injury: Considerations for rehabilitation. *British Journal of Occupational Therapy,* **58** 2, 55–60.
3   Chartered Society of Physiotherapy (1995) *Rules of Professional Conduct* CSP, London.
4   NHS Management Executive (1990) *A Guide to Consent for Examination and Treatment.* (HC(90)22 and HSG(92)32), Department of Health, London.
5   *Secretary of State for the Home Department* v. *Robb* [1995] 1 All ER 677.
6   *Leigh* v. *Gladstone* (1909) 25 TLR 139.
7   *Re M B (Caesarian Section)* The Times Law Report, 18 April 1997.
8   *St George's Healthcare National Health Service Trust* v. *S; R* v. *Collins and Others, ex parte S.* The Times Law Report, 8 May 1998.
9   Re C (Adult: Refusal of Medical Treatment) [1994] 1 All ER 819.
10   *F* v. *West Berkshire Health Authority and another* [1989] 2 All ER 545.
11   Practice Note [1993] 3 All ER 222 (replaces previous Practice Note issued 1989).
12   *R* v. *Bournewood Community and Mental Health NHS Trust, ex parte L* (HL) [1998] 1 All ER 634.
13   Law Commission (1995) Report No. 231 *Mental Incapacity* HMSO, London.
14   Lord Chancellor's Office (1997) Consultation Paper *Who Decides?* LCD, London.
15   NHS Management Executive (1990) *A Guide to Consent for Examination and Treatment.* (HC(90)22) Appendix B, Department of Health, London.
16   *Sidaway* v. *Bethlem Royal Hospital Governors* [1985] 1 All ER 643.
17   Jones, K. (1997) The Grain Store Analogy: Explaining rehabilitation theory to neurologically impaired patients and their families. *Physiotherapist,* **83**, 11, 575–7.
18   Mason, M. (1996) Letter to the editor: Facing the frightful facts. *Physiotherapy* **82**, 3, 216.
19   Chapman, J. & Langridge, J. (1997) Physiotherapy Health Education Literature. *Physiotherapy,* **83**, 8, 406–412.
20   Martlew, B. (1996) What Do You Let the Patient Tell You? *Physiotherapy,* **82**, 10, 558–65.
21   Armistead, J. (1997) An Evaluation of Initial Non-attendance Rates for Physiotherapy. *Physiotherapy,* **83**, 11, 591–6.

Chapter 8
Confidentiality

All physiotherapists, whether working in the public or private sector, have a duty to maintain the confidentiality of information obtained from or about the patient. This chapter explores the source of this obligation and the exceptions recognised in law to the duty[1]. The following topics are considered:

- The nature of the duty
- Exceptions to the duty of confidentiality
- Implications for the physiotherapist
- Link with ethical issues
- The future

The nature of the duty

The duty to respect patient confidentiality arises from a variety of sources which are set out in Figure 8.1.

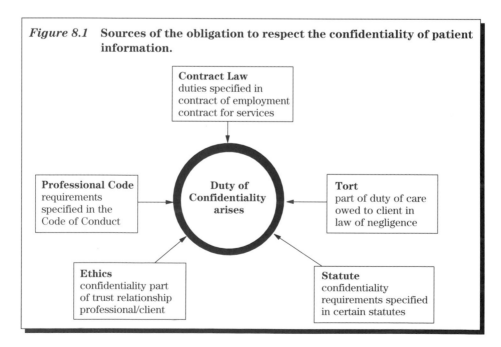

Figure 8.1   **Sources of the obligation to respect the confidentiality of patient information.**

Contract Law
duties specified in
contract of employment
contract for services

Professional Code
requirements
specified in the
Code of Conduct

**Duty of
Confidentiality
arises**

Tort
part of duty of care
owed to client in
law of negligence

Ethics
confidentiality part
of trust relationship
professional/client

Statute
confidentiality
requirements specified
in certain statutes

The Code of Professional Conduct

Each registered professional has certain professional obligations which are enforceable through the professional conduct machinery set up under the Council for the Professions Supplementary to Medicine (CPSM). Rule 3 of the *Rules of Professional Conduct* of the CSP sets out the duty of the physiotherapist in relation to confidentiality:

> 'Chartered Physiotherapists shall ensure confidentiality and security of information acquired in a professional capacity.'

The CSP has issued advice for physiotherapists[2] in the light of the publication of the Department of Health's guidance on the *Protection and Use of Patient Information*[3]. The CSP highlights the main principles to be followed and gives a list of sources for further reference. An annexe to the CSP guidance provides a model notice for patients relating to information and the patient's right of access to their health records.

Maintenance of high professional standards ideally requires the review of matters including patient information by persons other than the physiotherapist giving the treatment but Standard 24 of the CSP *Standards of Physiotherapy Practice*[4] provides in the quality assurance programme for the evaluation of clinical practice to be undertaken with due respect for patient confidentiality. Confidentiality is maintained throughout evaluation activities and clinical documentation is audited regularly.

The contract of employment/contract for services

The employed health professional also has an obligation to observe the confidentiality of patient information which derives from the contract of employment and is enforceable by the employer. This will usually be set out expressly in the contract of employment, but, even if the contract is silent on the topic, the courts may imply into it such a term. Should the health professional be in breach of this expressed or implied term, then the employer can take appropriate action through the disciplinary machinery. This may be simply counselling or an oral warning, or any of the stages in the disciplinary procedure may be invoked, depending on the circumstances. In serious cases, the employer may be considered justified in dismissing the employee. (In such a case if the employer has acted unreasonably and the employee has the necessary continuous service requirement (see Chapter 17) the employee could challenge the employer's action by an application to an industrial tribunal for unfair dismissal.)

Those who work as self-employed professionals do not have an obligation to an employer but they do have a contract for services with their patients which may impose conditions relating to confidentiality. Should the health professional be in breach of these contractual conditions, then the patient could bring an action in the civil courts and have the usual remedies for breach of contract (see Chapter 19 on the private practitioner).

The duty of care owed in the law of negligence

The health professional owes a duty to the patient to retain information given to her in confidence.

Case: *Furniss* v. *Fitchett*[5]

In this New Zealand case, the court upheld an action for damages in the tort of negligence for breach of confidence. A doctor treating the plaintiff had given to the patient's husband a letter about the patient's mental state, which was used by the husband's solicitor in matrimonial proceedings.

The doctor was held to be in breach of the duty of care which he owed to the patient.

Should the health professional be in breach of this duty, then the patient could bring an action against the employer of the health professional on the basis of its vicarious liability for the actions of an employee acting in course of employment.

One weakness of the patient's right of action in the law of negligence is that the patient has to prove harm. There may be potential, following unauthorised disclosure, for harm to arise, but until it does so arise the patient cannot obtain compensation. He might however obtain an injunction to prevent the disclosure.

Case: *X* v. *Y*[6]

The court ordered an injunction to be issued to prevent the disclosure by the press of the identity of doctors suffering from AIDS. Two general practitioners were diagnosed as having contracted AIDS. They received counselling in a local hospital while continuing with their medical practice. A journalist heard of the situation from an employee of the health authority and wrote an article for a national newspaper. The health authority sought an injunction to prevent any further disclosure of the information obtained from the patients' records. The judge granted the injunction on the grounds that the records of hospital patients, particularly those suffering from this appalling condition, should be as confidential as the courts could properly make them. He rejected the defendant's argument that it was in the public interest for the identify of these doctors to be known.

The judge did not however agree to the health authority's application for disclosure of the name of the employee who had given the information to the journalist. He held that the exceptions under section 10 of the Contempt of Court Act 1981 to the principle that the court cannot require disclosure from a journalist did not apply to the situation and the journalist was entitled to protect his source.

Another difficulty is that if a patient is wishing to preserve secrecy of information, then the danger of a court action is that the dispute will be brought into the open and the publicity will then defeat the patient's main objective. This perhaps explains why there are very few decided cases on confidentiality.

The duty set out in specific statutes

Figure 8.2 identifies the statutes which make it an offence to disclose specified information.

***Figure 8.2* Statutory prohibition against disclosure.**

- Abortion Regulations 1991 (made under the Abortion Act 1967)
- NHS (Venereal Disease) Regulations 1974
- Human Fertilisation and Embryology Act 1990 (as amended by the Human Fertilisation and Embryology (Disclosure of Information) Act 1992)
- Data Protection Act 1984 (due to be replaced when the Data Protection Act 1998 is brought into force with its subordinate legislation in 1999)

Where information is disclosed in breach of these statutory provisions, the holder of the records or the patient can initiate the appropriate enforcement machinery. In the case of unauthorised disclosure of information kept in computerised form, the Data Protection Registrar can remove from a data user his right to be registered under the Act and to hold personal information in computerised form. (See also Chapter 9 on the Data Protection Act provisions in relation to subject access.) Chris Austin[7] provides a useful summary of the law relating to confidentiality and computer held personal information in relation to occupational therapy.

The trust obligation between health professional and patient

This duty was acknowledged by the House of Lords[8] in the case known as 'the Spycatcher case'. It was accepted that as a broad principle a duty of confidence arises:

- if information is confidential; and
- comes to the knowledge of a person where he or she has notice, or is held to have agreed, that the information is confidential, (with the effect that it would be just that he or she should be precluded from disclosing the information); and
- it is in the public interest that the confidentiality should be protected.

Clearly these principles would apply to information which the physiotherapist was given by or about a patient. The principles were applied in the case of *Stephens* v. *Avery*[9].

Case: *Stephens* v. *Avery*

In this case concerning unconscionable disclosure the plaintiff and first defendant were close friends who freely discussed matters of a personal and private nature on the express basis that what the plaintiff told the first defendant was secret and disclosed in confidence. The first defendant passed on to the second and third defendants, who were the editor and publisher of a newspaper, details of the plaintiff's sexual conduct, including details of the plaintiff's lesbian relationship with a woman who had been killed by her husband. The plaintiff brought an action against the defendants claiming damages on the grounds that the information was confidential and was knowingly published by the newspaper in breach of the duty of confidence owed by the first defendant to the plaintiff.

In an action by the defendants to strike out the claim as disclosing no reasonable cause of action the defendants failed and appealed to the Chancery Division. They lost this appeal on the grounds that, although the courts would not enforce a duty of confidence relating to matters which had a grossly immoral tendency, information relating to sexual conduct could be the subject of a legally enforceable duty of confidence if it would be unconscionable for the person who had received information on the express basis that it was confidential subsequently to reveal that information to another.

Exceptions to the duty of confidentiality

All the sources of law which recognise that there is a duty of confidentiality also recognise that there will be exceptions where it is lawful to disclose confidential information. Thus Rule 3 of the CSP's *Rules of Professional Conduct* recognises exceptions to the duty of confidentiality.

'This information is not to be divulged to a third party without the written consent of the patient unless the Chartered Physiotherapist is directed to do so by a competent legal authority, such as a judge, or unless it is necessary to protect the welfare of the patient and the community.'

The main exceptions to the duty of confidentiality are shown in Figure 8.3.

Figure 8.3 **Exceptions to the duty of confidentiality.**

- Consent of the patient
- Disclosure in the clinical care or in the interests of the patient
- Court order:
  - subpoena
  - under the Supreme Court Act 1981
- Statutory duty to disclose
- Disclosure in the public interest

Consent of the patient

The duty of confidentiality is in the interest of the patient and the patient therefore can give consent to disclosure which without that consent would be unlawful. The patient should be competent to give consent. In the case of a mentally incompetent adult, consent to disclosure could be given on the patient's behalf in the patient's best interests by a representative guardian or carer of the patient. Where the patient is a child under 16 years, then the principles of the Gillick case would apply (see Chapter 23) and a mature competent child under 16 could give consent to disclosure of confidential information.

The consent of the patient or his representative would be a defence against any potential proceedings being brought against the health professional. It is essential that evidence is available that consent has been given. There are therefore considerable advantages in obtaining this consent in writing.

The patient has the right to withdraw consent unless the terms of the disclosure are contrary to this. For example a patient may agree that a video could be made about his care and treatment. Considerable expense may then be incurred for the video to be produced. The patient may then decide that he does not wish the video to be shown. Whether or not this can then be prevented will depend upon the terms on which his agreement to the disclosure was obtained.

Where the patient specifically refuses to give his consent to the disclosure of his diagnosis to others, such as his relatives, this request should as far as possible be respected under the duty of confidentiality and only if a specific exception to the duty applies could the information be passed on.

For clinical care or in the interests of the patient

Health professionals working in a multi-disciplinary setting need to share information about the patient in order to fulfil their duty of care to the patient. Indeed it could be said that if relevant information were not passed to other professionals caring for the patient and harm were to occur to the patient as a result of that failure, then the professional and her employer could be answerable to the patient in a negligence action.

Situation: Unknown information

A physiotherapist is asked to undertake treatment for a patient but is refused access to the medical records of the patient. She sees the patient in the OPD and the patient fails to inform her that she is pregnant. As a consequence of her treatment, the patient miscarries. Had the physiotherapist had access to the medical records she would have been aware of the pregnancy. Is the physiotherapist liable for the miscarriage?

In this situation, the physiotherapist should, as part of her examination of the patient, have inquired about a possible pregnancy. If she failed to do so, she would have been negligent. If she asked, but the patient was not honest, then there should be no negligence on the physiotherapist's part. However the fact that the physiotherapist does not have an automatic right of access to the patient's records is of concern.

Where information is disclosed to colleagues as part of the duty of care to the patient, care should be taken to ensure that it is relevant to and necessary for their responsibilities.

Situation: Telling colleagues

A mother, who is hemiplegic following a stroke, is refusing care for herself when she needs it to look after the child appropriately. She forbids the physiotherapist to discuss her needs with colleagues.

In this situation, in the interests of the child, the mother must accept that the child's interests require information to be made available about the mother's needs but only insofar as it is relevant to her ability to care for the child. It could be pointed out to the mother sensitively that, if because of her own needs she is unable to give the necessary care to the child, then action may have to be taken under the Children Act 1989 to secure the well-being of the child.

Court order

Subpoena

The court has the right to ensure that information relevant to an issue being decided before it is made available in the interests of justice. Both criminal and civil courts therefore have the right to issue a subpoena (see glossary) for the necessary information to be produced before it. Other quasi-judicial proceedings such as inquiries may also have a right to subpoena information depending upon the statutory provisions under which they are established.

Where a court requires information, a health professional cannot refuse to comply on the grounds that the information was received in professional confidence. The courts do not recognise any privilege from disclosure attaching to the doctor or other health professional, or even a priest. The only exceptions recognised by the courts to their right to order disclosure are: legal professional privilege and privilege on grounds of the public interest (e.g. national security).

Legal professional privilege This covers communications between clients and their legal advisers. The judge cannot order disclosure of such communications. The reason is that it is in the interests of justice for a client to be able to confide fully with legal advisers without fear that such communications could be ordered to be disclosed in court. Reports to legal advisers are also privileged from disclosure if the principal purpose for which they were written is in contemplation of litigation.

Sometimes there may be several purposes behind the preparation of a report, as in a report following a health and safety accident where the report can be used for both management purposes in order to prevent a similar accident arising again and can also be used for legal purposes. This was the situation in the case of *Waugh* v. *British Railways Board*[10]. where the House of Lords held that if the predominant purpose behind the report was for advice and use in litigation, then it will be privileged from disclosure.

However the court looks at the reality of the matter, not what is said.

In the case of *Lask* v. *Gloucester Health Authority*[11] the court considered the ruling in *Waugh* v. *British Railways Board* in the situation where the health authority claimed legal professional privilege in respect of confidential reports completed following an accident. However on the facts of the matter the court held that, in spite of declarations by the health authority and solicitors to this effect, the documents were not covered by legal professional privilege.

Public interest immunity is the other exception to the right of the judge to order disclosure of any document relevant to an issue before it. This covers such interests as the national security. The privilege from disclosure is given under the sworn affidavit of a Minister and can be overruled by the judge. Public interest immunity was considered by the Scott inquiry which recommended that immunity certificates should not be issued in criminal proceedings if the liberty of the subject was at stake.

Disclosure ordered under the Supreme Court Act 1981

This Act enables disclosure to be made where the case involves a claim for personal injury or death in two distinct circumstances:

(a) Under section 33 where disclosure can be ordered against a prospective *party* (the proposed plaintiff or defendant) *prior* to the writ/claim form being issued; and

(b) Under section 34 against a third party (i.e. not directly involved in the case) after the writ/claim form has been issued.

Under section 33 of the Supreme Court Act 1981, when disclosure is ordered against a person likely to be a party in a personal injury case before the writ/claim form is issued, it can be ordered to be made to the applicant's legal advisers and any medical or other professional advisers of the applicant or, if the applicant has no legal advisers, to any medical or other professional adviser of the applicant.

Situation: The physiotherapist as potential defendant

If a client is suing in relation to an incident during the care by a physiotherapist her records could be ordered to be disclosed to the legal advisers or professional advisers of the client while they are deciding whether or not to bring a case to court.

After litigation has commenced by the issue of a writ/claim form disclosure can be ordered under section 34 of the Supreme Court Act 1981 against a person who is not likely to be a party to a case, if that person has information likely to be relevant.

Situation: Disclosure ordered against a physiotherapist

The client of a physiotherapist is involved in a road traffic accident and sues the driver of the vehicle which caused the accident. This driver wished to have access to information about the client held by the physiotherapist relating to his care in order to determine the likely prognosis of the client. If, for example, there was concern that the patient was unlikely to make a full recovery as a result of the road accident, but that he suffered from severe disabilities anyway, these existing disabilities could affect both liability (whether the driver was 100% to blame) and quantum (the amount of compensation).

An order can be made in the action for disclosure of the client's records even though it is in breach of the duty of confidentiality and against the client's interests. If it is the client who caused the accident and who is being sued an order could similarly be made against the physiotherapist to show, for example, that the client should not have been driving, but only after proceedings have been begun by the issue of a writ/claim form.

The detailed Court Rules in accordance with which such applications are made are, at the time of writing, subject to change with the implementation of the Woolf Reforms in April 1999, but the draft rules indicate that the principles enshrined in the Act remain unaffected.

Statutory duty to disclose

Several statutes require disclosure to be made, whether or not the patient gives consent. They are shown in Figure 8.4.

Figure 8.4   **Statutory provisions requiring disclosure to be made.**

Notifications of communicable diseases
Public Health Act 1936
Public Health (Infectious Diseases) Regulations 1988 (SI 1988 No. 1546)
Public Health (Control of Disease) Act 1984
Public Health (Aircraft) Regulations 1979 (SI 1979 No. 1434)
Public Health (Ships) Regulations 1979 (SI 1979 No. 1435)

Notifications of abortions
Abortion Act 1967, section 2
Abortion Regulations 1991 (SI No. 499)

Notification of births and deaths
National Health Service Act 1977, section 124
National Health Service (Notification of Births and Deaths) Regulations 1982
   (SI 1982 No. 286)

Notification of poisonings and health and safety matters
Health and Safety at Work etc. Act 1974
Reporting of Injuries, Diseases and Dangerous Occurrences Regulations 1985
   (SI 1983 No. 2023)
Reporting of Injuries, Diseases and Dangerous Occurrences (Amendment)
   Regulations 1989 (SI 1989 No. 1457)

Disclosure for civil justice
Supreme Court Act 1981, sections 33 and 34 (see above)

Disclosure for criminal justice
Police and Criminal Evidence Act 1984
Prevention of Terrorism Acts
Road Traffic Act 1988, section 172

Where these Acts are relevant to the work of the physiotherapist she should be fully conversant with the statutory requirements on disclosure and ensure that any disclosure which she makes can be justified in law.

Disclosure in the public interest

This is the most difficult exception to the duty of confidentiality. Professional registration bodies all recognise that in certain circumstances, disclosure without the patient's consent and contrary to his wishes may be justified.

In one decided case[12] on the issue of disclosure in the public interest the Court of Appeal held that it was permissible for a psychiatrist who had been asked for a report by a patient who was seeking his discharge from detention under the Mental Health Act 1983 to send his report to the Mental Health Review Tribunal and the hospital without the consent of the patient.

Case: *W* v. *Egdell*

> W was detained in a secure hospital under sections 37 and 41 of the Mental Health Act 1983 following a conviction for manslaughter on the grounds of diminished responsibility. He had shot dead five people and two others required major surgery. He applied to a Mental Health Review Tribunal (MHRT) and obtained an independent medical report from Dr Egdell who formed the view that W was suffering from a paranoid psychosis rather than paranoid schizophrenia. In the light of this report W withdrew the application to the Tribunal. Dr Egdell had assumed that this report would be made available to the hospital and the Tribunal. He sought the permission of W to place his report before the hospital and he refused permission. Dr Egdell then sent the report to the managers asking them to forward a copy to the Home Secretary. He considered that his examination had cast new light on the dangerousness of W and it ought to be known to those responsible for his care and for the formulation of any recommendations for discharge.
>
> Subsequently the Home Secretary referred W to an MHRT under the rules which require a hearing to be held at least every three years. The Home Secretary sent a copy of Dr Egdell's report to the Tribunal. W then issued writs against Dr Egdell, the hospital board, the Home Secretary, the Secretary of State for Health and the Tribunal, seeking injunctions preventing the defendants from using this material and claiming damages for breach of confidentiality.

The trial judge held that the court had to balance the interest to be served by non-disclosure against the interest served by disclosure. Since W was not an ordinary member of the public but a detained patient in a secure unit, the safety of the public should be the main criterion. Dr Egdell had a duty to the public to place the result of his examination before the proper authorities, if in his opinion, the public interest so required. The public interest in disclosure outweighed W's private interest.

The Court of Appeal supported this reasoning and stated:

> 'A consultant psychiatrist who becomes aware, even in the course of a confidential relationship, of information which leads him, in the exercise of what the court considers a sound professional judgement, to fear that such decisions may be made on inadequate information and with a real risk of consequent danger to the public is entitled to take such steps as are reasonable in the circumstances to communicate the grounds of his concern to the responsible authorities.' (Lord Justice Bingham)

Other situations where disclosure in the public interest would be justified would include a situation where harm is occurring or likely to occur to a child or another person.

The multi-disciplinary report

Certain professional groups including the CPSM have participated with the British Medical Association and the Royal College of Nursing in drafting legislation to cover the use and disclosure of personal health information. In their report[13] public interest is defined as follows:

> 'It shall be lawful for a qualified health professional to disclose personal health information where:

(a) it relates to a patient for whom he [or she] has clinical responsibility, and

(b) in the opinion of that professional disclosure is necessary in the public interest.

Disclosure in the public interest is necessary only where:

(a) it relates to the prevention, detection or prosecution of a serious offence; or

(b) it relates to the protection of public safety; or

(c) failure to disclose would expose the patient or some other person to a real risk of death or serious harm.'

The draft legislation also provides further safeguards against unauthorised disclosure by suggesting that a decision on whether or not disclosure should be made:

'(i) Where the patient is being or has been treated in hospital as an in-patient or an out-patient under the care of a consultant, the disclosure decision must be taken by the consultant in charge of the patient's care; and
(ii) where the patient is not or has not been treated by a doctor, by the qualified health professional employed by or in contract with the health service body concerned who is responsible at the time of the decision for the particular aspect of the patient's care.'

This latter clause could clearly involve the physiotherapist. It would therefore be advisable for physiotherapists to ensure that a procedure is drawn up to cover those exceptional circumstances where they have to decide whether or not disclosure is justified in the public interest.

Draft legislation was introduced into the 1995–6 Parliamentary session but was not enacted.

Guidance from the NHS Executive

Following a consultation paper for the NHS on the confidentiality, use and disclosure of personal health information[14], the NHS Executive published guidelines[15] on the protection and use of patient information. The guidelines state that as well as being required for the prime task of delivering personal care and treatment, personal information about patients is also required for:

- assuring and improving the quality of care and treatment
- monitoring and protecting public health
- coordinating NHS care with that of other agencies
- effective health care administration, e.g. managing and planning services, contracting, auditing, risk management, investigating complaints
- teaching
- statistical analysis and research.

The Guidance states that patient information can be passed on in the following circumstances:

- with the patient's consent
- on a 'need to know basis' (i.e. for NHS purposes in the care and treatment of the patient or for the purposes set out above)
- as a result of statute or court order;
- if other reasons justify disclosure (e.g. the protection of the public – prevention of a serious crime or where there is a public health risk)

The NHS Executive bases the guidance on the EC Directive on Data Protection (1995) which member states had to implement by October 1998. It recognises that amendments to the guidance may be necessary following the legislation now enacted. The EC Directive permits the processing of health information where this is required

'for the purposes of preventive medicine, medical diagnosis, the provision of care or treatment or the management of health care services, and where those data are processed by a health professional subject under national law or rules established by national competent bodies to the obligation of professional secrecy or by another person also subject to an equivalent obligation of secrecy.' (Article 8, paragraph 3)

Implications for the physiotherapist

Julius Sims[16] discussed the duty of confidentiality in relation to the question as to whether a physiotherapist needed to know the HIV status of the patient. He concludes that except when progression to AIDS has occurred (in which case the diagnosis will be known to the therapist) a physiotherapist does not need to know a patient's HIV status. The reasons he gives are that

- a patient's HIV status does not determine the choice or effectiveness of therapy, and
- the adoption of universal precautions provides optimum protection against transmission of HIV and does not depend upon a knowledge of who is or is not seropositive.
- Nor could it be argued that the patient should know of the therapist's status since the chance of contracting HIV from an infected physiotherapist is so remote as to be virtually no risk.

A procedure is necessary for the physiotherapist to ensure that she preserves the confidential nature of information about the patient. This would also include safe storage of the records which she keeps and should also cover any sharing of records on a multi-disciplinary team basis. In addition the exceptions to the duty should be clarified so that the physiotherapist can be confident that she is acting within the law and retains the trust of the patient.

Figure 8.5 shows a checklist for ensuring that precautions are taken against any unauthorised disclosure.

Figure 8.5   Checklist for good practice in maintaining confidentiality.

- Are the records securely stored with restricted access?
- If access to the records or information is requested, who is making the request?
- What are their reasons for the request?
- What relationship do they have with the patient?
- Has the patient given consent?
- If not, why not?
- Is the patient under the care of a consultant?
- Has the consultant been asked to permit disclosure?
- Is there a duty in law to disclose?
- If so, under what category does the duty arise?
- What part, if any, of the information should be released to the person making the request?
- What should be recorded about the request and the response?

Link with ethical issues

This chapter has been concerned with the legal basis for the duty of confidentiality and the legal justifications for breaching that duty in specific situations. It has not been concerned with the moral or ethical dimensions. These are discussed in an article by Julius Sims[17]. He considers that it is rarely permissible to breach confidentiality in the client's own interests and cites an example of a therapist learning that a person wished to commit suicide. In such circumstances it is essential for an assessment to be made of the competence of the patient. If, for example, the patient is suffering from mental disorder and the physiotherapist failed to take action to protect the patient against these suicidal wishes, the physiotherapist would be failing in her duty of care to that patient. It is essential that an understanding of the legal situation should accompany any consideration of the ethical issues.

The future

At the time of writing, the European Directive on Data Protection[18] is still to be fully implemented. Member states had to comply with its provisions by 24 October 1998. It requires member states to establish a set of principles with which users of personal information must comply, gives individuals the right to gain access to information held about them and provides for a supervisory authority to oversee and enforce the law (see also Chapter 9 on access to health records). The Home Office Minister (George Howarth) has stated[19] that the set date cannot be made and the Directive will not be implemented till 1999.

Data Protection Act 1998

The Data Protection Act 1998 will not be brought into force until 1999, when the subordinate legislation is in place. Once in force the 1998 Act will repeal the Data Protection Act 1984. The Registrar has published a document entitled *The Data*

Protection Act 1998: An Introduction, and this is available from Publications, Office of the Data Protection Registrar, Wycliffe House, Water Lane, Wilmslow, Cheshire SK9 5AF.

Questions and exercises

1 Examine your practice in relation to passing on confidential information. What faults would you see in it?
2 To what extent can an employer enforce the duty of confidentiality amongst employees? Prepare a procedure for this.
3 What exceptions have you relied upon in passing on confidential information?

References

1 For further information see Darley, B., Griew, A., McLoughlin, K. & Williams, J. (1994) *How to Keep a Clinical Confidence* HMSO, London.
2 CSP Professional Affairs Department (1997) No. PA 37 (August 1997) *The Protection and Use of Patient Information.* CSP, London.
3 HSG(96) 18; LASSL(96) 5 (March 1997) *Protection and Use of Patient Information.* Department of Health, London.
4 Chartered Society of Physiotherapy (June 1993) *Standards of Physiotherapy Practice.* CSP, London.
5 *Furniss* v. *Fitchett* [1958] NZLR 396.
6 *X* v. *Y* [1988] 2 All ER 648.
7 Austin, C. (1996) Confidentiality, clinicians and confidentiality. *British Journal of Occupational Therapy* **59** 2, 62–4.
8 Attorney General v. *Guardian Newspaper Ltd (No 2)* [1988] 3 All ER 545.
9 *Stephens* v. *Avery and others* [1988] 2 All ER 477.
10 *Waugh* v. *British Railways Board* [1980] AC 521.
11 *Lask* v. *Gloucester Health Authority* The Times Law Report, 13 December 1985.
12 *W.* v. *Egdell* [1989] 1 All ER 1089; (CA) [1990] 1 All ER 835.
13 Multi-disciplinary Professional Working Group (1994) *An Explanatory Handbook of Guidance Governing Use and Disclosure of Personal Health Information.* British Medical Association, London.
14 Department of Health (1994) *Draft guidance for the NHS on the confidentiality, use and disclosure of personal health information* DoH, London.
15 HSG(96)18; LASSL(96)5 *Protection and Use of Patient Information.* Department of Health, March 1996.
16 Sims, J. (1997) Confidentiality and HIV Status. *Physiotherapy* **83** 2, 90–6.
17 Sims, J. (1996) Client confidentiality: ethical issues in occupational therapy. *British Journal of Occupational Therapy* **59** 2, 56–61.
18 European Directive on Data Protection Adopted by the Council of the European Union in October 1995.
19 Frances Gibb 'Data Protection law delayed' *The Times* 20 July 1998.

Chapter 9
Access to Records and Information

Patients have a statutory right to see their health records, whether they are held in computer or manual form and subject to only a few exceptions. The definition of health records includes records kept by the physiotherapist. The statutory right of access also applies to records held by those health professionals working in private practice, but here access might also be subject to conditions agreed in the contract between therapist and private patient. The contractual conditions cannot limit the statutory right. Separate statutory provisions cover the records held by those who work for social services departments (SSDs).

A physiotherapist's records may also become relevant to reports written by the patient's doctor for insurance or employment purposes and therefore come under the rules relating to disclosure of such reports[1]. An information paper prepared by the Professional Affairs Department of the CSP[2] provides guidance on the Access to Health Records Act 1990. It sets out the statutory provisions, an explanation of the individual's entitlement and the exclusions to these rights.

In addition to the statutory rights of access to health records and personal files kept by SSDs there is also a right at common law for the patient to receive, as part of the duty of care owed by the health professional to the patient, information which is relevant to decisions which the patient may be required to consider in relation to her treatment and care. The rights at common law of the patient to obtain information are set out in the leading case of *Sidaway*[3] considered in Chapter 7.

The following topics are considered in this chapter.

- Statutory rights
- Non-statutory access
- Access and the physiotherapist
- Access by others
- Conclusion

Statutory rights

The legislation giving statutory rights is as follows:

- Data Protection Act 1984 (to be superseded by the 1998 Act, see below)
- Access to Medical Reports Act 1988
- Access to Health Records Act 1990
- Access to Personal Files Act 1987
- Education (School Records) Regulations 1989

The Data Protection Acts 1984

The Data Protection Act 1984 gives rights of access to automated processed personal health information subject to the conditions laid down by statutory instrument[4]. Clarification is given of the statutory provisions by the Department of Health[5].

The Act covers only those records which consist of information relating to a living individual who can be identified from that information (or from other information in the possession of the data user), including any expression of opinion[6].

Principles

The Data Protection Act 1984 regulates the collection, processing and storage of information in automated form from which an individual can be identified. Data users are required to register with the Data Protection Registrar their recording and use of personal data and must comply with the Data Protection Act principles, as amended by the Data Protection Act 1998. These are shown below in Figure 9.1.

Figure 9.1 **Data Protection Act principles (as amended by 1998 Act).**

Personal data shall:

(1) be collected and processed fairly and lawfully and shall not be processed unless one of the conditions in Schedule 2 is met, and in the case of sensitive personal data, one of the conditions in Schedule 3;
(2) only be obtained for specified, lawful registered purposes and shall not be further processed in any manner incompatible with that purpose;
(3) be adequate and relevant and not excessive to the purpose for which they are held;
(4) be accurate and, where necessary, kept up to date;
(5) be held no longer than is necessary for the stated purpose;
(6) shall be processed in accordance with the rights of data subjects under this Act;
(7) appropriate technical and organisational measures shall be taken against unauthorised or unlawful processing of personal data and against accidental loss or destruction or damage to personal data;
(8) personal data shall not be transferred to a country outside the European Economic Area unless that country ensures an adequate level of protection for the rights and freedom of data subjects in relation to the processing of personal data.

Provisions on access

The data subject, i.e. the person about whom the information is recorded[6], has a right of access under the 1984 Act. He has the right to be informed by the data user as to whether any personal identifiable information about him is being held and if so he has the right to be supplied with a copy of that information[7].

Children have the right of access if they have the maturity to make a valid application. The concept of being 'Gillick Competent' would apply (see chapter 23).

The Act provided for regulations to be made to enable those who are responsible for the management of the affairs of an incompetent adult to have access, but no regulations have been passed. Regulations may be passed under the 1998 Act (see below) if the recommendations of the Law Commission on

Decision Making and the Mentally Incapacitated Adult are implemented[8] (see Chapter 22 on those with learning disabilities and Chapter 24 on the elderly).

Exceptions

Under statutory instrument, the access provisions are modified in the case of access to personal health records[9]. This applies to data held by a health professional or data held by a person other than a health professional where the information constituting the data was first recorded by or on behalf of a health professional. Health professional is defined as shown in Figure 9.2.

Figure 9.2   Definition of health professional[10].

- registered medical practitioner
- registered dental practitioner
- registered chemist
- registered optician
- registered pharmaceutical chemist or druggist
- registered nurse, midwife or health visitor
- registered chiropodist
- dietitian
- art or music therapist employed by a health authority
- scientist employed by a health authority as head of department

- occupational therapist
- orthoptist
- physiotherapist
- clinical psychologist
- child psychotherapist
- speech therapist
- osteopath
- chiropractor

Access is not permitted where disclosure:

- would be likely to cause serious harm to the physical or mental health of the data subject; or
- would be likely to reveal to the data subject the identity of another individual (who has not consented to the disclosure of the information) either as a person to whom the information or part of it relates or as the source of the information, or enable that identity to be deduced by the data subject either from the data itself or from a combination of that data and other information which the data subject has or is likely to have.

This second exception does not, however, apply where the other individual is a health professional who has been involved in the care of the data subject and the information relates to him in that capacity.

The data user, who is not a health professional, is required to consult the appropriate health professional before permitting or refusing access. The appropriate health professional is defined as:

- the medical practitioner or dental practitioner who is currently or was most recently responsible for the clinical care of the data subject in connection with the matters to which the information which is the subject of the request relates; or
- where there is more than one such practitioner, the practitioner who is the most suitable to advise on the matters to which the information which is the subject of the request relates; or
- where there is no practitioner available falling within subparagraph a or b, a

health professional who has the necessary experience and qualifications to advise on those matters.

If the exclusion provisions apply, the data user does not have to notify the applicant that information is being withheld. It is sufficient for the data user to notify the applicant that there is no information being held which has to be revealed to the data subject.

Procedure for application
The application is made in writing to the data user, i.e. the person who holds the personal data, giving sufficient information for the relevant data and the subject user to be identified, together with the appropriate fee.

Rights of the data subject

- Unless the exclusion provisions discussed above apply, the data subject is entitled to be supplied with a copy of the information requested within 40 days of the date on which the application, giving all the necessary information is received.
- If the information supplied to the data subject is inaccurate he or she can request that the information is rectified or erased and has the right to enforce this in the Court.
- If the inaccuracy causes distress to the data subject, then the data subject has the right to claim compensation for the harm suffered. The data user has a defence if the inaccurate information was received from the patient or a third person or if the data user took such care as was reasonably required in the circumstances to ensure the accuracy of the data at the material time.
- If the data subject is refused the information, he or she can either make an application to the County or High Court or to the Data Protection Registrar for the enforcement of the statutory rights.

The Data Protection Act 1998
The Data Protection Act 1998 was passed in accordance with the EC Directive (see Chapter 8) but will not be brought into force until 1999 when the subordinate legislation required to give it effect will be in place. It will repeal and replace the 1984 Act. The basic principles are the same but there are subtle differences of emphasis and terminology. The Registrar has published a document entitled *The Data Protection Act 1998: An Introduction* which is available from the Office of the Data Protection Registrar (see address list) and other guidance is being produced.

The Access to Medical Reports Act 1988

Basic principles
This Act enables a patient to see and if necessary suggest corrections where an insurance company or employer requests a medical report from the patient's own doctor for insurance or employment purposes. The records to which the doctor might refer may include information received from physiotherapists.

The right of access can be withheld in similar circumstances to those stated above. Therefore if, in the unlikely circumstances that the physiotherapist is concerned that any information is likely to cause serious harm to the physical or mental health of the patient or identify a third person who has requested not to be identified, then she should ensure that the information which she passes to the doctor is suitably annotated.

Access to Health Records Act 1990

Principles
After the implementation of the Data Protection Act 1984 granting access to automated personal health records, an anomaly existed in that there was a statutory right to identifiable personal information held on computerised records, but not to that held in manual form. Since many health records were and still are held in manual form the statutory right had little impact. Legislation was therefore introduced to enable patients to have access to such health records held in manual form.

The Access to Health Records Act 1990 came into force on 1 November 1991 and only applied to records kept after that date, although earlier records could be shown if that were necessary to make sense of those kept after that date. Guidance was issued by the Department of Health[11].

Holder of the records
The Act gives the applicant the right to seek access from the holder of the records. This is defined as:

- in the case of a record made by the general practitioner, the general practitioner or (where there is no GP) the Health Authority;
- in the case of the provision of health services by the health service body on whose behalf the record is held;
- in any other case, the health professional who made the record.

Health professional
This is defined in exactly the same way as under the Data Protection Act 1984 (see Figure 9.2 above).

Health record
A record is defined as a health record if:

- it consists of information relating to the physical or mental health of an individual who can be identified from that information, or from that and other information in the possession of the holder of the record; and
- it has been made by or on behalf of a health professional in connection with the care of that individual.

Who can apply
The following have the right of access:

- the patient;
- a person authorised in writing to make the application on the patient's behalf;
- where the patient is a child (a person under 16 years), a person having parental responsibility for the child;

- where the patient is incapable of managing his own affairs, a person appointed by the court to manage his affairs;
- where the patient has died, the personal representative(s) (see glossary) of the patient or any person who may have a claim arising out of the patient's death.

Access under this last subsection can be prevented if the record includes a note, made at the patient's request, that he or she did not wish access to be given on such an application. Any information need not be disclosed if it is not relevant to any claim (e.g. in connection with disease caused by his work environment) which may arise from the patient's death.

If the applicant is a child (i.e. a person under 16 years), then the holder must be satisfied that the patient is capable of understanding the nature of the application. If a person with parental responsibility is applying the patient must either consent to the application or the patient must be incapable of understanding and the giving of access would be in his best interests. (Refer to Chapter 23 for the law relating to children.)

Procedure
The patient has the right to make an application for access to a health record or any part of a health record. The application is made to the holder of the record who is required to seek the observations of the health professional by or on behalf of whom the record was made. No fee can be charged unless access is required to records made more than 40 days before the application. A charge can however be made for postage and copying. The 40 day period is calculated from an acceptable application. If the applicant has provided insufficient information, then the holder has 14 days within which to write to the applicant asking for more details.

Nature of access
Where an application is made, the holder of the record must (unless the exceptions exist) allow the applicant to inspect the record or a part of the record and if requested supply a copy of the record or extract.

Exclusions
The holder of the records can refuse access on the same grounds as exist in relation to computerised records, i.e. if any part of the health record would disclose:

- information likely to cause serious harm to the physical or mental health of the patient or of any other individual; or
- information relating to or provided by any other individual, other than the patient, who could be identified from that information (unless that individual has consented) or is a health professional who has been involved in the care of the patient).

Access can also be refused if:

- the health records were made before 1 November 1991 (unless access is necessary in order to make intelligible any part of the subsequent record to which access is required to be given); or

● where the record would show that an individual might have been born as a result of infertility treatment[12].

Right to correction of inaccurate records
Section 6 of the 1990 Act enables a person who considers that any information contained in a health record or part of a health record is inaccurate to apply to the holder of the record for the necessary correction to be made. If the holder is satisfied that the information is inaccurate he may make the necessary correction. If he is not so satisfied he must make a note, in the part of the record containing the disputed information, of the matters in respect of which the information is considered to be inaccurate. In both cases he must supply the applicant with either a copy of the correction or the note. A fee cannot be charged. The Act defines 'inaccurate' as meaning 'incorrect, misleading or incomplete' (section 6(3)).

Request to clarify and explain
Where the information contained in a record or extract which is inspected or copied for the applicant is expressed in terms which are not intelligible without an explanation, an explanation of those terms shall be provided with the record or extract, or supplied with the copy (section 3(3)). This provision prevents health professionals hiding behind professional jargon to keep information secret from the patient.

Means of enforcement
A person with a statutory right of access under the 1990 Act can apply to the County Court or the High Court if the holder has failed to comply with any requirement under the Act. The court must be satisfied that the applicant has fulfilled any requirements laid down by the Secretary of State.

Protection of those with rights of access
Section 9 of the 1990 Act makes any contractual term which compels an individual to supply to another person a copy of a health record to which he has been given access under this Act void. Thus no-one can be compelled to show the record to another person. (This does not of course prevent the court requiring the holder of the record to disclose health information under a sub-poena.)

Access to Personal Files Act 1987

Provisions comparable to those under the Access to Health Records Act 1990 have been enacted in respect of housing and social services records to enable the person in respect of whom the records are held to obtain access. However access can be withheld if serious harm would be caused to the physical or mental health of the applicant. The fact that the right of access is subject to different statutory procedures can cause difficulties where there is a unified record system in existence with social services records and health records being held on the same file, since the holders of the records differ according to whether they are health records or social services records. (See Chapter 12 on record keeping.)

Education (School Records) Regulations 1989

These regulations enable manual records on pupils held by maintained schools to be open to access.

Non-statutory access

There appear to be few formal applications made under the statutory provisions, which suggests that health professionals are disclosing the records without requiring the patient to make a formal application. It should be remembered that the existence of statutory rights of access for the patient does not mean that the patient necessarily has to apply formally for access. There may be many reasons why the health professional agrees to informal access of the patient to his records and this could then be arranged. There is the possibility that greater openness with the patient over access to records and information may make the patient less suspicious and there will be even fewer formal applications for access under the statutory provisions.

It has, however, been established that, if the statutory provisions do not apply, the patient does not have an absolute right of access at common law[13]. The Court of Appeal stated that a doctor or health authority was entitled to deny access to the records by the patient on the ground that their disclosure would be detrimental to him.

Access and the physiotherapist

It is seldom that secrecy of information from the patient can be justified in the case of the treatment provided by the physiotherapist. There are very few situations where the physiotherapist would feel that serious harm could arise to the physical or mental health of the patient if access were to be permitted.

Orders to withhold information

Sometimes however the problems which can arise are not of the physiotherapist's making as the following situation illustrates.

Situation: Orders to withhold information

A consultant physician treating a patient has diagnosed multiple sclerosis. It is his view that the patient could not yet cope with this diagnosis and he therefore instructs the multi-disciplinary team caring for the patient that she should not be told. The physiotherapist takes part in a pre-discharge assessment of the patient and accompanies her home to decide if she could cope with living on her own. During the visit the patient raises with the physiotherapist her concerns about her illness and asks the physiotherapist directly if she has multiple sclerosis. What is the legal situation?

Although the physiotherapist is a personally accountable registered professional who should use her own discretion in making health decisions, she may also be part of the multi-disciplinary team usually headed by the consultant responsible for the care and treatment of the patient. In this case her concerns about openness and disclosure to the patient should have been raised as soon as she was aware of the restrictions ordered by the consultant and she should have taken up this with him then. However in the situation which occurs she has the following options:

- to refuse to say and suggest that the patient should have an appointment to discuss with the consultant her diagnosis and treatment;
- to answer the patient honestly and ignore the consultant's orders;
- to lie to the patient.

It would be hoped that the third option would be unacceptable to all health and social services professionals. The first option would probably be appropriate in most cases. The second option may be justified in exceptional circumstances. However if the physiotherapist follows this line, then she must be prepared to justify her actions:

- before disciplinary proceedings should the consultant report her to her managers and they decide to take such action;
- in civil litigation, if the patient reacts to this information by attempting to take (or succeeding in taking) her own life and the employer of the physiotherapist is sued for its vicarious liability for the harm caused by her;
- in professional conduct proceedings if it is decided that she is guilty of infamous conduct (the present definition but due to change – see Chapter 4) as a registered professional.

It may be that before all three forms of hearings, she is able to justify her actions as being in the best interests of the patient. She should ensure that her records are comprehensive and explain clearly why she took the decisions which she did. In deciding whether it is appropriate to ignore the consultant's direction she should be mindful of the fact that there is no absolute duty to disclose everything to the patient. Under the statutory provisions there is a right of exclusion from access which the holder of the records can exercise on the basis of the advice of the health professional concerned and at common law the House of Lords in the *Sidaway* case recognised the right of therapeutic privilege, i.e. to withhold information from the patient in exceptional circumstances when it is justified as being in the best interests of that patient.

Nevertheless the GMC has recently advised registered medical practitioners that they should ensure that patients are given full information about their condition and that those who fail to tell patients the truth about their treatment risk being struck off. The new guidelines are issued in the updated *Good Medical Practice* booklet issued by the GMC[14]. These follow a Court of Appeal decision in a case brought by the father of a boy suffering from Addison's Disease who claimed that doctors should have informed him about his son's condition. The Court of Appeal held that doctors were not under a legal obligation to tell the truth and therefore could not be sued for concealing the failures that led to the child's death. The father, Will Powell, has indicated his intention to take the case to the European Court.

A distinction may also have to be made between those physiotherapists who work for social services, where the patient may not be directly under a consultant and the general practitioner is therefore the lead medical practitioner responsible for the clinical care of the patient, and those physiotherapists who work in health care, where there would usually be an identifiable consultant in charge of the patient's care.

Truth telling

'Truth telling in occupational therapy'[15] by Rosemary Barnitt is an excellent analysis of the ethical issues which arise in deciding whether or not the patient should be given the full information. The principles also apply to physiotherapy. The article shows the difficulties which can arise in a multi-disciplinary team over who controls the truth telling. She concluded that there was a clear need for simple policies and procedures to be established around truth telling in health care settings, and for these to be made available to all participants in the treatment transaction. Her research was based on a postal questionnaire across England and Wales. As shown above, there is a right recognised both by statute and at common law for information to be withheld from the patient in exceptional circumstances if it would cause serious harm to the mental or physical condition of the patient.

Situation: Telling the patient

> A physiotherapist received a referral form for a patient whose diagnosis was Parkinson's Disease. She told the patient that she was visiting to assist him following his diagnosis of Parkinson's Disease. He stated bluntly that he did not have Parkinson's.

In this situation, the physiotherapist was wrong-footed because she assumed that the patient had been told and had accepted the diagnosis. She could only attempt to retrieve the situation by glossing over the diagnosis and concentrating on any weaknesses which the patient had.

Diagnosis not given to the physiotherapist

A variant of the above situation would be where the physiotherapist is not herself told of the patient's diagnosis. Problems can then arise for the physiotherapist when she does not know the medical condition of a referral – how for example can she decide on priorities? Can the doctor be forced to disclose? What happens if the patient does not want the physiotherapist to get in touch with the doctor?

In such a situation each case would have to be treated on its merits and many different legal principles apply. The duty in relation to confidentiality is discussed in Chapter 8 where it is noted that providing personal patient information to the multi-disciplinary team caring for the patient is a justifiable exception to that duty since it would be in the interests of the patient.

Another issue which arises in the situation where the doctor is refusing to give the physiotherapist patient information is that of the standard of care to be provided by the physiotherapist. If she is kept in ignorance of certain information about the patient's condition, she may make some grave errors of judgment which could cause harm to the patient. Her right to have the relevant information to care appropriately for the patient is clear and she should bring up any such issue with the multi-disciplinary team. It is more difficult in the community, where a physiotherapist working for social services may not be a member of such a team and it may be the GP who is refusing to give the necessary information. It might have to be explained to the GP by senior management that, unless specific information is made available, priorities cannot be set reasonably nor the appropriate care given.

Access by others

Statutory rights of persons other than the patient under the 1990 Act are discussed above. Other rights of access including those of the courts and where certain statutes require information to be disclosed are considered in Chapter 8 on confidentiality.

Conclusion

The impact of statutory rights of access has led to greater openness between patient and health professional. Informal sharing of information is important and the practice by some NHS Trusts, as an income generation method, that the patient should be compelled to take the formal statutory route in order to obtain access is unsupportable. Patient's Charters and the impact of the White paper on the NHS[16] are both likely to improve access to information by the patient.

 Questions and exercises _____

1 A client asks for sight of the clinical records you are keeping on her. What action do you take and what considerations do you take into account?
2 Explain to a colleague the legal procedure under the Access to Health Records Act 1990 which enables a patient to have sight of her records.
3 In what circumstances do you consider that it would cause serious harm to the physical or mental health of the patient to see her records?

References

1 For more detailed information see: Cowley, R. (1994) *Access to Medical Records and Reports, a Practical Guide* NAHAT/Radcliffe Medical Press, Oxford.
2 CSP Professional Affairs Department (1991) No. PA 2 (January 1995) *Access to Health Records* CSP, London.
3 *Sidaway* v. *Bethlem Royal Hospital Governors* [1985] 2 WLR 480.
4 Data Protection (Subject Access Modification) (Health) Order 1987 SI No. 1903 of 1987.
5 HC(87)14 *Data Protection Act 1984: Modified Access to Personal Health Information* and HC(89)29 *Access to Health Records Act 1990: Health Service Guidance*.
6 Data Protection Act 1984 section 1(3).
7 Data Protection Act 1984 section 21.
8 Law Commission (1995) Report No. 231 *Mental Incapacity* HMSO, London.
9 Data Protection (Subject Access Modification) (Health) Order 1987 SI No. 1903 of 1987.

10 Schedule 1 of Data Protection (Subject Access Modification) (Health) Order 1987 SI No. 1903.

11 HSG(91)6 *Access to Health Records Act*.

12 Access to Health Records (Control of Access) Regulations 1993 SI No. 746 of 1993.

13 *R* v. *Mid Glamorgan Family Health Services Authority, ex parte Martin* [1993] 137 SJ 153; (QBD) The Times Law Report 2 June 1993; *upheld by* (CA) The Times Law Report 16 August 1994; [1994] 5 Med LR 383.

14 General Medical Council (1998) *Good Medical Practice*. (revised 1998) GMC, London.

15 Barnitt, R. (1994) Truth Telling in Occupational Therapy. *British Journal of Occupational Therapy*, **57** 9, 334–40.

16 DoH (1997) *The New NHS: Modern, Dependable*. HMSO, London.

Section C
Accountability in the Civil and Criminal Courts

Chapter 10
Negligence

Litigation is increasing as the expectations of clients in relation to health care grow and the publicity about awards of compensation raises hopes of vast settlements. In July 1998 it was reported that the NHS was facing a £2.3 billion bill for negligence payouts[1]. At present there are few reported cases of negligence involving physiotherapy services but this does not mean that the physiotherapist can ignore the implications of civil actions being brought.

The employed physiotherapist is unlikely herself to be sued personally. This is because employers are indirectly responsible in law for the wrongful acts of their employees whilst an employee is acting in course of employment. This is known as the vicarious liability of the employer and is explained further below. However the private practitioner who does not have an employer must ensure that she has the necessary insurance cover to pay out any compensation claims brought against her.

Even if the physiotherapist is an employee she still needs to have an understanding of the law relating to negligence so that she is appropriately prepared to defend any allegations against her.

This chapter covers the following topics:

- Civil actions
- Principles of negligence
- Vicarious and personal liability distinguished
- Defences to an action
- Calculating compensation
- Examples of situations involving physiotherapists
- Liability for students and unqualified assistants
- Care of property
- Documentation
- Future developments

Civil actions

These include those actions which are brought in the civil courts by an individual or organisation, usually with the aim of obtaining compensation or other remedy which the court is able to order. The main group of civil actions affecting health professionals are called torts i.e. civil wrongs excluding breach of contract.

Within the group various causes of action are included – negligence, trespass, breach of statutory duty, defamation, nuisance and others. In each case the burden will usually be upon the person bringing the action (known as the plaintiff/claimant) to establish on a balance of probabilities the existence of each of the elements which make up each cause of action. Thus in an action for trespass to the person (see Chapter 7) the plaintiff/claimant must show that there was a direct interference or touching of her person and that it was without her consent or other lawful justification.

Principles of negligence

This is the most common tort, being actions brought in situations where the plaintiff/claimant alleges that there has been personal injury or death, or damage or loss of property caused by another. Compensation is sought for the loss which has occurred. To succeed in the action the plaintiff/claimant has to show the following elements:

- that the defendant owed to the person harmed a duty of care;
- that the defendant was in breach of that duty;
- that the breach of duty caused reasonably foreseeable harm to the plaintiff/claimant.

These four elements – duty, breach, causation and harm are discussed below.

Duty of care

The law recognises that a duty of care will exist where one person can reasonably foresee that his or her actions and omissions could cause reasonably foreseeable harm to another person. A duty of care will always exist between the health professional and the client, but it might not always be easy to identify to which people such a duty extends. For example, would a physiotherapist have a duty of care to report that the neighbour of a client appears to be requiring the assistance of the community team?

Situation: A duty of care?

A physiotherapist is visiting a client who has just been discharged from hospital and is told that the neighbour has not been seen for a few days and there are concerns about her health. Could the physiotherapist say 'that person is not my client and so I am not going to take any further action'? It could happen, that the neighbour dies and the relatives, on hearing that the physiotherapist had been told of possible problems, commence a civil action for failure to fulfil the duty of care. Would the allegation that a duty of care existed be upheld?

There is no decided case on the point, but it is likely that the courts would recognise a duty of care on the part of a health professional as existing in such circumstances. However this then gives rise to other such questions as whether the physiotherapist has a duty of care when she is on holiday and discovers that a person nearby is in need of help. The usual legal principle is that there is no duty to volunteer services unless a pre-existing duty exists. It is likely that the courts would not recognise a duty as arising in a holiday situation. There may however be a professional duty recognised by the registration body (see Chapter 4).

In the case of *Donoghue* v. *Stevenson*[2] the House of Lords defined the duty of care owed at common law (i.e. judge made law).

> 'You must take reasonable care to avoid acts or omissions which you can reasonably foresee would be likely to injure your neighbour. Who then in law is my neighbour? The answer seems to be persons who are so closely and directly affected by my act that I ought reasonably to have them in contemplation as being so affected when I am directing my mind to the acts or omissions which are called in question.'

Despite there being such a straightforward definition laid down by the House of Lords there is often a difficulty in deciding how far and to whom, precisely, the duty of care extends. Cases are decided on their particular facts.

In a case involving the escape of Borstal boys who caused serious damage to a yacht[3], the House of Lords held that a duty of care was owed by the Home Office to any persons who were injured or whose property was damaged as a result of the institution's failure to keep the boys under proper control. A footballer owes a duty of care to other players and a tackle which was judged an intentional foul and caused an injury to another player was held to be a breach of that duty of care[4]. In contrast the Court of Appeal held that a fire brigade did not owe a duty of care to an owner or occupier merely by attending a fire[4a].

The issue may be of importance to physiotherapists in the context of referrals – at what point does the physiotherapist owe a duty of care to a client? Immediately after a referral or only after the referral has been accepted? Negligence relating to referrals and priority setting is discussed below.

Specific situations where the disputes over the existence of a duty of care might arise include:

- Conflict between different health professionals and social services staff e.g. the boundaries between nurses and physiotherapists on discharge of patients from continuing care. This is considered in Chapter 18 on community care.
- What is the duty of care to a person who refuses to leave hospital? Can he be compelled to leave a hospital bed;
  - if the hospital is being closed;
  - if he no longer needs NHS help; or
  - if relatives refuse to move him?

This is also considered in Chapter 18.

- What is the duty of care if people wish to take their own discharge? Can health professionals refuse to let people take their own discharge when they could cause harm to themselves at home? This is considered in Chapter 7 on consent.
- In what circumstances does the physiotherapist have a duty of care to the carer? This would be answered in law on the basis of the principles set out in the *Donoghue* v. *Stevenson* case quoted above.

- Does a physiotherapist who works in occupational health have a duty of care to report to the employers if she becomes aware of a pattern of repetitive strain injury (RSI) type symptoms arising from a particular new task in the workplace, even if such a duty is not specifically set out in her job description.

It is probable that the answer to the question in this last situation is, 'yes'. The job description is not a contractual term, and an implied term in the contract of employment requires the employee to act with reasonable care and skill in fulfilling her duty of care. In the circumstances described here the duty of care would include a responsibility to report.

Breach of duty

Determining the standard of care

In order to determine whether there has been a breach of the duty of care, it will first be necessary to establish the required standard. The courts have used what has become known as the 'Bolam test' to determine the standard of care required by a professional. In the case from which the test took its name[5] the court laid down the following principle to determine the standard of care which should be followed:

> 'The test is the standard of the ordinary skilled man exercising and professing to have that special skill.' (McNair, page 121)

The Bolam Test was applied by the House of Lords in a case[6] where negligence by an obstetrician in delivering a child by forceps was alleged:

> 'When you get a situation which involves the use of some special skill or competence, then the test as to whether there has been negligence or not ... is the standard of the ordinary skilled man exercising and professing to have that special skill. If a surgeon failed to measure up to that in any respect (clinical judgement or otherwise) he had been negligent and should be so adjudged.'

The House of Lords found that the surgeon was not liable in negligence and held that an error of judgment may or may not be negligence. It depends upon the circumstances.

This standard of the reasonable professional man following the accepted approved standard of care can be used to apply to any professional person – architect, lawyer or accountant, as well as any health professional. The standard of care which a physiotherapist should have provided would be judged in this way. Expert witnesses would give evidence to the court on the standard of care they would expect to have found in the circumstances giving rise to the claim. These experts would be respected members of the profession of physiotherapists, possibly head of a physiotherapy department or training college (see Chapter 13).

In a civil action, the judge would decide, in the light of the evidence which has been given to the court, what standard should have been followed.

Experts can, of course, differ and a case may arise where the expert giving evidence for the plaintiff states that the accepted approved standard of care was not followed by the defendant or its employees whereas in contrast the expert evidence for the defendant states that a reasonable standard of care was followed. Where such a conflict arises the House of Lords in the case of *Maynard* v. *West Midlands Regional Health Authority*[7] has laid down the following principle:

> 'It was not sufficient to establish negligence for the plaintiff to show that there is a body of competent professional opinion that considered the decision was wrong, if there was also a body of equally competent professional opinion that supports the decision as having been reasonable in the circumstances.'

The determination of the reasonable standard of care has been more recently considered by the House of Lords in the case of *Bolitho* v. *City Hospital Hackney*[8]. In this case the House of Lords stated that:

> 'The use of these adjectives – responsible, reasonable and respectable – [in the Bolam case] all show that the court has to be satisfied that the exponents of the body of opinion relied upon can demonstrate that such opinion has a logical basis ... [T]he judge before accepting a body of opinion as being responsible, reasonable or respectable, will need to be satisfied that, in forming their views, the experts had directed their minds to the question of comparative risks and benefits and had reached a defensible conclusion on the matter.'

> '[I]t will very seldom be right for a judge to reach the conclusion that views genuinely held by a competent medical expert are unreasonable.'

Setting standards in physiotherapy practice

The CSP has given guidance on how to set standards[9]. It emphasises that those developing standards must consider:

- Who are the standards for?
- What will the standards be used for?
- Who will audit the standards?

It stresses the need for standards to be realistic, understandable, measurable and achievable. The document envisages that standards will be drafted by each of the clinical interest groups and these will be submitted to the Quality Unit of the Professional Affairs Department for comment. The final draft will be submitted to the CSP Professional Practice Committee (PPC) with a recommendation that PPC approves the document for publication and inclusion in the Standards Pack. Clearly evidence on standards given by experts from the physiotherapy profession would refer to these agreed standards.

The White Paper[10] which is discussed in Chapter 17 is likely to lead to increasing emphasis on standard setting. Bodies have been set up such as the National Institute of Clinical Excellence, the Commission for Health Improvement and the National Standards Frameworks and these are there to give guidance on standards to be achieved in all sectors of hospital and community care. Physiotherapists will be expected to follow the results of clinical effectiveness research in their treatment and care of the patients. Patients will be able to use these national guidelines to argue that inadequate care has been provided.

Judy Mead of the Professional Affairs Department of the CSP is at the time of writing drafting a briefing paper for chartered physiotherapists on clinical governance which will include guidance on clinical effectiveness and research based practice. Reference should also be made to her book on evidence based practice[11].

Has there been a breach of the duty of care?

Once it has been established in court what the reasonable standard of care should have been, the next stage is to decide whether what took place was in accordance with the reasonable standard, i.e. has there been a breach of the duty of care. Evidence will be given by witnesses of fact as to what actually took place. The role of such witnesses is considered in Chapter 13.

Difficulties can arise in establishing the standard of care, especially in circumstances where the technique gives rise to complications. For example Darren Rivett and Peter Milburn[12] discuss the complications which can arise from spinal manipulative therapy. Their findings from research in New Zealand suggest that serious complications from the manipulative therapy may constitute a hitherto unrecognised substantial proportion of all spinal troubles. They recommend further research to identify the rate of particular complications and identify hazardous techniques. Should such complications arise and a patient seek compensation, expert evidence would be required to show that a reasonable standard of care was followed despite these effects. (See the Case of *Maynard* above for the situation where there is a responsible body of opinion in favour of and against a procedure.) It would also be necessary to show that the patient was informed of the significant risks of substantial harm before the treatment commenced (see Chapter 7).

Causation

The plaintiff must show that not only was there a breach of the duty of care, but that this breach of duty caused actual and reasonably foreseeable harm to the plaintiff. This requires both

- factual causation to be shown, and also
- evidence that the type of harm which occurred was reasonably foreseeable.

Factual causation

There may be a breach of the duty of care and harm but there may be no link between them. The following is the classic case[13] illustrating an absence of factual causation.

Case: *Barnett* v. *Chelsea HMC*

Three night watch men drank tea which made them vomit. They went to the casualty department of the local hospital. The casualty officer, on being told of the complaints by a nurse, did not see the men, but told them to go home and call in their own doctors. Some hours later one of them died from arsenical poisoning. The court held that

- the casualty department officers owed a duty of care in the circumstances; and
- the casualty doctor had been negligent in not seeing them; but

- even if he had, it was improbable that the only effective antidote could have been administered in time to save the deceased.

Therefore the defendants were not liable. The patient would have died anyway.

The onus is on the plaintiff to establish that there is this causation link between the breach of the duty of care and the harm which occurred. In the following case[14], the plaintiff failed initially to establish causation although ultimately the House of Lords ordered a new hearing on the issue and at the end of the day, faced with more protracted litigation, the parties agreed to a settlement.

Case: *Wilsher* v. *Essex Area Health Authority*

A premature baby was being treated with oxygen therapy. A junior doctor mistakenly inserted the catheter to monitor the oxygen intake into the vein rather than an artery. A senior registrar when being asked to check what had been done failed to notice the error. The baby was given excess oxygen. The parents claimed compensation for the retrolentalfibroplasia that the baby suffered, but failed to prove that it was the excess oxygen which had caused the harm. They therefore failed in their claim.

It was agreed that there were several different factors which could have caused the child to become blind and the negligence in question was only one of them. It could not be presumed that it was the defendant's negligence which had caused the harm.

It has also been difficult for claimants to establish causation when suing for compensation for harm which it is claimed has resulted from vaccine damage. In the case of *Loveday* v. *Renton and another*[15] a claim was brought against the Wellcome Foundation who made vaccine against whooping cough, and against the doctor who administered it, seeking compensation for brain damage which was alleged to have been caused by the vaccine. The case failed because the judge held that the plaintiff had not established on a balance of probabilities that the pertussis vaccine had caused the brain damage.

Subsequently, however, in an Irish case brought against the Wellcome Foundation and others for vaccine damage[16] it has been held that causation as well as breach was established. The High Court had dismissed the plaintiff's claim because of the lack of proof of causation, but on appeal the Irish Supreme Court held that the Wellcome Foundation was liable for the negligent manufacture and release of a particular batch of triple vaccine and that the brain damage was caused as a result. It referred the case back to the High Court on the amount of compensation and in 1993 the court approved an award of £2.75 million as compensation for the brain damage sustained in September 1969. The award was so high because it included the cost of care for the 24 years since the injury occurred and also the cost of future care which, in cases of brain damage, can be very high.

Reasonably foreseeable harm

The harm which might arise may not be within the reasonable contemplation of the defendant so that, even though there is a breach of duty and there is harm, the defendant is not liable. For example a physiotherapist may have ordered the wrong equipment for a person at home and therefore be in breach of the duty of care, but the client may have suffered harm because she used the equipment in an inappropriate way.

Case: *Jolley v. Sutton London Borough Council*[17]

> Some children found a boat abandoned on grass beside council housing. The local authority had a duty under the Occupier's Liability Act 1957 (see Chapter 11) to any visitor to ensure the area was safe. In the High Court the plaintiff was awarded £633 770 (taking into account contributory negligence of 25%) for the injuries he sustained when the boat, which some children had propped up with a car jack so that they could repair it, collapsed on top of him crushing his back.

However the Court of Appeal found in favour of the defendant council and the award was withdrawn. This was because, although it was reasonably foreseeable that injuries could have occurred in the event of children playing on the boat, the injuries sustained by the plaintiff were not reasonably foreseeable and therefore the defendants were not liable for them. The Council had not disputed that it was negligent, but simply claimed it was not liable because the accident was of a different kind from anything which it could have reasonably foreseen.

New intervening cause

It may also happen that any causal link between the plaintiff's breach of duty and the harm suffered by the client is interrupted by an intervening event.

Situation: Intervening act

> A physiotherapist failed to make an appropriate assessment for the discharge of the patient from the department, but the patient was injured in a road accident as a result of another person's negligence and died from her injuries.

In this situation the negligence of the physiotherapist has not caused the death of the patient so her employer would not be vicariously liable.

Harm

To succeed in an action for negligence plaintiffs or their representatives must establish that they have suffered harm which the court recognises as being subject to compensation. Thus personal injury, death and loss or damage to property are the main areas of recognisable harm. In addition the courts have ruled that nervous shock (now known as post traumatic stress syndrome) can be the subject of compensation within strict limits of liability (and where an identifiable medical condition exists). A test of proximity to the defendant's negligent action or omission has been set by the House of Lords[18].

Some of the types of harm covered by the effect of personal injury are illustrated below in the section showing how compensation is calculated.

Vicarious and personal liability distinguished

As stated above it is unlikely that an employed physiotherapist will be sued personally since the employer would be vicariously liable for her actions.

To establish the vicarious liability of the employer the plaintiff must show:

- the employee
- was negligent or was guilty of another wrong
- whilst acting in course of employment.

An independent practitioner would have to accept personal and professional liability for her actions but she may also be vicariously liable for the harm, caused during the course of employment, by anyone she herself employs.

Each of the elements shown above must be established. It follows that:

- the employer is not liable for the acts of his independent contractors (i.e. self-employed persons who are working for him on a contract for services) unless he is at fault in selecting or instructing them; and
- the employer may challenge whether the actions were performed in the course of employment.

For example, a physiotherapist may have undertaken a training in a complementary medicine such as aromatherapy. If she decided to use these new skills whilst at work without the agreement, express or implied, of the employer and through her use of the remedies caused harm to the client, her employer might refuse to accept vicarious liability on the grounds that she was not acting in the course of employment. (See Chapter 27 on complementary therapies.)

The physiotherapist may also undertake extra-curricular activities with patients such as horse-riding or going to a commercial gym. Would these activities be considered to be in the course of employment so that if the physiotherapist were negligent, the employer would be vicariously liable for this negligence? It is not possible to generalise since it all depends upon the circumstances. Thus a physiotherapist who in her own time returned to work to give her clients assistance with horse riding might be considered by the employer to be doing this on her own account and not on its behalf. However it would be different, if this activity were included in the client's treatment plan and there was an expectation that the physiotherapist would provide attendance. Similarly, if it is agreed that the physiotherapist should accompany the client on a day trip, even though it is her day off, it may still be considered to be in the course of employment.

Where such uncertainties are likely to arise it is wise to clarify such issues in advance with the employer, so that the physiotherapist knows whether she ought to obtain private insurance cover for such activities or notify her existing insurer about their taking place. An independent physiotherapist in private practice should ensure that she notifies her insurers of the exact content of her work and whether it involves possibly risky activities (see Chapter 19 on the private practitioner).

Defences to an action

The main defences to an action for negligence are listed below:

- Allegations of fact are disputed.
- It is denied that all elements of negligence are established.
- The defendant alleges contributory negligence on the part of the claimant.
- The defendant claims exemption from liability.
- The time set for bringing a claim has expired.
- The defendant alleges the claimant voluntarily assumed the risk.

Disputed allegations of fact

Many cases will be resolved entirely on what facts can be shown to exist. Thus the effectiveness of the witnesses for both parties in establishing the facts of what did or did not occur will be the determining factor in who wins the case. Reference should be made to Chapter 12 on record keeping and Chapter 13 on witnesses in court for further discussion on the nature of evidence and the role of the witnesses. In theory, it might appear before the hearing at court that one party has a particularly strong case but, unless the facts on which that case rests can be proved in court, the actual outcome of the case might be that the opponent wins.

Basically every case depends on proper hard evidence and whether the witnesses of fact (either about the event or about the extent of the injuries), including the parties themselves, can be believed.

Elements of negligence not established

The plaintiff must establish that all elements required to prove negligence are present, i.e. duty, breach, causation and harm. If one or more of these cannot be established then the defendant will win the case.

Contributory negligence

If the client is partly to blame for the harm which has occurred then there may still be liability on the part of the professional but the compensation payable might be reduced in proportion to the client's fault. In extreme cases such a claim may be a complete defence if 100% contributory negligence is claimed. In determining the level of contributory negligence, the physical and mental health and the age of the client would be taken into account.

Situation: Contributory negligence

A physiotherapist made a negligent assessment of a person's needs but, in addition, the client failed to give the physiotherapist vital information relevant to those needs. Harm subsequently befell the client as a result of the assessment being inaccurate.

In an action brought by the client the client's contribution to that harm is taken into account.

The Law Reform (Contributory Negligence) Act 1945 enables an apportionment of responsibility for the harm which has been caused which may result in a reduction of damages payable. The Court can reduce the damages 'to such extent as it thinks just and equitable having regard to the claimant's share in the responsibility for the damage' (section 1(1)).

One of the most frequent examples of contributory negligence being taken into account is in road traffic accidents where the injuries sustained by the plaintiff are greater because he or she was not wearing a seat belt. (For contributory negligence by a child see Chapter 23.)

Exemption from liability

It is possible for people to exempt themselves from liability for harm arising from their negligence but the effects of the Unfair Contract Terms Act 1977 means that this exemption can only apply to loss or damage to property. A defendant cannot exclude liability for negligence which results in personal damage or death, either by contract or by a notice.

Where exemption from liability for loss or damage to property is claimed by the defendant, it must be shown by the defendant that it is reasonable to rely upon the term or notice which purported to exclude liability. The relevant provisions of the Unfair Contract Terms Act 1977 are shown in Figure 10.1.

Figure 10.1   Unfair Contract Terms act 1977 – sections 2 and 11 (extracts).

2(1) A person cannot by reference to any contract term or to a notice given to persons generally or to particular persons exclude or restrict his liability for death or personal injury resulting from negligence.

2(2) In the case of other loss or damage, a person cannot so exclude or restrict his liability for negligence except in so far as the term or notice satisfies the requirement of reasonableness.

[The 'reasonableness' test is explained in section 11]

11(3) In relation to a notice (not being a notice having contractual effect) . . . it should be fair and reasonable to allow reliance on it, having regard to all the circumstances obtaining when the liability arose or (but for the notice) would have arisen.

11(5) It is for those claiming that a contract term or notice satisfies the requirements of reasonableness to show that it does.

Limitation of time

Actions for personal injury or death should normally be commenced within three years of the date of the event which gave rise to the harm or three years from the date on which the person had the necessary knowledge of the harm and the fact that it arose from the defendant's actions or omissions.

Exceptions

There are however some major qualifications to this general principle and these are shown in Figure 10.2.

Figure 10.2   **Situations where the limitation of time can be extended.**

- Those suffering from a disability:
  - Children under 18 years – the time does not start to run until the child is 18 years.
  - Those suffering from a mental disability – time does not start to run until the disability ends. In the case of those who are suffering from severe learning disabilities or brain damage this may not be until death.
- Discretion of the judge. The judge has a statutory power to extend the time within which a plaintiff can bring an action for personal injuries or death if it is just and equitable to do so.

The implications of the rules relating to limitation of time are that in those cases which might come under one of the exceptions to the three year time limit, records should be kept and not destroyed. This is particularly important in the case of children and those with learning disabilities. For example in the case of *Bull* v. *Wakeham*[19] the case was brought 18 years after the plaintiff's birth. In a news item report in 1995[20] a man then 33 years old obtained compensation of £1.25 million because of a failure to diagnose severe dehydration a few weeks after his birth.

Knowledge

Plaintiffs are assumed to have the necessary knowledge (and so the 'clock' starts running) when they know or it is reasonable to expect them to know the following facts:

- that the injury in question was significant;
- that the injury was attributable in whole or in part to the act or omission which is alleged to constitute the negligence, nuisance or breach of duty;
- the identity of the defendant;
- (if it is alleged that the act or omission was that of a person other than the defendant) the identity of that person and the additional facts supporting the bringing of an action against them.

Knowledge that any acts or omissions did or did not, as a matter of law, involve negligence, nuisance or breach of duty is irrelevant. The plaintiff cannot bring an action out of time if he knew all the facts more than three years ago but has only just found out they could give rise to a claim.

A person is not fixed with knowledge of a fact ascertainable only with the help of expert advice so long as he has taken all reasonable steps to obtain and, where appropriate, to act on that advice.

Voluntary assumption of risk

Volenti non fit injuria is the latin tag for the defence that a person willingly undertook the risk of being harmed.

In a case[21] where a rugby player was injured following a tackle which he alleged threw him against a concrete wall it was held that, even if there had been any liability under the Occupier's Liability Act 1957 (which the court did not find – see Chapter 11), the player must be taken to have willingly accepted the risk of playing on the field, which complied with the regulations.

It is unlikely to succeed as a defence in an action for professional negligence since the professional cannot contract out of liability where harm occurs as a result of her negligence (see the Unfair Contract Terms Act considered above). However it may be relevant to the physiotherapist who undertakes potentially risky activities with a client, such as horse-riding, gymnastics or certain types of dance. Such activities may have an element of danger about them and, if the risks are explained to the client and the client has the competence to assume the risk of harm arising, then this may be a successful defence to a claim against the physiotherapist that she was negligent in proposing a risky activity. However where the client lacks the mental competence to make such a decision, then there is a duty of care placed upon the physiotherapist to take all reasonable care, according to the Bolam test, that harm would not occur. This may entail not undertaking such an activity (see Chapter 24 for risks in the care of the elderly). It is unlikely that the courts would hold that a mentally incompetent adult voluntarily assumed the risk of being harmed as a result of the negligence of the physiotherapist.

Calculating compensation

In some cases of negligence, liability might be accepted by the defendant, but there might still be disagreement between the parties over quantum, i.e. the amount of compensation. Alternatively there might be agreement over the amount of compensation and liability alone might be disputed. In others, both liability and quantum might be in dispute.

Physiotherapists are sometimes called as expert witnesses to give evidence of assessment in cases, where there is a dispute over quantum. This is further discussed in Chapter 13.

An example of a case giving details of a compensation calculation is shown below.

Case: *Misell* v. *Essex County Council*[22]

Mr Misell, a coal conveyer operator, fell from his motorcycle, whilst negotiating a corner of a country road, maintained by Essex County Council. He suffered a severe arm injury which resulted in substantial loss of the use of that arm; he lost his job and had been out of work ever since.

On the question of quantum, the following was awarded:

General Damages	£40 000
interest accruing	£1 600
Loss of earnings to date	£47 695
Travelling expenses	£200
interest	£4 328
Future loss	£119 383.66

Future loss was made up of the following:

Loss of future earnings	£104 190
Additional costs attributable to the injury	£8 438
Additional one off expenditure	£6 755.66

The future loss of earnings was based on the fact that he was then 50 years old with no prospect of obtaining paid employment during his pre-retirement age life. A multiplier of 7.8 was set.

The additional costs attributable to the injury were based on a calculation of £937.50 per annum to which a multiplier of 9 was fixed.

The court in its calculation of compensation takes into account the fact that the award is being made at once and therefore the plaintiff is benefiting from the ability to obtain interest on the lump sum. Calculations are made as to what interest can be expected. It is difficult to balance matters fairly but in a recent case the House of Lords has ruled that, in the award of compensation, victims should not be expected to speculate on the stock market and therefore lower levels of return based on index-linked government securities can be used as the basis of calculation[23]. The effect of this ruling will be to increase the capital amount awarded to victims. In the case itself James Thomas, a cerebral palsy victim as a result of negligence at birth, was awarded £1 285 000 by the High Court judge, but in a very controversial decision this was reduced by the Court of Appeal by £300 000 on the basis that the capital could be invested in higher return (but more risky) equities. The House of Lords restored the original amount.

Requirements for ongoing physiotherapy treatment can be included in the compensation claim and, if they are disputed, it will be essential for a physiotherapist to give expert evidence on the matter (see Chapter 13).

In a case where the plaintiff a senior psychiatric registrar suffered a cardiac arrest and irreparable brain damage following a minor gynaecological operation the High Court awarded £249 239. This sum included the costs of one full time and two part time physiotherapists five times per week. The Court of Appeal did not overturn the award[24].

Examples of situations involving physiotherapists

Failures in assessment

Assessment of the client's needs is the first step for a physiotherapist in developing a treatment plan. It is now clear that the physiotherapist would have a duty to use her own professional judgment in determining the client's clinical situation and what physiotherapy treatments were indicated. If the expressed reason for referral by a doctor differed from the physiotherapist's assessment, the latter would have a duty to notify the doctor that in her judgment different treatments were required. She should not professionally undertake treatment which in her view is not clinically indicated: a defence of obeying orders would not suffice if harm were caused to the client as a consequence of this.

The CSP has included in its *Standards of Physiotherapy Practice*[25] standards for assessment. It defines assessment as:

'A continuous process by which the acquisition of relevant, quantified and other data will result in the formulation of a treatment plan related to goals which have been actively set with the patient'.

Standard 10 covers the initial assessment. The criteria for standard 10 compliance include written evidence on a database consisting of:

- a clinical examination of the patient;
- pertinent information gathered from the patient and other relevant sources; and
- a problem list which demonstrates appropriate interpretation and analysis of that database.

If no further investigations are required then there must be written evidence that the reasons for this have been explained to the patient and carer.

Standard 11 requires written evidence of agreed, problem orientated and related treatment plans.

Failures in communication

Failures in communication can also give rise to liability should the physiotherapist fail to pass on information or if she has failed to communicate appropriately with other health professionals or the client and carers. An understanding of practitioner/client and practitioner/practitioner interaction is therefore essential to ensure real communication[26].

Unknown contra-indications

For example, it is now increasingly the practice for metal staples to be used in the repair of hernias[27]. Physiotherapists who use short wave diathermy (SWD) over a hip should be aware if metal staples have been used since metal within the magnetic field is a contra-indication. Therefore if a physiotherapist, in ignorance of the metal staples inside the patient, used SWD and caused the staples to heat and harm the patient, the patient would have grounds for an action. The fact that the physiotherapist was not aware of the staples would not be an adequate defence if any reasonable physiotherapist, in following the Bolam test, would have discovered this information prior to using such a treatment.

Bad news

Policies are necessary to ensure that 'bad news' is communicated in an appropriate way.

Case: *AB and Others* v. *Tameside & Glossop Health Authority*[28]

This case involved notifying persons that they had been treated by an HIV positive health worker. It was alleged by 114 of the patients who had been so notified that the two defendant health authorities were negligent in choosing to inform patients by letter as opposed to face to face, and moreover that the facilities offered by the letter were not properly provided. The High Court judge found in favour of the plaintiffs on the grounds:

- that the health authorities did not exercise due care in that they should have realised that the best method of communicating such news was face to face; and
- that there was a foreseeable risk that some vulnerable individuals might suffer psychiatric injury going beyond shock and distress.

The health authorities appealed. Court of Appeal found for the defendants on the facts of this particular case, but confirmed that in law there was a duty on the defendants to take such steps as were reasonable to inform patients of such news, having regard to the possibility of psychiatric injury.

Overhearing

Patients (and relatives) overhearing careless or insensitive discussion is an issue throughout health care.

A stroke patient has described how he heard doctors writing him off as a hopeless case as he lay in hospital unable to respond[29].

In this case the patient made a partial recovery with some movement in his left hand and, computer-aided, has written an account of his experience. There would be the possibility of legal action if he were able to show that harm has occurred as a result of this lack of thought by the doctors.

Many physiotherapists may forget that their unconscious patients may be able to hear and they therefore need to beware of what they say to their colleagues and to relatives.

Rationing and setting priorities

Rationing in physiotherapy services

The CSP has provided information on the rationing of physiotherapy services[30]. It notes that physiotherapy has always been rationed by lack of referral, lack of resources or lack of available expertise. Amongst the issues which it asks physiotherapists to consider are:

- The duty of care to patients (see above)
- Rules of professional conduct (see Chapter 4)
- Efficacy of treatment (see below)
- Delegation of physiotherapy tasks (see below)
- Prioritising of services (see below).

Prioritising

The CSP information leaflet on rationing considers a number of options in reviewing working practices to make the most effective use of existing resources. It recognises however that it may be necessary to reduce the breadth of service offered.

'This then ensures that those patients who are accepted for treatment receive a safe, optimum service. Often it is necessary to withdraw the service to one section or category of patient.'

The CSP recommends that management should be notified about the decisions which have had to be made. The Association of Chartered Physiotherapists in Management (ACPM) believe that

'It is the purchaser's responsibility, not the provider, to make decisions about cuts if they have to be made, and to take the consequences. If there is to be rationing, it must be patient focused, not profession focused'.

The determination of priorities is as much a part of the duty of care owed by a physiotherapist as is the assessment and the provision of care. Thus if a physiotherapist was at fault in failing to recognise the priority which should be given to a client following a carefully carried out assessment, and no reasonable physiotherapist following the accepted standard of care (i.e. the Bolam test) would have made a similar decision, the physiotherapist or her employer may be liable in negligence should harm befall the client as a consequence.

Referrals and information
The proper determination of priorities cannot be done unless there is full information about a referral. Failure to obtain the full information about a referral can cause many problems for the physiotherapist. Sometimes it may not be possible to make a judgment on priorities unless the patient has been seen.

■ What is the situation if a physiotherapist is unable to follow these standards?

Situation: referrals

A physiotherapist receives referrals regularly from doctors with little information about the patient's diagnosis. There is a waiting list for physiotherapy services. What should the physiotherapist do?

In this situation it is impossible for the physiotherapist to make any determination on priorities without adequate information from the person referring. This should be made clear to those referring and a referral form should be designed and the necessary information obtained before an assessment of priorities is made. When the physiotherapist actually sees the patient she would, of course, have to make her own examination and take a case history and determine the treatment plan and the priority which is assigned to that patient.

■ What is the situation in the case of a self-referral, where the client is not prepared to allow the physiotherapist to make contact with her doctor?

In such circumstances, the physiotherapist should make it clear to the client that, unless she has contact with the client's doctor over pre-existing medical conditions and existing treatment, she cannot fulfil her duty of care to the client according to the approved standard of care. Ultimately the physiotherapist could advise that it would be hazardous to treat the client without the full information and therefore may have to refuse the referral. She should of course make every effort to discover what are the reasons for the client's objection to the information being passed on.

Inadequate time to see patient

■ Where does the physiotherapist stand legally if she has only time to see an in-patient for five minutes in a day when she believes professionally that he should be seen for 30 minutes?

The physiotherapist has a duty to provide a reasonable standard of care to each individual patient. If the five minutes is too short to ensure that the patient is appropriately treated, then the physiotherapist has a duty to inform her manager that, because of pressure of work, she is not providing a reasonable standard of care. It may be that there is a need to reassess priorities and some patients may have to be omitted entirely from the service. Similar problems occur in out-patients where a physiotherapist could consider that a patient should be seen three times per week but in practice can only offer an appointment once a week. Again the allocation of resources to patients must be made according to the reasonable standards of care as set out in the Bolam test. The physiotherapist would have a professional duty to ensure that any concerns about the availability of resources are taken up with management.

Situation: Reduced service

A physiotherapist is only able to see an out-patient once a week instead of a preferred frequency of three times per week. Five years later the patient declares an intention of suing the NHS trust for failures to provide adequate physiotherapy, which he alleges has delayed his full recovery.

On these facts it would firstly be important to check if the time limits set by law for bringing an action have been breached (see above). If an action is brought the physiotherapist would have to show that the patient received a reasonable standard of care, even though ideally additional sessions would have been of benefit. There may be evidence that the treatment plan included exercises for the patient to undertake at home to offset the reduced number of sessions and failure on the client's part do to so could reduce any liability on the part of the health authority or Trust (see Contributory negligence above). Clearly the records kept by the physiotherapist will be of vital importance in determining the facts and whether the reasonable standard of care was followed.

Where a patient is given instructions for after-care treatment including exercises to be undertaken, there is considerable advantage in ensuring that this is in writing. For example in the case brought by Frank Cunningham[31] (see Chapter 13), there was a dispute as to whether he was given written instructions following application of plaster about the circumstances in which he should return to hospital. The hospital said he was, but Mr Cunningham denied this. A tear off slip signed by the patient may be useful in such disputes.

Resourcing

It is important that resources are used effectively. A recent announcement by the Department of Health[32] stated that patients failed to turn up for 5.5 million appointments out of a total of 40 million between 1996 and 1997. On average this results in a waste of £275 million. More effective methods of making appointments in a physiotherapy department might improve the rate of non-attenders and hence the use of physiotherapy resources.

In determining the standard of care which should be followed in resourcing a department reference could be made to such works as that by Joyce Williams on staffing levels[33]. This mentions the duty of care in the context of negligence and setting staffing levels: workload levels should be monitored regularly and unacceptable levels defined. The action to be taken in dealing with unmet need at that point should also be stated: e.g. to refer back, to prioritise, and to record in the patient's notes that treatment was not given or reduced and the reason for this.

> 'As a basic principle therapists should not accept responsibility for a workload or an individual patient if they are unable to fulfil their duty of care by providing adequate effective treatment in a reasonable time period.'

Physiotherapists must clearly distinguish between services which are reduced as a result of pressure from resources and those where any increase would not benefit the patient's condition. For example, in one case[34] concerning special needs, the local authority and health authority gave evidence that, although the child was receiving the maximum physiotherapy treatment which they were able to provide, there was no guarantee that increased physiotherapy would actually improve L's physical condition.

Inter-professional practice

Communication between health and social services professionals is essential in ensuring that the client receives the appropriate standard of care. This is particularly important where one person is designated as the key worker on behalf of the multi-disciplinary team (see below). However the Court of Appeal[35] has stated that the courts do not recognise a concept of team liability and it is therefore for each individual professional to ensure that her practice is according to the approved standard of care. Nor should a professional take instructions from another professional which she knows would be contrary to the standard of care which her profession would require.

The sharing of records is considered in Chapter 12.

■ Where the physiotherapist has strongly advised a certain course of action what is the situation if her advice is then ignored?

She should ensure that her recommendations are in writing and that she keeps a copy. She would still have a duty to take all reasonable precautions to prevent the client suffering harm. This would include consultation with her managers. If it is clear, that the client is in danger, steps may have to be taken to ameliorate this. It would be professionally unacceptable for the physiotherapist to deny responsibility for the case just because her advice was ignored.

Home visits

Physiotherapists are confronted with many potential legal situations arising from a home visit, such as:

- What if the client refuses to return to hospital, against the advice of the physiotherapist?
- What if the physiotherapist advised against the immediate discharge of the client but her advice is not followed?
- Can the physiotherapist enter private accommodation without the owner or client being present?
- In what circumstances could the physiotherapist insist upon having an escort when accompanying a client on a home visit?

These questions are considered in Chapter 7 on consent, Chapter 11 on health and safety and rights of occupation and Chapter 18 on community care.

Key worker system

The physiotherapist may be appointed as the key worker for an individual patient/client and work with other members of the multi-disciplinary team in the care of the patient. In such a situation, she should ensure that she works within her sphere of competence and knows her own limitations, bringing the other members of the team into the direct care of the patient where their professional expertise is required. As is discussed above, the courts do not recognise any concept of team liability. The scope of professional practice of the physiotherapist is discussed in Chapter 4.

Negligent advice

There can be liability for negligence in giving advice but the plaintiff would have to show that it was clear to the defendant that he or she would rely upon the advice and in so doing had suffered reasonably foreseeable loss or harm[36]. An example can be seen from the following situation.

Situation: Failure to give clinical advice

A physiotherapist did not warn a patient that until his condition improved he should avoid contact sports. He later returned to the department with further injury and stated that he was holding the physiotherapist responsible for not warning him to avoid such sporting activity.

In a situation like this the advice given to the patient by the physiotherapist would be judged by the reasonable standard of the profession in those circumstances, which would include the knowledge she had of his activities, how thoroughly she had taken note of such background information, and any general warning given which could be deemed to include specific warnings. In addition there may be an element of contributory negligence if it would have been reasonable to expect the patient to refrain from activities which could obviously worsen his condition.

Situation: Advice ignored

> The physiotherapist gives appropriate advice relating to the post-operative care of a patient, but the patient ignores this. Is the physiotherapist responsible for any harm which occurs?

The answer is that, provided that the information was given and understood by the patient, then the physiotherapist would not be liable. The patient would be 100% responsible for the harm. If however the patient was mentally incapacitated, then this fact should be taken into account by the physiotherapist in giving the information, and it may be necessary to communicate with a relative or carer as well, the need to act in the best interests of the patient overriding issues of confidentiality.

In circumstances where the same information is frequently given it may be of help if the information is put in writing in a simple leaflet for the patient. The physiotherapist should note in her records that the leaflet has been given out and in certain circumstances could obtain the signature of the patient that the leaflet has been received.

References

If a negligently written reference is provided liability can arise, either to the recipient of the reference (if in reliance upon that reference he has suffered harm[37]) or to the person who is the subject of the reference.

Situation: Providing a reference

> A physiotherapist is asked to provide a reference for a patient who has a mental health problem. The patient asks the physiotherapist not to refer to the history of mental illness. What is the position if the physiotherapist gives the reference without mentioning the mental illness, the patient obtains the post, and then the employer blames the physiotherapist for an inaccurate reference which has led to harm?

If the mental health of the patient was relevant to the use the recipient would make of the reference, then it should have been mentioned in a reference and, if it is omitted, the physiotherapist could be liable for negligent advice. In such circumstances she should have told the patient that, if she gave a reference, it would have to include a mention of the mental illness. This is a difficult area, since many persons who have suffered mental ill health may find that they are discriminated against without justification. The physiotherapist should, if uncertain, consider consulting her line manager for advice on whether the job in question requires mental health information and she should also look very carefully at the person specification and job description which should come with the request for a reference or which the patient himself should have or could ask for.

There can also be liability to the person on whose behalf the reference is given if the reference is written without reasonable care and if 'harm' or pecuniary loss occurs to the subject of the reference as a result of potential employers relying upon an inaccurate and misleading reference[38].

Every care should be taken to ensure that any reference is written accurately in the light of the facts available.

Volunteering help

Many physiotherapists volunteer to use their skills to assist in a great variety of situations, on an unpaid basis and outside the course of their employment (for example many will volunteer to assist disabled persons to ride horses) but this can in itself lead to difficulties. Unfortunately it does not follow that, because the help has been volunteered, the recipients, in their gratitude, will ignore any harm which arises from negligence. In recent years there have been successful cases brought against a referee in rugby match[39] and against a mountain rescue guide.

Case: *Cattley v. St John Ambulance Brigade*[40]

The St John Ambulance Brigade were sued by a person helped by two of their members on the grounds that these volunteers had caused the victim further harm. The person claiming compensation was 15 at the time of the accident. He had been competing in a motor cycle scramble for school boys. He came off his bike and was treated at the track by two brigade members. He suffered from cracked ribs and also compression fractures of the sixth and seventh dorsal vertebrae which had damaged the spinal cord and caused incomplete paraplegia. He claimed that the spinal injury was aggravated by the negligent examination and treatment offered him by the St John Ambulance personnel in the period immediately after the fall. It was alleged that he had been lifted to his feet causing further damage to his already injured spinal cord.

The question arose, was there a duty of care owed and if so what was the standard? The judge found no difficulty in holding that there was a duty of care and he held that the standard should be an adaptation of the Bolam test. Did the first aider act in accordance with the standards of the ordinary skilled first aider exercising and professing to have the special skills of a first aider?

In applying this test the judge rejected the version of events given by the boy and his father and held that all the evidence pointed to the fact that at all times the first aiders had acted in accordance with the ordinary skill to be expected of a properly trained first aider i.e. not to move a victim of suspected fracture. The claim was therefore rejected but the legal principle was established that even a volunteer has to act in accordance with a certain standard of care.

Situation: Holidays for terminally ill children

A physiotherapist belonged to an association which raised moneys for holidays for terminally ill children. She used two weeks of her holiday to accompany the children with friends and other health professionals. She is concerned that she does not have any insurance cover for this work. What is her situation?

Anyone volunteering help should ensure that they do have insurance cover for their actions. In volunteering help outside the physiotherapist would probably not be covered in law by the vicarious liability of her employer (see above) and therefore, were any harm to arise as a result of her negligence, the physiotherapist could then face litigation and, if the plaintiff succeeded, damages would be awarded against her personally. It is essential that such volunteers check with the CSP that they have insurance cover for the voluntary activities which they undertake, making expressly clear the nature of their voluntary help and any associated risks.

In the light of decided cases and situations such as discussed above, the following would appear to be essential requirements for any physiotherapist volunteering help. She should:

- determine her competence to assist;
- identify the standard of care required;
- ensure that this standard of care is followed;
- check that she has the appropriate insurance cover;
- ensure that any necessary records are kept of the activity.

Instructing clients

Physiotherapists, even those who are not tutors, may find that they are expected to take classes. Often they may have had no training in teaching and instructing others. However they would still be expected to follow a reasonable standard in explaining treatments and exercises to clients. If they are negligent in this and as a result of that negligence harm occurs then their employer could be vicariously liable.

Situation: Taking classes

A physiotherapist takes classes in the following topics: shoulder, back, neck, and ankle. She instructs from five to ten people at a time and finds that it is an effective use of her time. Unfortunately, during one of the ankle classes, one of the patients in attempting to carry out the instructions, tripped very badly and now requires further surgery. She is blaming the physiotherapist and threatening to sue the trust.

In this situation, the procedure followed by the physiotherapist and the instructions which she gave will be compared with the reasonable, safe and competent practice which could be expected from a physiotherapist in that situation, given the reasonably foreseeable risks relating to each client.

Liability for students and unqualified assistants

Exactly the same principles apply to the delegation and supervision of tasks as to the carrying out of professional activities. The professional delegating a task should only do so if she is reasonably sure that the person to whom she is delegating is reasonably competent and sufficiently experienced to undertake that activity safely in the care of the patient. At the same time the professional must ensure that the person delegated to has a sufficient level of supervision to ensure that she herself is reasonably safe in carrying out that delegated activity.

Should harm befall a client because an activity was carried out by a junior member of staff, a student or a physiotherapy assistant, it is no defence to the client's claim to argue that the harm occurred because that person did not have the ability, competence or experience to carry out that task reasonably safely[41].

Situation: Too inexperienced

A physiotherapist, recently qualified, was attending a patient on the ward. The patient was on IV antibiotics. The physiotherapist agreed to take the patient for a walk in the grounds. He disconnected the IVs and went with the patient for 10 minutes in the sunshine. On his return he reconnected the drip. Unfortunately he set it at the wrong speed so that the patient received four hours of the drug in half an hour.

In this situation there is no doubt that the physiotherapist has been negligent and therefore, if the patient has suffered harm, the Trust will be vicariously liable for the actions of the physiotherapist. The fact that he was only recently qualified cannot be used as a defence. Clearly senior staff also have a responsibility that junior staff do not act outside their experience and competence.

The CSP Assistants List

The Chartered Society of Physiotherapy has included a code of conduct for physiotherapy assistants in its *Rules of Professional Conduct*[42]. The code covers the topics shown in Figure 10.3.

***Figure 10.3* Code of Conduct for Physiotherapy Assistants.**

(1)   Status of physiotherapy assistants
(2)   Scope of practice
(3)   Relationships with physiotherapists
(4)   Relationships with patients
(5)   Confidentiality
(6)   Relationships with professionals and carers
(7)   Advertising
(8)   Sale of goods
(9)   Standards of conduct

The Chartered Society of Physiotherapy keeps a register of Assistants but this does not confer membership of the CSP. Assistants who fail to conform to the Code of Conduct can nevertheless be disciplined by the CSP. Examples of conduct which could lead to disciplinary action by the CSP include:

● criminal convictions;
● disciplinary proceedings by an employer (dismissal by an employer will be

automatically followed by the assistant being removed from the CSP Assistants list);

- abuse of occupational privilege or skills; and
- personal conduct derogatory to the reputation of the CSP.

Delegation criteria

Advice is also given by the CSP on when to delegate tasks[43]. It suggests that the criteria shown in Figure 10.4 should be followed in delegation.

Figure 10.4 **CSP recommended criteria for delegation.**

(1) Assessment of the patient by a Chartered Physiotherapist (CP)*
(2) The CP to identify the physiotherapy management programme for the patient
(3) The CP to monitor the progress and reassess
(4) The CP to only delegate tasks to assistants judged to be competent
(5) This judgment to be based on:

- the known training and experience of the assistant
- the diagnosis, stability and severity of the patient's overall condition
- the patient's predicted response to the programme
- the physical accessibility of the supervising physiotherapist
- the availability of appropriate supervision in the event of a crisis or emergency.

*In certain circumstances the assistant may be the first point of contact with the patient and the CSP guidance sets out the procedures to be followed in this case and when a physiotherapist is not readily accessible.

Concern over the use of unregistered assistants is likely to grow as the skill-mix of qualified registered staff and support staff changes and more work is undertaken by persons who are not registered practitioners. Physiotherapists have a responsibility to ensure both that the activities which they delegate are appropriate for that person and that she is given proper supervision. Assistants in turn have a responsibility to ensure that they 'confine themselves to tasks delegated to them by the physiotherapists for which they have established and maintained their competence'[44].

Liz Saunders carried out an audit of physiotherapy services in an OPD three years after the implementation of a change in skill-mix and increased delegation to assistants[45]. It was found that the systematic approach to delegation had succeeded in terms of costs and patient satisfaction with no loss of quality of service. In her paper she suggests a seven point strategy for delegation:

- Ensure competence of assistant
- Give formal instructions to assistant
- Give explanation to patient
- Arrange appointments
- Supervise assistant
- Ensure communication links are understood
- Inform assistant of outcome of episode of care.

Liability for harm

■ If the physiotherapist ensures that there is appropriate delegation, what is the situation if the unqualified person causes harm to the client?

If the physiotherapist has acted reasonably in following the approved standard of professional practice according to the Bolam test, she would not be liable in negligence. However the person undertaking the delegated activity would be liable and the employer would be vicariously liable for this individual's negligence, subject, of course, to the harm occurring as a reasonably foreseeable result of the negligent act or omission (see above).

Non-registered junior staff in the multi-disciplinary team

There is a danger that the real contribution which can be made to care planning and multi-disciplinary decision making by persons such as physiotherapy assistants, technicians and support workers may not be recognised or may be treated dismissively. Many support workers develop a close rapport with clients and it is essential that any relevant information which they possess should be made known to the team and listened to.

Chapter 4 of the inquiry report about the homicide committed by Jason Mitchell[46], a mentally disordered person, is concerned with assessments on Jason made by professional staff in disciplines other than psychiatry and nursing and points out:

'They contained observations and insights into Jason Mitchell's thoughts and feelings which were rarely recorded in the medical and nursing notes and which could present a different perspective on his case. They tended to be recorded in detail, but were marginalised.'

Attention is drawn in the report to the contribution of a technical instructor in the occupational therapy department at West Park Hospital whose report on Jason Mitchell is given in full as an addendum to the chapter. The Inquiry noted that her report was not included in the Mental Health Review Tribunal papers. In general her report had been ignored or discounted by the doctors central to the care and treatment of Jason Mitchell but in the Inquiry's view, 'the material in her report ought to have prompted at least an assessment, if not a further therapeutic involvement, with a qualified and experienced clinician, possibly a psychologist'. The Inquiry concluded:

'Jason Mitchell's case illustrates how contributions from an unqualified member of staff were disregarded, and consequently how important data were put out of sight and mind. Nothing relevant to the assessment and treatment of a patient should be ignored, whatever its origins.'

Generic or specific assistants?

Jane Langley[47] in an article in *Physiotherapy* discusses the moves to include physiotherapy assistants with a core body of non-professional workers in order to provide a flexible, cost-effective workforce able to help a range of professionals. She stresses the importance of considering the needs of the patients and the importance of using the resources available to a physiotherapy service to the best effect. It is of course essential, whether general or specific assistants are used, to ensure that they are capable of performing the tasks delegated to them and the appropriate level of supervision is provided to meet their needs. Clearly the more specialist the tasks to be delegated, the more useful it is to have specific assistants.

Analysis of task delegation

The management of delegation to physiotherapy assistants is discussed by Liz Saunders[48] who suggested a functional analysis model to determine issues arising in delegation: tasks are analysed to determine whether sub-tasks are knowledge, rule or skill based and thus suitable or not for delegation. The four stages which are identified are:

- Examination of the current system
- Identification of the level of delegation
- Establishment of the new procedure for delegation
- Monitoring the new system.

As a result of a systematic analysis of task delegation, management can adjust physiotherapist–assistant ratios to create appropriate skill-mix for the area. Saunders also considers the training implications of delegation following the task analysis.

It is essential that delegation is on a personal basis and takes into account the individual assistant's personal knowledge, experience, skill and training.

Care of property

Failure to look after another person's property could lead to criminal prosecution, e.g. theft, or a civil action for trespass to goods, or negligence in causing loss or damage to property.

In an action for negligence, the person who has suffered the loss or damage to property must establish the same four elements which must be shown in a claim for compensation for personal injury, i.e. duty, breach, causation and harm.

Situation: Breaking china

> A physiotherapist, visiting a patient at home, knocked a piece of china off a dresser. The carer stated that it was a very valuable piece of Spode and would have to be replaced. Where does the physiotherapist stand?

Clearly the physiotherapist has a duty of care in relation to the property of the patient. However it may not be entirely her fault that the accident occurred. Was the china in a sufficiently safe place in relation to its value? Would it have been possible for a person taking care still to have knocked it? If the answers are affirmative then this may amount to contributory negligence by the patient. The employer of the physiotherapist would be vicariously liable for the loss since she was acting in the course of employment.

Where, however, property is left in the care of a person (the bailee) then, should the property be lost or damaged, the burden would be on the bailee to establish how that occurred without fault on his or her part. It should be noted that liability for loss or damage to property can be excluded if such an exclusion is reasonable (see the Unfair Contract Terms Act above).

Receipt of gifts from clients is discussed in Chapter 4 on professional conduct.

Documentation

In every area of professional practice, it is essential to ensure that comprehensive clear records are kept in the interests of patient care and also for the defence of the practitioner in the event of any dispute or complaint. In a case in 1994[49], the plaintiff claimed that, during a physiotherapy treatment session, he felt something go wrong with the lower part of his spine and alleged negligence on the part of the physiotherapist. The judge and Court of Appeal both found that he was firstly exaggerating his claims and secondly had not proved the necessary causal link. However the defendants' case was not helped by the paucity of notes of the physiotherapists and they were fortunate that this did not affect the findings of the judge. Reference should be made to Chapter 12 on record keeping.

Future developments

Weaknesses of the present system

The would-be litigant faces several difficulties set out below.

Payment into court
The defendant may pay a sum 'into court', proffering settlement of the dispute, which the plaintiff is advised is too little. The plaintiff could therefore continue with the claim but if, eventually, the judge (who will be unaware of the payment in) awards the same or less than the payment into court, then the plaintiff must meet the defendant's costs. These may exceed the amount of compensation awarded.

Lack of funds to pursue litigation
Legal aid is being phased out from personal injury litigation and the system of conditional fees is being introduced into the English judicial process. The plaintiff is able to negotiate with a solicitor payment on a 'no win – no fee' basis, i.e. if the plaintiff loses the solicitor does not charge any fees. Costs of the successful defendant would still be owing and insurance protection is proffered to meet these and other costs not covered by the agreement with the solicitor. The impact on personal injury claims in health cases is not yet clear.

Slow court procedures
Cases can take many years to come to court and be resolved. Lord Woolf in his report *Access to Justice* noted the many hindrances to speedy court processes, of which disputes between experts was one. He has recommended the introduction of a case management approach which is considered below (see also Chapter 13).

No fault liability

These considerable weaknesses in the present system of obtaining compensation for personal injury have led to suggestions that a system of 'no fault' liability should be introduced. In this system as the result of an arrangement between insurance companies, employers and the state, a compensation fund exists from which payment is made to the injured person without the need to prove that the defendant (or his employees) had been at fault. Under the present system compensation is only paid where liability on someone's part can be established and as a result, if liability is disputed through the appeal system, an award made by a lower court may even be withdrawn. This happened to Justin Jolley (see above) when the Court of Appeal decided that the Sutton Council were not, after all, legally liable to compensate him for his particular injuries which left him wheelchair bound.

The Pearson Report[50] which considered reforms in 1978 did not recommend no fault liability in the case of medical negligence, but recommended that we should on the whole retain our present system of liability by establishing fault, except in some specific circumstances (e.g. vaccine damage and for volunteers in medical research). Attempts to introduce a no fault liability system such as exists in New Zealand, Finland and Sweden have failed, but there are strong calls for its introduction.

Alternative dispute resolution (ADR)

An alternative which is being considered by the Department of Health is the introduction of alternative forms of dispute resolution such as mediation or arbitration. These have the advantage of a cheaper, speedier, resolution and there is much to recommend any system which ensures that any money paid out is to the benefit of the person who has suffered the harm, rather than to the benefit of the lawyers.

Lord Woolf's reforms of the civil justice system (see below) go a little way towards this with 'pre-action protocols' that require the parties to attempt settlement before any writ/claim form is issued.

The Woolf reforms

The present system of obtaining compensation for personal injuries is extremely unsatisfactory. It is slow, expensive, uncertain and by no means ensures that justice is done or seen to be done.

In June 1995 Lord Woolf issued an interim report on access to justice[51]. This included recommendations to change our system of obtaining compensation for personal injuries. It was followed in January 1996 by a consultation document[52] with papers covering the following issues:

- Fast track
- Housing
- Multi-party actions
- Medical negligence

- Expert evidence
- Costs.

The Final Report was published in July 1996[53].

Lord Woolf's interim report contained a new procedural framework for civil litigation of which the central feature is a new system of case management with the courts rather than the parties taking the main responsibility for the progress of cases.

The fast track paper suggested that defended cases would be allocated for the purposes of case management by the courts to one of three tracks:

- Small claims
- A new fast track with limited procedures and reduced costs
- A new multi-track (for more complex cases over a certain financial limit). However certain exceptions to the fast track were recommended and these included medical negligence cases.

The Consultation Paper on medical negligence cases considers that these should benefit from the proposed reforms on the following grounds:[54]

- More informative pleadings should help to define the real issues at an earlier stage and speed up the progress of cases.
- Case management should encourage a less adversarial approach and enable cases to settle on appropriate terms at an earlier stage.
- Extended summary judgment may help prevent unmeritorious cases being pursued or defended too long.
- Improved training and greater specialisation should help judges to identify weak cases, to narrow and determine issues and to limit the scope of evidence.
- Increased use of split trials (i.e. dealing with liability and quantum at different trials) will limit unnecessary work on quantum in cases where liability is in issue and might not be established.
- Greater emphasis on early definition of issues between experts should encourage a less adversarial approach and reduce cost and delay. (The recommendations relating to expert witnesses are discussed in Chapter 13.)

The final report from Lord Woolf was published in July 1996 and was accompanied by a draft of the general rules which will form the core of a single, simpler procedural code to apply to civil litigation in the High Court and county courts. His specific proposals on medical negligence include:

- Training health professionals in negligence claims
- The GMC and other regulatory bodies to consider the need to clarify their professional conduct responsibilities in relation to negligence actions
- Improvement of record systems to trace former staff
- The use of alternative dispute mechanisms
- A separate medical negligence list for the High Court and county courts
- Specially designated court centres outside London for handling medical negligence cases
- Reducing delays by improving arrangements for case listing
- Investigation of improved training in medical negligence for judges

- Standard tables to be used where possible to determine quantum
- Practice guidance on the new case management
- A pilot study to consider medical negligence claims below £10 000.

The NHS litigation authority

The NHS litigation authority[55] exercises functions in connection with the establishment and the administration of the scheme for meeting liabilities of health service bodies to third parties for loss, damage or injury arising out of the exercise of their functions. Guidance on NHS indemnity for clinical negligence claims has been issued by the NHS Executive[56]. Following the audit of the NHS accounts, the Head of the National Audit Office announced in 1998 that £300 million had been paid out to meet negligence claims, that a further £1 billion had been set aside and that this was unlikely to be sufficient and further liabilities could amount to a further £1 billion[57].

The Law Commission recommended changes to the present system relating to the quantifying of damages for personal injury[58] in 1996 and has suggested, amongst other recommendations, that the NHS should be able to recover the costs arising from the treatment of road traffic and other accident victims. It is estimated that this might bring in £120 million to the NHS but more radical measures will be necessary to make any serious reduction in the present costs of the NHS.

It remains to be seen if the ever increasing sums claimed in compensation for personal injuries can be met through the pooling of liability administered by the clinical negligence scheme for trusts. If not, radical changes may have to be made.

Questions and exercises

1 Explain the difference between vicarious liability and personal liability.
2 Take any situation where harm nearly occurred to a client, and work out what the client would have had to prove to obtain compensation if he had suffered an injury.
3 How would you define the reasonable standard of care in relation to any chosen treatment provided by yourself?
4 Prepare a protocol to ensure safe delegation to and supervision of a physiotherapy assistant.
5 What would you take into account in determining your liability in relation to voluntary activities?

References

1 Ian Murray 'NHS faces £2.3 billion bill for negligence payouts' *The Times* 21 July 1998, page 8 (reporting on National Audit Office NHS accounts July 1998).
2 *Donoghue* v. *Stevenson* [1932] AC 562.
3 *Home Office* v. *Dorset Yacht Co Ltd* (HL) [1970] 2 All ER 294.
4 McCord v. *Swansea City AFC Ltd* (1997) *The Times* 11 February 1997; CL 1997 3780.

4a *Capital & Countries plc* v. *Hampshire County Council* (CA) [1997] WLR 331.

5 *Bolam* v. *Friern Hospital Management Committee* [1957] 1 WLR 582.

6 *Whitehouse* v. *Jordan* [1981] 1 All ER 267.

7 *Maynard* v. *West Midlands Regional Health Authority* (HL) [1985] 1 All ER 635.

8 *Bolitho* v. *City and Hackney Health Authority* [1997] 3 WLR 1151; [1997] 4 All ER 771.

9 CSP Professional Affairs Department (1996) No. 16 (February 1996) *How to ... Set Standards.* CSP, London.

10 DoH (1997) White Paper *The New NHS – Modern, Dependable* HMSO, London.

11 Mead, J. (1998) *Evidence Based Health Care: A practical guide for therapists.* Butterworth Heinemann, London.

12 Rivett, D.A. & Milburn, P. (1997) Complications arising from spinal manipulative therapy in New Zealand. *Physiotherapy* **83** 12, 626–32.

13 *Barnett* v. *Chelsea Hospital Management Committee* [1968] 1 All ER 1068.

14 *Wilsher* v. *Essex Area Health Authority* (CA) [1986] 3 All ER 801; (HL) [1988] 1 871.

15 *Loveday* v. *Renton and another* (1998) *The Times* 31 March 1988.

16 *Best* v. *Wellcome Foundation and others* [1994] 5 Med LR 81; discussed in *Medico Legal Journal* **61** 3, 178.

17 *Jolley* v. *Sutton London Borough Council* (CA) The Times Law Report 23 June 1998.

18 *Alcock* v. *Chief Constable of South Yorkshire* (HL) [1992] 1 AC 310.

19 *Bull* v. *Wakeham* 2 February 1989 Lexis Transcript.

20 Jeremy Laurance 'Man handicapped as a baby 33 years ago wins £1.25m' *The Times* 15 November 1995, page 5.

21 *Simms* v. *Leigh Rugby Football Club Ltd* [1969] 2 All ER 923.

22 *Misell* v. *Essex County Council* (QBD) (1994) 93 LGR 108.

23 *Wells* v. *Wells*; *Thomas* v. *Brighton HA*; *Page* v. *Sheerness Steel Co Plc* (HL) [1998] 3 All ER 481.

24 *Lim Poh Choo* v. *Camden and Islington Health Authority* [1979] 1 All ER 332.

25 Chartered Society of Physiotherapy (June 1993) *Standards of Physiotherapy Practice.* CSP, London.

26 Jenkins, M., Mallett, J., O'Neill, C., McFadden, M. & Baird, H. (1994) Insights into 'practice' communication: An interactional approach. *British Journal of Occupational Therapy,* **57** 8, 297–302.

27 Tetley, M. (1994) Personal View: A SWD contra-indication Trap. *In Touch* No. 71, 40–41.

28 *AB and Others* v. *Tameside & Glossop Health Authority* [1997] 8 Med LR 91.

29 Nigel Hawkes '"Hopeless" patient overheard prognosis' *The Times* 5 April 1996.

30 CSP Professional Affairs Department (1997) No. PA 30 (July 1997) *Rationing of Physiotherapy Services.* CSP, London.

31 *Cunningham* v. *North Manchester Health Authority* (CA) [1997] 8 Med LR 135.

32 James Landale 'No-Show patients cost NHS £275 million' *The Times* 15 September 1998.

33 Williams, J. (undated) *Calculating staffing levels in physiotherapy services* PAM-PAS, Rotherham.

34 *Hereford County Council* v. *L* 4 September 1997 (QBD) Lexis Transcript.

35 *Wilsher* v. *Essex Area Health Authority* (CA) [1986] 3 All ER 801.

36 *Hedley Byrne and Co Ltd* v. *Heller and Partners Ltd* (HL) [1963] 2 All ER 575.

37 *Hedley Byrne and Co Ltd* v. *Heller and Partners Ltd* (HL) [1963] 2 All ER 575.

38 *Spring* v. *Guardian Assurance PLC and others* Times Law Report, 8 July 1994.

39 *Smolden* v. *Whitworth* (1996) *The Times* 23 April 1996; CL 1996 4534; (CA) *The Times* 18 December 1996.

40 *Cattley* v. *St John's Ambulance Brigade* (QBD) 25 November 1989 (unreported but see Griffiths, G. (1990) in: *Modern Law Review* 1990 **53** 255.)

41 *Wilsher* v. *Essex Area Health Authority* (CA) [1986] 3 All ER 801.

42   Chartered Society of Physiotherapy (1995) *Rules of Professional Conduct.* CSP, London.

43   CSP Professional Affairs Department (1996) No. PA 6 (January 1996) *When to Delegate Tasks.* CSP, London.

44   Chartered Society of Physiotherapy (1995) *Rules of Professional Conduct of the CSP: Code of Conduct of Physiotherapy Assistants.* CSP, London.

45   Saunders, E. (1998) Improving the practice of delegation in physiotherapy. *Physiotherapy* **84** 5, 207–15.

46   Blom-Cooper, E. *et al.* (1996) *The Case of Jason Mitchell: Report of the Independent Panel of Inquiry* Duckworth, London.

47   Langley, J. (1996) General or Specific Assistants. *Physiotherapy* **82** 11, 605.

48   Saunders, E. (1996) Managing Delegation to Physiotherapy Assistants: application of a Functional Analysis Model. *Physiotherapy* **82** 4, 246–52.

49   *Jago* v. *Torbay Health Authority* 23 May 1994 (CA) Lexis Transcript.

50   Lord Pearson (1978) *Royal Commission on Civil Liability and Compensation for Personal Injury* (The Pearson Report) HMSO, London.

51   Lord Woolf (June 1995) *Interim Report on Access to Justice Inquiry*, HMSO, London.

52   Lord Woolf (January 1996) *Access to Civil Justice Inquiry Consultation Paper*, HMSO, London.

53   Lord Woolf (July 1996) *Final Report Access to Justice*, HMSO, London.

54   Paragraph 13 'Medical negligence in the new system' in: Lord Woolf (July 1996) *Final Report Access to Justice*, HMSO, London.

55   *National Health Service Litigation Authority (Establishment and Constitution) Order 1995* SI No. 2800 of 1995.

56   HSG(96)48 *NHS Indemnity: Arrangements for Clinical Negligence claims in the NHS.*

57   Ian Murray 'NHS faces £2.3bn bill for negligence payouts' *The Times* 21 July 1998.

58   Law Commission (1996) *Damages for Personal Injury: medical, nursing and other expenses* HMSO, London.

Chapter 11
Health and Safety

The physiotherapist works in a potentially dangerous environment, whether in a domestic setting or in hospital therapy centres and workshops. This chapter covers the basic principles of law relating to the health and safety at work, taking examples from physiotherapy practice. The topics to be covered are as follows:

- Health and Safety at Work etc. Act 1974
- Risk assessment
- Manual handling
- Reporting risks, injuries etc.
- Occupier's liability and consumer protection
- Employment matters
- Special areas

Many of these areas are covered in the Health and Safety information manual prepared by the Industrial Relations Department of the CSP[1]. Issues relating to insurance are considered in Chapter 15.

Health and Safety at Work etc. Act 1974

Enforcement

The Health and Safety at Work etc. Act 1974 (HASAW) is enforced through the criminal courts by the Health and Safety Inspectorate which has the power to prosecute for offences under the Act and under the Regulations and which also has powers of inspection and can issue enforcement or prohibition notices. Inspectors are not liable for any economic loss suffered by the organisation as a result of their issuing a notice[2].

Since the abolition of the Crown's immunity in relation to the health and safety laws (by the National Health Service Amendment Act 1986) prosecutions and notices can be brought against the health authorities. Trusts do not enjoy any immunity from health and safety legislation. Social services departments can also be prosecuted.

Basic employer/employee duties

The basic duty on the employer is set out in Figure 11.1.

> **Figure 11.1   Duty under the HASAW.**
>
> **Section 2(1)**. It shall be the duty of every employer to ensure, so far as is reasonably practicable, the health, safety and welfare at work of all his employees.

Section 2(2) of the 1974 Act gives examples of the various duties which must be carried out but these do not detract from the width and comprehensiveness of the general duty.

The Act also places a specific responsibility upon the employee. This is shown in Figure 11.2.

> **Figure 11.2   Employer's statutory duty under section 7 of HASAW.**
>
> It shall be the duty of every employee while at work –
>
> (a)   to take reasonable care for the health and safety of himself and of other persons who may be affected by his acts or omissions at work; and
>
> (b)   as regards any duty or requirements imposed on his employer or any other person . . ., to co-operate with him so far as is necessary to enable that duty or requirement to be performed or complied with.

It is also a criminal offence for any person to interfere with health and safety measures (see Figure 11.3).

> **Figure 11.3   HASAW – section 8.**
>
> No person shall intentionally or recklessly interfere with or misuse anything provided in the interests of health, safety or welfare in pursuance of any of the relevant statutory provisions.

General health and safety duty of employer to non-employees

Under section 3 of the 1974 Act the employer has a general duty of care to persons not in his employment (see Figure 11.4).

> **Figure 11.4   HASAW – section 3.**
>
> The employer has a duty to conduct his undertaking in such a way as to ensure, so far as is reasonably practicable, that persons not in his employment who may be affected thereby are not thereby exposed to risks to their health and safety.

This duty would therefore cover patients, visitors and the general public.

The Court of Appeal has recently held[3] that the employer was not guilty of an offence under section 3 if an employee was negligent and caused harm to others, provided the employer had taken all reasonable care in laying down safe systems of work and ensuring that the employees had the necessary skill and instruction and were subject to proper supervision, with safe premises, plant and equipment. However, if a civil claim were brought, the employer would be liable to pay any compensation found to be due under the principle of vicarious liability (see glossary and Chapter 10).

Safety Representatives and Safety Committees Regulations 1977

These regulations (SRSC) brought into force the requirement in HASAW that employers should permit safety representatives appointed by the recognised trade union to inspect the workplace, get information held by the employer relating to health, safety or welfare and have paid time off for training and carrying out their functions. Each employer is required to set up a health and safety committee to consider matters relating to health and safety. Further information on the powers and responsibilities of safety representatives and the role of the committees is set out in the information manual prepared for safety representatives by the Industrial Relations Department of the CSP[4].

For those workplaces which are not covered by SRSC the Health and Safety (Consultation with Employees) Regulations 1996 require employers to consult with workers or their representatives on all matters relating to employees' health and safety.

Regulations under HASAW

New regulations came into force on 1 January 1993 as a result of European Directives. These are shown in Figure 11.5.

Figure 11.5 **Health and Safety Regulations.**

- Management of Health and Safety at Work Regulations 1992 (SI No. 2051)
- Provision and Use of Work Equipment Regulations 1992 (SI No. 2932)
- Manual Handling Operations Regulations 1992 (SI No. 2793)
- Workplace (Health, Safety and Welfare) Regulations 1992 (SI No. 3004)
- Personal Protective Equipment at Work Regulations 1992 (SI No. 2966)
- Health and Safety (Display Screen Equipment) Regulations 1992 (SI No. 2792)

Figure 11.6 shows the areas covered by these regulations relating to the management of health and safety at work.

The Management of Health and Safety at Work Regulations 1992

Of the regulations that came into force in 1993, the Management of Health and Safety at Work Regulations are the most far reaching in that they apply to all work environments and both employers and the self-employed. Figure 11.6 shows the areas covered by these Regulations.

Figure 11.6   Management of Health and Safety at Work Regulations 1992.

(1)   Commencement and interpretation
(2)   Areas exempt from the rules, i.e. sea-going ships and sea-board activities
(3)   Risk assessment
(4)   Health and safety arrangements
(5)   Health surveillance
(6)   Health and safety assistance
(7)   Serious and imminent danger and danger areas
(8)   Information for employees
(9)   Co-operation and co-ordination
(10) Persons working for outside undertakings and self-employed persons
(11) Capabilities and training
(12) Employees' duties
(13) Temporary workers and other specialist categories
(14) Exemption certificates
(15) Exclusion of liability
(16) Extension outside Great Britain
(17) Modification of the Safety Representatives and Committees Regulations

---

The Code of Practice

A Code of Practice has been approved in conjunction with these regulations[5]. This Code does not have legal force but as the preface states:

> 'Although failure to comply with any provision of this Code is not in itself an offence, that failure may be taken by a Court in criminal proceedings as proof that a person has contravened the regulation or sections of the 1974 Act to which the provision relates.'

It goes on to say:

> 'In such a case, however, it will be open to that person to satisfy a Court that he or she has complied with the regulation or section in some other way.'

but the burden of proof (see glossary) is clearly laid on the defendant (albeit at the lower civil case standard of being on a balance of probabilities), a reversal of the normal circumstances in a criminal case.

Risk assessment

Not all the provisions in the Management of Health and Safety at Work Regulations can be covered in detail in a book like this, but Regulation 3 on risk assessment will be selected to be looked at in detail.

The law

Figure 11.7 sets out the basic requirement as specified in Regulation 3(1).

Figure 11.7 **Regulation 3(1).**

Every employer shall make a suitable and sufficient assessment of –

(a) the risks to the health and safety of his employees to which they are exposed whilst they are at work; and
(b) the risks to the health and safety of persons not in his employment arising out of or in connection with the conduct by him of his undertaking,

for the purpose of identifying the measures he needs to take to comply with the requirements and prohibitions imposed upon him by or under the relevant statutory provisions.

The duty also applies to physiotherapists in private practice. Figure 11.8 sets out Regulation 3(2).

Figure 11.8 **Regulation 3(2).**

Every self-employed person shall make a suitable and sufficient assessment of –

(a) the risks to his own health and safety to which he is exposed whilst he is at work; and
(b) the risks to the health and safety of persons not in his employment arising out of or in connection with the conduct by him of his undertaking,

for the purposes of identifying the measures he needs to take to comply with the requirements and prohibitions imposed upon him by or under the relevant statutory provisions.

There is a duty under Regulation 3(3) to review the assessment when there is reason to suspect that it is no longer valid or there has been significant change in the matters to which it relates.

Where more than five people are employed there must be a record of the findings of the assessment and any group of employees identified as being especially at risk (Regulation 3(4)).

The guidance

The guidance in the Code of Practice emphasises that risk assessment must be a systematic general examination of work activity, with a recording of significant findings, rather than a reactive procedure.

Definition of risk and aims of assessment

The definition of risk includes both the likelihood that harm will occur and its severity. The aim of risk assessment is to guide the judgment of the employer or self-employed person as to the measures they ought to take to fulfil their statutory obligations laid down under HASAW and its regulations.

The key words 'suitable' and 'sufficient' are defined in the guidance as being a risk assessment that:

'(a) should identify the significant risks arising out of work . . .

(b) should enable the employer or the self-employed person to identify and prioritise the measures that need to be taken to comply with the relevant statutory provisions.

(c) should be appropriate to the nature of the work and such that it remains valid for a reasonable period of time.'

How the risk assessment is to be carried out

Figure 11.9 sets out the requirements of a valid risk assessment set out in paragraph 16 of the Code.

Figure 11.9   Requirements of valid risk assessment.

(a)   In particular a risk assessment should ensure that all relevant risks or hazards are addressed:

    (i)   the aim is to identify the significant risks in the workplace. Do not obscure those risks with an excess of information or by concentrating on trivial risks;

    (ii)   in most cases, first identify the hazards, i.e. those aspects of work (e.g. substances or equipment used, work processes or work organisation) which have the potential to harm;

    (iii)   if there are specific Acts or Regulations to be complied with, these may help to identify the hazards;

    (iv)   assess the risks from the identified hazards; if there are no hazards there are no risks . . .

    (v)   be systematic in looking at hazards and risks . . .

    (vi)   ensure all aspects of the work activity are reviewed.

(b)   address what actually happens in the workplace or during the work activity;

    (i)   actual practice may differ from the works manual . . .

    (ii)   think about the non-routine operations . . .

    (iii)   interruptions to the work activity are a frequent cause of accidents . . .

(c)   ensure that all groups of employees and others who might be affected are considered . . .

(d)   identify groups of workers who might be particularly at risk: for example young or inexperienced workers, those who work alone, any disabled staff;

(e)   take account of existing preventive or precautionary measures . . .

It may be possible for several employers engaged in the same activity to share model risk assessments.

Recording

The record should represent an effective statement of hazards and risks which then leads management to take the relevant action to protect health and safety. It should be in writing unless in computerised form and should be easily retrievable. It should include:

- the significant hazards;
- the existing control measures in place; and
- the persons who may be affected by those risks.

Preventive and protective measures
The following principles apply:

- If possible avoid the risk altogether.
- Combat risks at source rather than by palliative measures.
- Whenever possible, adapt work to the individual.
- Take advantage of technological and technical progress.
- Risk prevention measures need to form part of a coherent policy and approach having the effect of progressively reducing those risks that cannot be prevented or avoided altogether.
- Give priority to those measures which protect the whole workplace and all those who work there, and so yield the greatest benefit.
- Workers, whether employees or self-employed, need to understand what they need to do.
- The avoidance, prevention and reduction of risk at work needs to be an accepted part of the approach and attitudes at all levels of the organisation and to apply to all its activities, i.e. the existence of an active health and safety culture affecting the organisation as whole needs to be assured.

Risk management and the physiotherapist

For the most part, the physiotherapist would share common health and safety hazards with other hospital, community or social services based employees and thus models of risk assessment and management which applied to other health professionals would also apply to physiotherapy. Thus hazards relating to the safety of equipment, cross-infection risks, safe working practices or to violence at work would all apply to physiotherapists who should be involved in the system of the assessment of risk.

Moreover the nature of physiotherapy involves the physiotherapist regularly weighing risk against benefit as clients are pushed to the limits of what they can achieve in the restorative process. Each physiotherapist should therefore be able to carry out a risk assessment of health and safety hazards in relation to clients as well as for colleagues, carers and the general public.

Manual handling

Back injuries have been recognised as a major reason for sickness and staff retiring early on grounds of ill health. Whilst there are no reported cases of claims brought by physiotherapists, they are vulnerable to the possibility of back injury because of the work which they undertake in the movement of clients and the lifting of equipment. It is essential therefore that they should have a good understanding of the regulations relating to manual handling and the duties of the employer and of themselves.

Legal duties are placed upon employers in relation to manual handling by the Manual Handling Regulations and also as a result of the duty of the employer under the contract of employment to take reasonable care of the health and safety of an employee.

Manual Handling Regulations and guidance

Regulations were introduced in 1992 as a result of an EC directive (see Figure 11.5) Figure 11.10 sets out the content of the regulations. The Royal College of Nursing and the National Back Pain Association in their *Guide to the Handling of Patients*[6] point out that there are discrepancies between the EC Framework Directive[7] and the UK Regulations and that the former imposes a higher duty on employers closer to that of 'practicality' rather than 'reasonable practicability', but this issue is yet to be tested in the ECJ.

Figure 11.10   **Manual Handling Regulations 1992.**

(1)   Commencement
(2)   Interpretation
(3)   Disapplication of the Regulations
(4)   Duties of employers
     (1) (a) Avoidance of manual handling
        (b) (i)   Assessment of risk
           (ii) Reducing the risk of injury
           (iii) The load – additional information
     (2) Reviewing the assessment
(5)   Duty of employees
(6)   Exemption certificates
(7)   Extension outside Great Britain
(8)   Repeals and revocations

Schedule 1: Factors to which the employer must have regard and questions he must consider when making an assessment of manual handling operations.

The list shown in Figure 11.10 constitutes the regulations which have been enacted under HASAW. In addition guidance on manual handling is offered by the Health and Safety Executive[8]. The guidelines are not themselves the law and the booklet advises that they

> 'should not be regarded as precise recommendations. They should be applied with caution. Where doubt remains a more detailed assessment should be made.'

A working group set up by the Health and Safety Commission has produced a booklet on *Guidance on Manual Handling of Loads in the Health Services*[9]. This document is described as 'an authoritative document which will be used by health and safety inspectors in describing reliable and fully acceptable methods of achieving health and safety in the workplace.'

Part of this health services specific guidance material relates to staff working in the community.

In addition physiotherapists should be aware of the guidance issued by the Professional Affairs Department of the CSP[10]. A joint statement on manual handling has been issued by the CSP, RCN and COT[11] which aims at preventing any conflict between the different health professionals over manual handling of patients. It sets out the principles which should be followed and calls upon its members to discuss and resolve any areas of disagreement on the methods to be used in the handling of individuals or groups of patients. The professional bodies also would like to collect evidence of problems with the implementation of safer handling policies.

Content of the Regulations

The duty under the regulations can be summed up as follows:

- If reasonably practicable avoid the hazardous manual handling.
- Make a suitable and sufficient assessment of any hazardous manual handling which cannot be avoided.
- Reduce the risk of injury from this handling so far as is reasonably practicable.
- Give both general indications of risk and precise information on the weight of each load; and indicate the heaviest side of any load, where the centre of gravity is not positioned centrally.
- Review the assessment.

Avoiding the risk
By Regulation 4(1)(a) each employer *shall*

'so far as is reasonably practicable, avoid the need for his employees to undertake any manual handling operations at work which involve a risk of their being injured.'

The *Guidance* asks the question, as an example of this, whether a treatment can be brought to a patient rather than taking the patient to the treatment. It may be that in the case of physiotherapy it would be very difficult to remove the risk of injury entirely without reducing patient choice to unacceptable levels or denying the patient any therapeutic handling (see below).

Carrying out the assessment
By Regulation 4(1)(b) Each employer *shall*

'where it is not reasonably practicable to avoid the need for his employees to undertake any manual handling operations at work which involve a risk of their being injured ... make a suitable and sufficient assessment of all such manual handling operations to be undertaken by them, having regard to the factors which are specified in column 1 of Schedule 1 to these Regulations and considering the questions which are specified in the corresponding entry in column 2 of that Schedule.'

Schedule 1 is set out as shown in Figure 11.11.

Figure 11.11   Schedule 1 of Manual Handling Regulations 1992.

Factors to which the employer must have regard and questions he must consider when making an assessment of manual handling operations.

Column 1	Column 2
Factors	*Questions*
1. The tasks	e.g. do they involve holding or manipulating loads at a distance from the trunk?
2. The loads	e.g. are they: heavy; bulky or unwieldy etc.?
3. The working environment	e.g. are there space constraints preventing good posture; uneven slippery or unstable floors etc.?
4. Individual capability	Does the job require unusual strength, height etc.?
5. Other factors	e.g. is movement or posture hindered by personal protective equipment or by clothing?

Appendix 2 of the Regulations gives an example of an assessment check list:

- Section A covering the preliminary stage;
- Section B the more detailed assessment where necessary; and
- Section C identifying the remedial action which should be taken.

Taking appropriate steps to reduce the risk

By Regulation 4(1)(b)(ii), where it is not reasonably practicable to avoid manual handling operations involving a risk of employees being injured each employer *shall*

'take appropriate steps to reduce the risk of injury to those employees arising out of their undertaking any such manual handling operations to the lowest level reasonably practicable.'

For example, in carrying out the assessment of risk and deciding how to minimise the risk, it could be decided, in the circumstances of that particular case, to install a hoist. This may include the possibility of installing a hoist for a domiciliary confinement, even though only temporarily.

Situation: Oswestry Frame

A patient needs to be lifted into an Oswestry Frame but this would involve the physiotherapist in manual handling. On its own the frame would cost about £500 but if it is fitted with a mechanised hoist attachment it could cost over £3000. Can the physiotherapist refuse to use the frame if it is not fitted with a hoist?

The risk assessment in these circumstances should take account of the reasonable possibility of avoiding any manual handling. The requirement imposed by the regulations is not absolute, but rather a matter of what is reasonably practicable. All the circumstances must be taken into account. It may be possible that in some cases the patient can move into the standing frame without involving the physiotherapist in manual handling. The additional cost involved in purchasing the hoist would have to be judged against other priorities as part of the assessment.

Giving general and specific information
By Regulation 4(1)(b)(iii) where it is not practicable to avoid the need to undertake manual handling:

> 'Each employer shall ... [T]ake appropriate steps to provide any of those employees who are undertaking any such manual handling operations ..., where it is reasonably practicable to do so, precise information on:
> (aa)   the weight of each load, and
> (bb)   the heaviest side of any load whose centre of gravity is not positioned centrally.'

Review
Regulation 4(2) requires the employer to review the assessment:

> '(a)   if there is reason to suspect that it is no longer valid; or
> (b)   there has been a significant change in the manual handling operations to which it relates;
> and where as a result of any such review changes to an assessment are required, the relevant employer shall make them.'

It is in the interests of all physiotherapists to ensure that the employer is reminded when a review becomes necessary under the above provisions.

Temporary staff

The duty which is owed by the employer is owed not only to employees but also to temporary staff such as agency or bank staff who are called in to assist. All such employees are entitled to be included in the risk assessment process, since, as has been seen, the assessment must take into account the individual characteristics of each employee. Physiotherapists who are unusually small in height or not so strong as the average might require special provisions in relation to manual handling.

Physiotherapists in private practice

Independent physiotherapists are not employees and as self-employed persons would be responsible for carrying out the assessments and taking the necessary precautions for themselves and any staff whom they employ. Where they work alongside employed physiotherapists, they should ensure that the NHS Trust takes into account hazards to their health and safety and that the agreement which they have with the NHS Trust reflects this duty.

Enforcement

■ What action can be taken if the employer ignores these regulations?

The regulations are part of the health and safety provisions which form part of the criminal law. Infringement of the regulations can lead to prosecution by the Health and Safety Inspectorate. The Inspectorate has the power to issue enforcement or prohibition notices against any corporate body or individual. A health authority no longer enjoys the immunity from the criminal sanctions which it once did as a crown authority and therefore these enforcement provisions are available against it. Similarly an NHS Trust is subject to the full force of the criminal law.

■ What if the carer or client refuses to use a hoist?

If a risk management assessment for manual handling in a patient's home indicates that a hoist is necessary to prevent harm to any carer/professional, then the professional can insist that when she visits the home she will use a hoist. If the patient refuses to be placed in a hoist, she can advise the patient that the only way of safely moving her/him is by a hoist, and if the patient continues to refuse, then the patient can be told that support and assistance will not be provided if it endangers the health and safety of the professionals. She can also advise the carer on the reasons why a hoist is necessary, but of course she cannot enforce the use of the hoist by the carer. If the carer ignores the instructions, fails to use the hoist and injures her back, then there should be no liability on the staff who gave her the correct guidance.

■ What remedies exist for compensation?

Breach of the regulations can be a basis of a civil claim for compensation unless the regulations provide to the contrary. Section 47 of HASAW, however, prevents breach of certain duties under the Act being used as the basis for a claim in the civil courts. Breach of the regulations can however be the basis of a civil claim for compensation unless the regulations provide to the contrary. Nevertheless, even where what is alleged is a breach of the basic duties, a physiotherapist who suffered harm as a result of the failure of the employer to take reasonable steps to safeguard her health and safety could sue in the civil courts on the basis of the employer's duty at common law (see below).

The statutory duty to ensure the Act is implemented is paralleled by a duty at common law placed upon the employer to take reasonable steps to ensure the employee's health and safety. Contracts of employment should state clearly the duty upon the employer to take reasonable care of the employee's safety and also the employee's duty to co-operate with the employer in carrying out health and safety duties under the Act, the Regulations and at common law. It is, of course, in the long term interests of the employer to prevent back injuries thereby reducing the incidence of sickness and absenteeism and also avoiding payment of substantial compensation to his injured employees.

Training

This is essential to ensure that staff have the understanding to carry out the assessments and to advise on lifting and the appropriate equipment. Regular monitoring should take place to ensure that the training is effective and the policies for review are in place. There is also a duty on the employer to ensure that staff who are not expected to be regularly involved in manual handling are aware of the risks of so doing.

An example is a case where a social worker succeeded in a claim against the County Council that employed her[12].

Case: *Colclough* v. *Staffordshire County Council*

The plaintiff was employed as a social worker in the elderly care team. Her duties consisted largely of assessing clients for residential placement and other needs. She was called out to an elderly man's home after referral from his GP. When she arrived she gained access with a neighbour, only to find the man halfway out of his bed. He was in a very distressed state and she felt it was important for him to be lifted back into the bed as she was worried about him being injured. The neighbour, who had some nursing experience, told the social worker how to lift the man. As both of them attempted to lift the man, who weighed around 15 stone, the social worker sustained a lumbar spine injury. She sued on the grounds that the employers had failed to provide her with any training and/or instruction in lifting techniques. The employers denied liability on the ground that it was not a normal part of a social worker's duties to undertake any lifting tasks. They alleged that she should have summoned some assistance from the emergency services.

The judge held that it was reasonably foreseeable that the plaintiff would be confronted with emergency situations when working as a social worker in the elderly care team. Although the situation which arose was most unusual, the employers were under a duty to warn her that she should not lift in such circumstances. This duty did not go so far as to impose upon the employer in these circumstances a duty to provide a long training course but certainly to bring to the notice of social workers the risks of lifting. Her claim succeeded without a finding of contributory negligence (see glossary).

The implications of this decision are that even staff who are not expected to be involved in manual handling as part of their work must be trained in risk awareness in order to protect them should they ever be in the situation where they could be endangered through manual handling.

Lifting and instructing others

Physiotherapists may be asked to instruct others such as carers, clients or other health or social service employees in operations involving manual handling and compliance with the regulations. Before they instruct others they should be sure that they receive the necessary additional training to undertake the task of instruction since failure to instruct competently could in itself give rise to an action in negligence if harm should occur as a result of negligent instructions (see Chapter 10 on negligent advice). The CSP has given advice to physiotherapists who are approached to undertake instruction in patient handling[13]. The guidance emphasises

- the importance of the competence of the physiotherapists to teach manual handling,
- the necessity of ensuring that appropriate resources in terms of management support, time, venue and equipment are provided, and
- that the training should be part of a planned, ongoing and updated programme (not an *ad hoc*, one-off session).

It recommends a ratio of one tutor to six students for practical sessions and sets out the essential elements of any training programme. As in all situations where there is the potential for litigation full records should be kept and the information which the CSP recommends should be recorded is set out in Figure 11.12.

Figure 11.12 **Documentation and manual handling training.**

- the names of trainees, their qualifications and job titles
- the sessions attended by each
- the length of each session
- a full and accurate note of contents of each session
- a record and copy of any handouts
- the signature of each participant countersigned by trainer
- a note of those who failed to attend

The CSP has also given similar advice on the training for manual handling of inanimate loads[14]. It recommends that physiotherapists should pass on to management any problems which are revealed in discussions about lifting processes together with any positive suggestions for their amelioration.

Failures to instruct by agencies

Sometimes physiotherapists become aware that agency staff have not been instructed in manual handling techniques. It would be reasonable practice in this situation for the physiotherapist to ensure that senior management of the agency were informed so that steps could be taking to provide formal training for agency staff.

Therapeutic handling

It is sometimes argued that therapeutic lifting e.g. in orthopaedic wards to facilitate early mobilisation does not come under the manual handling regulations. There are however no grounds for this assertion. The definition of manual handling is:

'any transporting or supporting of a load (including the lifting, putting down, pushing, pulling, carrying or moving thereof) by hand or by bodily force.'

and this would therefore include therapeutic situations.

'No lifting policy' and therapeutic handling

The first requirement of any manual handling policy is to avoid any manual handling where it is reasonably practicable to do so. Clearly, if this were to be implemented in the therapeutic regime, patients would never get mobilised following strokes and orthopaedic or other trauma. The physiotherapist should ensure that a risk assessment is carried out which takes into account both the needs of the patient to become mobile and also dangers that staff face in promoting this mobilisation. Guidance is provided by the CSP on treatment involving manual handling[15]. It emphasises that therapeutic handling may involve the taking of calculated risks but that it is appropriate and essential if the patient's prompt progress towards optimal function is not to be impeded or stopped.

Lifting extremely heavy persons

This is of considerable concern to physiotherapists. An extremely heavy person is defined by E. Fazel[16] as 25 stone (130 kg) or over. In a case study of the problems encountered following an emergency admission, the author analyses the possible action which could be taken, including reviewing the equipment which is available. The implications for other services such as the Fire Brigade and funeral directors are considered and a protocol for the safe handling of extremely heavy patients is supplied.

The legal issues arising are significant. Staff cannot cease to provide services for such persons, but the consequences in terms of costs and effort in minimising the risk of harm are considerable.

Physiotherapists, manual handling and the courts

(See also Chapter 13 on these issues.)

Recent years have seen an increase in litigation in respect of back injuries when failures in fulfilling health and safety duties in respect of manual handling are alleged. The physiotherapist may be a witness of fact or expert witness (see Chapter 13). As a witness of fact she may have to give evidence in respect of her involvement in training the individual concerned (see above), or in carrying out a risk assessment or as a witness to the alleged incident.

The records of a physiotherapist concerning the patient who is involved in a manual handling situation may be relevant in determining the risks to any staff involved in manual handling. Thus in *Bowfield* v. *South Sefton (Merseyside) Health Authority*[17], (in respect of a manual handling incident) records taken by physiotherapists during multi-disciplinary rounds were important in determining the extent to which the plaintiff employee would have been aware of any limitations on the patient's part. (A decision in favour of the employee was overturned by the Court of Appeal.)

Reporting risks, injuries etc.

RIDDOR 1995

The Reporting of Injuries, Diseases and Dangerous Occurrences Regulations 1995 came into force on 1 April 1996 replacing earlier statutory instruments. The lists of reportable diseases and occurrences were updated. It is legally possible for reports to be made by telephone.

Encouraging others to report accidents

Situation: Failure to report

> A physiotherapist is visited by a patient for treatment and is told that the injury occurred in an accident at work. The physiotherapist asks if the patient reported it and is told that she did not. Should the physiotherapist take any action?

In the above situation, unless the physiotherapist worked with the patient or had some responsibilities for the accident, it is not the duty of the physiotherapist to report the incident. However she should make every effort to persuade the patient to report it herself, wherever it took place.

In a case heard in 1987[18] the plaintiff gave evidence that she had to go into hospital because of her back for in-patient treatment, and that the physiotherapist there asked her whether she had reported the accident and told her that she was silly not to have done so. She (i.e. the plaintiff) said of that

> 'I didn't really know who to report it to, and the physiotherapist said I'd have to go to court. I'd seen a lot of doctors who knew about the fall, none of them had ever advised me to make a claim.'

It is important that the physiotherapist should give clear information to clients about the need for them to report industrial accidents to their employers. Physiotherapists should also know to whom clients can be referred to obtain information on criminal injury compensation.

Whistle blowing

The additional protection against dismissal of employees who report health and safety hazards given by the Trade Union Reform and Employment Rights Act 1993 was consolidated in the Employment Rights Act 1996. The Public Interest Disclosure Act 1998 is intended to strengthen further protection given to employees who report health and safety hazards. This is considered in Chapter 17 on employment.

Occupier's liability and consumer protection

Occupier's Liability Act 1957

This Act places a duty of care upon the occupier (of whom there may be several) to take reasonable care of his visitors to ensure that they are safe for the purposes for which they are permitted to be on the premises. The Act is enforceable in the civil courts if harm has occurred.

Occupier

The occupier would be the person in control of the premises. This would normally be the NHS Trust in respect of hospital property and the ward sister would be acting as the agent of the occupier in respect of the safety of her ward. The Physiotherapist Manager could be deemed the occupier of the physiotherapy department. There can however be several occupiers. For example if painters employed by independent contractors come onto the premises they may also be in occupation of the premises and could be responsible for harm which occurs as a result of their lack of care.

Visitor

A visitor is a person on the premises with the express or implied consent of the occupier. In the context of hospitals the term would therefore include patients, staff, visitors, tradesmen or any one else with a *bona fide* reason to be there and who is not excluded by the occupier (see below).

The nature of the duty owed

The duty is set out in section 2(2) of the Act and Section 2(3) clarifies the duty further in relation to specific circumstances as shown in Figure 11.13.

Figure 11.13   The Occupier's Liability Act 1957 sections 2(2) and (3).

2(2) The common duty of care is a duty to take such care as in all the circumstances of the case is reasonable to see that the visitor will be reasonably safe in using the premises for the purposes for which he is invited or permitted by the occupier to be there.

2(3) The circumstances relevant for the present purpose include the degree of care, and of want of care, which would ordinarily be looked for in such a visitor, so that (for example) in proper cases –

(a)   an occupier must be prepared for children to be less careful than adults; and
(b)   an occupier may expect that a person, in the exercise of his calling, will appreciate and guard against any special risks ordinarily incident to it, so far as the occupier leaves him free to do so.

The Occupier's Liability Act 1957 and children is considered in Chapter 23.

The physiotherapist and premises in the community

Where a physiotherapist is visiting private homes, the occupier may be the owner of the house who is also in occupation, or the occupier may be a tenant. If the physiotherapist is injured on the premises it will depend upon how the injury occurred as to who would be liable: thus if she is injured as the result of a frayed rug, the person in occupation (whether tenant or owner) would be liable; if she were injured as a result of a structural defect then the owner or landlord would be liable depending upon the nature of the tenancy agreement.

The occupier has the right to ask any visitor to leave the premises. Should the visitor fail to leave, then she becomes a trespasser and the occupier can use reasonable force to evict her. If, therefore, the physiotherapist should be asked by a client or carer to leave she should go. Should she be concerned for the well being of the client, she should ensure that social services are notified so that appropriate action can be taken. Where there is a clash between carer and client and the former asks her to leave but the latter wants her to stay, the physiotherapist has to decide on the basis of the specific circumstances: the rights of the client to occupation as compared with those of the carer, and the specific needs of the client. Where the physiotherapist considers it prudent to leave the premises she must discuss with her manager how best the client's needs can be met.

The Occupier's Liability 1984

The 1957 Act does not cover the situation relating to trespassers. Until the 1984 Act was passed the law relating to the nature of the duty owed to a trespasser was according to the common law (i.e. the decisions of judges – see Chapter 2).

Whether or not a duty is owed by the occupier to trespassers, in relation to risks on the premises, depends upon the following factors set out in section 1(3) and shown in Figure 11.14.

Figure 11.4 **The Occupier's Liability Act 1984 – section 1(3).**

(a) [if the occupier] is aware of the danger or has reasonable grounds to believe that it exists;
(b) [if the occupier] knows or has reasonable grounds to believe that the other is in the vicinity of the danger concerned or that he may come into the vicinity of the danger (in either case, whether the other has lawful authority for being in that vicinity or not); and
(c) the risk is one against which, in all the circumstances of the case, [the occupier] may reasonably be expected to offer the other some protection.

In applying these factors to decide if a duty is owed to a trespasser, it would be rare for a duty to be owed to a mentally competent adult. It is, however, more likely that a duty will be owed to a child trespasser. Thus, for example, if a child on hospital premises is expressly told that he cannot go through a particular door or into another section of the hospital and he disobeys those instructions, then he becomes a trespasser for the purposes of the Occupier's Liability Acts. Although not protected by the 1957 Act, it is likely that a duty to the child would then arise under the 1984 Act depending on the child's age and understanding.

The nature of the duty owed to trespassers
Once it is held that a duty of care is owed to a trespasser, the 1984 Act by section 1(4) defines the duty as follows:

'The duty is to take such care as is reasonable in all the circumstances of the case to see that he does not suffer injury on the premises by reason of the danger concerned.'

The duty can be discharged by giving warnings, but in the case of children this may have limited effect – it would depend upon the age of the child.

The Consumer Protection Act 1987

This enables a claim to be brought where harm has occurred as a result of a defect in a product. It is a form of strict liability in that negligence by the supplier or manufacture does not have to be established. The plaintiff will however have to show that there was a defect. These issues are considered further in Chapter 15 on the law relating to equipment. See also PA 4 *Equipment Safety and Product Liability* produced by the CSP[19]. The work of the Medical Devices Agency is also relevant and is considered in detail in Chapter 15.

The Control of Substances Hazardous to Health Regulations 1994

All health workers have responsibilities under the COSHH Regulations. The physiotherapist who uses different substances in her work should be specifically alert to the need to ensure that the regulations are implemented.

The five stages of assessment set out in the *Guide* issued by the Health and Safety Executive[20] are shown in Figure 11.15.

Figure 11.15   Stages in COSHH assessment.

(1)   Gather information about the substances, the work and the working practices
(2)   Evaluate the risks to health
(3)   Decide what needs to be done
(4)   Record the assessment
(5)   Review the assessment

There must be clarity over who has the responsibility for carrying out the assessment, but the guidance emphasises the importance of involving all employees in the task.

All potentially hazardous substances must be identified. These will include domestic materials such as bleach, toilet cleaner, window cleaner, and polishes, and office materials such as correction fluids, as well as the medicinal products in the treatment room and materials and substances used in physiotherapy.

An assessment has to be made as to whether each substance could be inhaled, swallowed, absorbed or introduced through the skin, or injected into the body (as with needles). The effects of each route of entry or contact and the potential harm must then be identified. There must then be an identification of the persons who could be exposed and how.

Once this assessment is complete, decisions must be made on the necessary measures to be taken to comply with the Regulations and on who should undertake the different tasks. In certain cases, health surveillance of the employees is required if there is a reasonable likelihood that the disease or ill-effect associated with exposure will occur in the workplace or hospital environment concerned. Physiotherapists should be particularly vigilant about any substances used in their activities and cleaning fluids and ensure that a risk assessment is undertaken and its results implemented.

Mangers should ensure that the employees are given information, instruction and training. Records should show what the results of the assessment are, what action has been taken and by whom, and regular monitoring and review of the situation.

The Health and Safety Commission (HSC) has published a Consultative Document proposing new Control of Substances Hazardous to Health Regulations to replace those of 1994. The proposals are designed to provide further protection for workers, by providing a mechanism to speed up the introduction of new Maximum Exposure Limits and for approving changes to the list. Further details of the proposals can be obtained from the HSC (see list of addresses).

Employment issues

Common law duty implied in the contract of employment

Some of the terms in the contract of employment are implied by the law. These include the obligation of the employer to safeguard the health and safety of the employee by

- employing competent staff,
- setting up a safe system of work, and
- maintaining safe premises, equipment and plant.

The employee needs to obey the reasonable instructions of the employer and must take reasonable care in carrying out the work. Thus, as has been seen in the discussion on manual handling above, the employee may have a claim for breach of contract by the employer if back injuries result from failure on the employer's part in not providing appropriate training or equipment.

Statutory requirements

The employer's duty at common law to take reasonable care to safeguard the employees against the reasonable foreseeable possibility of harm arising from work related disorders is paralleled by the duties laid down in the Health and Safety at Work etc. Act 1974, and under the Regulations relating to Manual Handling (see above), the Management of Health and Safety at Work, Display Screen Equipment and the other regulations listed in Figure 11.5.

The Employer's Liability (Defective Equipment) Act 1969
Where

- the employee suffers personal injury in the course of employment as a consequence of a defect in equipment, and

- the equipment is provided by the employer for the purposes of his business, and
- the defect is attributable wholly or partly to the fault of a third party,

then the employee can recover compensation from the employer on the grounds that the injury is deemed to be also attributable to the employer. The employer can raise any contributory negligence by the employee as a defence in the action and can recover a contribution or indemnity from the third party.

The advantage of the Act is that it saves the employee from having to ascertain the identity of the third party and bringing an action directly against them.

Employers' Liability (Compulsory Insurance) Act 1969

This requires all non-crown employers to be covered by an approved policy of insurance against liability for bodily injury or disease sustained by an employee and arising out of and in course of employment. Despite the abolition of crown immunity, Schedule 8 of the NHS and Community Care Act 1990 preserves the immunity of health authorities and trusts from this Act, but local authorities are bound by it, as are private hospitals and also private practitioners who may be employers.

Effect of failure by the employer

The employer's failure to take reasonable care of the health, safety or welfare of the employee could result in the following actions by the employee:

- action for breach of contract of employment; and/or
- action for negligence, where the employee has suffered harm (the employee could also use as evidence any breach of specific health and safety regulations); and/or
- application to the industrial tribunal claiming constructive dismissal (see glossary and Chapter 17) if it can be shown that the employer is in fundamental breach of the contract of employment.

Examples of cases brought in relation to the employer's duty of care at common law are the manual handling case above and the stress case outlined below.

Special areas

Animals

A physiotherapist may be concerned with danger from dogs kept by clients and carers and needs to know what her rights are in this respect.

- Could she refuse to attend a client because there is an aggressive animal in the house?
- What are her rights if she is injured?

If a client or carer has an animal which the owner does not have under control and, as a consequence, a visiting physiotherapist is injured, then the physiotherapist may be able to claim compensation under the Occupier's Liability Act 1957 above. She would need to establish that the owner as occupier of the premises failed to take reasonable care to ensure that she was safe. The fact that it was known that the animal could be aggressive would place upon the occupier a clear duty to protect visitors from it.

Where it is known that an aggressive animal is on the premises then the owner can be warned that, unless the animal is kept under control, the physiotherapy department cannot provide a service to the client in that home. This would of course be an extreme situation, but the employer has a duty to take reasonable care of its employees and cannot therefore force the employee to enter a dangerous situation or take unreasonable risks.

Violence

Violence in the health services
Unfortunately there are more and more reports of attacks on health service employees, not just from strangers in the streets but also from carers and even clients. The rules relating to the terms of service of general practitioners enable them to arrange for the removal from their list of any patient who threatens violence to them. There have been reported cases of harm to physio and other therapists. Thus in a case in 1983[21] a voluntary patient at a mental hospital was charged with assault occasioning actual bodily harm to an occupational therapist employed at the hospital and an occupational therapist was killed by a mentally ill patient in the Edith Morgan Unit at Torbay. An inquiry was set up following this death[22] (see further Chapter 21).

The Industrial Relations Department at the CSP has prepared a *Health and Safety Briefing Pack on Violence at Work*[23] which gives practical advice to CSP safety representatives and other members. The briefing note quotes the results of a survey carried out in 1996 which covered 10% of working CSP members and shows the low numbers who feel that there are appropriate policies in place. Only 18% had training on dealing with violence and aggression; over 70% were not aware of any methods in place so that staff whereabouts are known. Extrapolating from the survey figures 20% of physiotherapists and assistants have been physically assaulted by a client, two thirds of the CSP members surveyed reported occasional face-to-face verbal aggression from clients and almost half experienced aggression over the telephone, from clients, relatives or the public.

Making statements
If a physiotherapist is involved in violence or witnesses a violent incident, she should make sure that a report and statement are completed. Thus in one case[24] where unfair dismissal was alleged two physiotherapists witnessed an assault by a member of staff, when a blow or blows were struck. They made statements to that effect (see chapter 13). A consultant who examined the victim saw no visible sign of bruising or assault except a slight red mark on the right cheek and but for the contemporaneous statements of the two physiotherapists there would have been no independent evidence of the assault.

Avoiding being a victim

Will Geddes and Mark Pepper give practice advice to physiotherapists to avoid being a victim, emphasising that awareness and avoidance are the keys to not being a victim[25]. The authors suggest that in the domiciliary situation a physiotherapist should:

- know their escape route and the layout of the house;
- know whether the front door is locked; and
- know where the keys are.

In the practice setting the authors suggest that:

- the treatment room door be kept open;
- the key be kept in the outside of the door;
- a latch lock be fitted to the outside of the door; and
- the position of the treatment couch allows easy access to the door.

Generally it is important that the physiotherapist should:

- ensure someone knows where she is;
- avoid being in confined spaces (e.g. a bathroom) with strangers;
- carry a personal alarm;
- know where there is a panic button; and
- carry a mobile phone.

Further advice is given to physiotherapists on the problems of violence and working alone by Mora[26] in various papers in *Physiotherapy*.

The employer's role

The employer has a duty to take reasonable care of the physiotherapist in relation to reasonably foreseeable violence. A risk assessment would therefore be required of this possibility and as a result any reasonable means to protect the employee should be adopted.

■ Is it possible to remove the risk altogether?

If the answer to this is 'yes' but, for example, only by stopping all home visits by physiotherapists, this would not be 'reasonably practicable' in the term of the Regulations.

■ What preventive action or protective measures can be taken?

The answer to this might include the provision of mobile phones, two way radios, and personal alarms; or, in very dangerous areas or on visits to clients who present a threat, physiotherapists going in pairs or accompanied by another person. In the institutional setting, protective measures may include more staffing, higher levels of supervision of difficult to manage patients and special security measures, such as close circuit TV monitors.

■ What reviews should be undertaken and why?

Regular reviews of any situation are necessary to ascertain if the nature of the risk has changed (e.g. is the district more violent than it was formerly assessed to be? Has the nature and condition of patients in a hospital ward deteriorated?)

and the success of any previous measures taken to prevent harm to physiotherapists. The question should be raised of whether any further measures are necessary

This type of analysis will relate not only to the physiotherapists but could be part of a wider assessment of all health professionals into which the physiotherapist could have an input.

Reference should be made to the guidance prepared by the Health and Safety Commission[27]. This gives practical advice for reducing the risk of violence in a variety of settings and emphasises the importance of commitment from highest levels of management. It was reported in October 1998[28] that North West Durham Health Care Trust are to meet the full legal costs and provide emotional and professional support for all health care staff who take court action against an assailant in cases where the Crown Prosecution Service fails to pursue the offender. It might be questioned, however, why the CPS is failing to prosecute; if the reason is the unlikelihood of securing a conviction, it may be that the health care professional would not succeed even though the standard of proof required in civil cases is lower. Perhaps more emphasis should be placed on encouraging the CPS to fulfil its function.

Monitoring potentially violent situations is essential and the physiotherapist should play her full part to bring any concerns to the attention of the management and ensure that action is taken.

Situation: Fear of violence

> A physiotherapist visited a patient in his home following a stroke. She felt threatened by his attitude but found difficulty in defining exactly the reason for her fears. Should she record her concerns?

This is a situation with which many physiotherapists could identify. The feeling of fear is almost intuitive, but the physiotherapist would have a duty to ensure that her colleagues were warned of potential dangers. She might therefore record in her notes that it may be advisable for a second person to accompany the physiotherapist for the next house call. The duty of confidentiality owed to the patient (see Chapter 8) would be subject to an exception in the public interest where a physiotherapist needed to warn colleagues about a fear of violence from a particular patient. This might give rise to something of a dilemma since the patient has access as of right to the health care notes. However in extreme cases access to this section of the notes could be withheld on the ground of the risk of causing serious harm to the patient or another (see Chapter 8).

Stress

The 'Stress Check' campaign

The extent of stress amongst therapists was shown in a survey carried out by *Therapy Weekly*. It commenced a 'Stress Check' campaign in October 1992 and attracted a massive response. Simon Crompton analysed the results in a *Stress Check* booklet[29] and showed that over half of the respondents had considered leaving work within the previous year. The factors most likely to affect respondents were:

- having too much to do;
- concern at changes in NHS/social services;
- inadequate resources; and
- interruptions.

The booklet published by *Therapy Weekly* provides a workbook which gives a guide for self-help, including an analysis of coping styles, suggestions for setting up staff support and an inventory of local and national resources for further information and advice. A charter it proposes for therapists is shown in Figure 11.16 based on the Staff Support Charter from the National Association for Staff Support. *The Stress Check* suggests ways for checking stress, covering the workload, rewards and use of time.

Figure 11.16   **Therapist's Charter.**

- Managers should plan to minimise stress and maximise support.
- All staff have a right to support, both formal and informal.
- All staff should be aware of what stresses them, and find ways of coping.
- All staff should be aware that they can contribute to a caring culture where stress can be recognised, prevented or supported.
- Every workplace needs a clear policy on stress and staff support and all staff should have a copy.
- Every workplace needs a named individual to take care of staff support.
- All staff should be aware that managers endorse their right to ask for help.
- Every workplace should ensure access to training in stress awareness and personal development.
- Every workplace should have good communications (both ways) so that all staff understand each other's goals, needs and problems.
- All staff should ensure they are genuinely consulted, fully informed and free to express their own views on management plans.

The CSP guidance
The Industrial Relations Department of the CSP has issued as part of its guidance on health and safety a briefing paper for safety representatives on stress[30]. This discusses the causes of stress at work and its effects, sets out the law which applies and gives guidance on negotiating to prevent stress.

The employer's duty in law
Concern with stress at work is now recognised as part of the employer's duty in taking reasonable care of the health and safety of the employee.

Case: *Walker* v. *Northumberland County Council*[31]

A social work manager dealing with child abuse obtained compensation when his employer failed to provide the necessary support in a stressful work situation after he returned to work following an earlier absence due to stress. The employer was not liable for the initial absence, but that put it on notice that the employee was vulnerable and its failure to provide the assistance it was acknowledged he needed was a breach of its duty to provide reasonable care for his health and safety as required under the contract of employment.

Reference should also be made to Chapter 10 on negligence, Chapter 15 on equipment issues and Chapter 16 on transport issues.

Sexual and other harassment

Balancing privacy and protection

It is essential that physiotherapists are sensitive to the dangers of sexual harassment and make every effort to avoid potentially difficult situations. On the one hand they must preserve the patient's privacy and dignity (see below) but on the other hand they must ensure that they are chaperoned in any situation which could lead to accusations of harassment or impropriety by the physiotherapist or where the physiotherapist is herself (or himself) at risk.

The standards of the CSP require the patient's privacy and dignity to be respected at all times (Standard 1) and Standard 17 requires treatment areas to provide privacy, security and comfort with curtaining/screening provided to ensure visual privacy for patients and a separate room for individual examinations, interviews or treatments of a particularly personal nature.

Situation: sexual harassment

> To his embarrassment a male physiotherapist discovered that a female patient appeared to have a 'crush' on him and sent him affectionate letters. He did not wish to appear rude to her, but found it difficult to maintain his professional distance.

In the above situation, the male physiotherapist should ask his senior to remove him from being involved in the treatment of that patient. The patient may well be upset by the move but it should be explained to her that the physiotherapist could not continue to care for her and fulfil his professional obligations.

The Prevention of Harassment Act 1997

The Prevention of Harassment Act 1997 can also provide some protection in the workplace if an individual considers that they are subject to unreasonable unwanted attention.

The Act creates the following:

- A criminal offence of harassment (section 1) which is defined as a person pursuing a course of conduct which amounts to harassment of another and which he knows or ought to know amounts to harassment of the other (the reasonable person test (see glossary) is applied).
- A civil wrong whereby a person who fears an actual or future breach of section 1 may claim compensation including damages for anxiety and financial loss.

- The right to claim an injunction (see glossary) to restrain the defendant from pursuing any conduct which amounts to harassment.
- The right to apply for a warrant for the arrest of the defendant if the injunction has not been obeyed.
- An offence of putting people in fear of violence, where a person on at least two occasions causes by his conduct another person to fear that violence will be used against them.
- Restraining orders made by the court for the purpose of protecting the victim of the offence or any other person from further conduct amounting to harassment or to fear violence.

Certain defences are permitted in the Act including that an individual is preventing or detecting crime.

Bullying at work

Guidance is provided by the Industrial Relations Department of the CSP[32] on bullying at work. It defines bullying as:

'Offensive, abusive, intimidating, malicious or insulting behaviour or abuse of power, which makes the recipient feel upset, threatened, humiliated or vulnerable, undermines their self-confidence and may cause them stress.'

It discusses the different types of bullying and its causes and quotes the case of Janet Ballantyne. In June 1996 Unison negotiated for her an out-of-court settlement of £66 000 as compensation for the stress that she had suffered as a residential social worker. Bullying issues were central to her stress and compensation was paid for the anxiety, depression and panic attacks which were caused by the style of her abusive manager. The CSP briefing note suggests ways of negotiation to prevent bullying at work. It is hoped that any member of the CSP who is reported to be a bully would be subject to professional conduct proceedings.

In another profession £100 000 was accepted in an out-of-court settlement by a teacher who alleged that he had been bullied by the head teacher and other staff, when he was teaching in a school in Pembrokeshire[33]. Dyfed County Council denied negligence. He suffered a minor breakdown in October 1996 and was returned to the same school although he had asked for a transfer. He claimed that he was isolated, ignored and subjected to a series of practical jokes. He then suffered a second nervous breakdown. It was claimed that a support plan worked out for him by the Council had not been properly implemented. The lessons for managers from this case are obvious.

Repetitive strain injury (RSI)

This conditions is also now known as Occupational Overuse Syndrome (OOS). Physiotherapists should be aware both for themselves and their clients of the legal implications of RSI. An analysis of the legal issues in RSI has been undertaken by Karen Barker[34] who discusses the dramatic increase in the reported incidence of work related upper limb disorder (WRULD).

RSI and the courts

Even though in an early case a judge was quoted out of context as declaring that repetitive strain injury had no place in medical books[35], RSI has been recognised for the purpose of compensation in health and safety cases. Thus in the case of *Bettany* v. *Royal Doulton UK Ltd*[36] the High Court found that repetitive work causing only pain with no other associated symptoms could be classed as an overuse injury caused by the plaintiff's work (although on the actual facts of the case the employers were not found to be in breach of the duty of care owed to the plaintiff – they had warned her of the dangers, had introduced a system of reporting problems and had moved her to lighter work). Likewise £40 000 was awarded by the court to a legal secretary on the grounds that she had sustained physical injury, even though there was an absence of objective clinical signs[37]. In a case in May 1998 it was reported[38] that five women workers at the Midland bank were awarded a total of £50 000 after a judge ruled that their part time jobs processing cheques at high speed were responsible for giving them RSI. This was another case of 'diffuse' RSI where the victims suffer disabling pains but no specific injuries can be diagnosed. The women said that even though part time they had to work under intense pressure processing cheques and other information into computers against strict time limits. Workers who achieved four key strokes per second earned gold stars and more payment.

Reversing the trend

A recent House of Lords decision, however, may make it more difficult to obtain compensation for RSI. On 25 June 1998 the House of Lords[39] rejected claims that a secretary who was sacked after she developed a form of repetitive strain injury should be able to sue her employers. It overruled the Court of Appeal decision that Ann Pickford should be allowed to make a claim against Imperial Chemical Industries. The Court of Appeal (reversing the High Court decision) had found that ICI was negligent in failing to warn her of the need to take breaks during her work using a word processor and gave her the right to take her case back to the High Court for an assessment of damages, which she estimated at £175 000. In a majority judgment (four to one) the House of Lords decided that ICI did not need to warn her about the dangers of repetitive strain injury because typing took up at a maximum only 75% of her workload. To impose a warning which might cause more harm than good would be undesirable since it might be counter-productive. The House of Lords also questioned whether she had proved that the pain was organic in origin. She had been sacked in 1990 after taking long periods off work because of pain in both hands. She claimed that the injury had been caused by the very large amount of typing at speed for long periods without breaks or rest periods. The House of Lords said that it could reasonably have been expected that a person of her intelligence and experience would take rest pauses without being told.

The House of Lords held that the Court of Appeal should not have overruled the findings of the High Court Judge, since he had ample evidence before him to justify his decision that in the plaintiff's case the giving of warnings was unnecessary even though typists in another department had been given warnings.

It also held that RSI as a medical term was unhelpful. It covered so many conditions that it was of no diagnostic value as a description of disease. On the other hand PDA4 (Prescribed disease A4) had a recognised place in the Department of Health and Social Security's list for the purposes of industrial injury, meaning a cramp of the hand or forearm due to repetitive movements such as those used in any occupation involving prolonged periods of handwriting or typing.

One of the lessons from this case, therefore, is that the physiotherapist should be wary of using such terms as RSI about a patient's condition unless she has clear medical evidence for it.

Physiotherapists, RSI and giving evidence

Physiotherapists may become involved in the legal situation in several ways. They may be caring for clients suffering from this disability and so be asked to be witness of fact in terms of any litigation in which the client may be involved.

Alternatively a physiotherapist may be asked to provide an independent expert opinion on an RSI case not involving one of her patients. The physiotherapist should be careful to act within the scope of her competence in giving an opinion about whether a patient is suffering from RSI. There may for example be a value in witnessing the function which was carried out by the patient within the work situation, seeing the actions which were involved, the speed, position and movements of the patient. The physiotherapist should be aware that if she gives negligent advice to a patient and the solicitor or provides a report which is inaccurate she could be liable for that negligence. (See Chapter 10 on negligent advice and Chapter 13 on giving evidence in court for discussion on this topic.)

Special equipment and research

The dangers of RSI from using a mobile telephone are pointed out by Sally Roberts[40]. The condition is known variously as 'pressure palsy' or 'mobile phone user's shoulder droop'. She considers equipment which is available to prevent the condition.

Alison Smith has reported[41] on the results of experiments (in both a laboratory and field setting) with a small number of people which show that keyboard operators tend to find working with an arm rest more comfortable than having no support. However the results are not conclusive and more research is required. She concluded that the Relax Arm may offer benefits to many OOS sufferers, but should not be distributed to sufferers without careful consideration of their individual condition.

Jeff Boyling[42] reports on recent research confirming RSI as having a pathological cause. He states that the CSP has asked for RSI to be counted among the conditions to be included in the National Service Frameworks proposed in the Government's NHS White Paper to guarantee national standards of diagnosis and treatment. Industrial records show that RSI affects 200 000 people a year, costing industry £400 million a year.

Conclusions

A risk management strategy is at the heart of any policy relating to health and safety, not just for employees but also for the clients and general public. Regular monitoring of the implementation of a risk management policy should ensure that harm is avoided and that a quality service is maintained for the public. This should be accompanied by clear, comprehensive documentation. The Health and Safety Executive in 1998 launched a discussion document[43] to reduce the numbers of employees suffering from work related ill health. The aim is to produce a strategy which is shared with other organisations and to make recommendations to the Health and Safety Commission for Great Britain. The consultation paper is being accompanied by meetings across the country.

 Questions and exercises

1 Undertake a risk assessment of your department.
2 Show the differences between the implementation of the Health and Safety at Work etc. Act by the Health and Safety Inspectorate and a case brought by an employee for compensation because of breach of the duty to care for the health and safety of an employee by the employer.
3 A physiotherapist reports that a house she visits is in a dangerous condition. What should her employer do?
4 A client complains that a hoist recently provided has broken. What actions lie against the manufacturers? (Refer also to Chapter 15 on equipment)

References

1 CSP Industrial Relations Department (undated) *Health and Safety: Safety Representatives Information Manual.* CSP, London.
2 *Harris* v. *Evans and another* (CA) The Times Law Report, 5 May 1998.
3 *R* v. *Nelson Group Services (Maintenance) Ltd* (CA) The Times Law Report, 17 September 1998.
4 CSP Industrial Relations Department (undated) *CSP Safety Representatives Information Manual.* CSP, London.
5 Health and Safety Commission (1993) *Management of Health and Safety at Work: Approved Code of Practice.* HMSO, London.
6 The Royal College of Nursing and the National Back Pain Association (1997) *Guide to the Handling of Patients,* 4th edn. NBPA with the RCN, London.
7 EC Directive 90/269/EEC (on the minimum health and safety requirements for the manual handling of loads – fourth individual directive within the meaning of Article 16(1) of Directive 89/391/EEC).
8 Health and Safety Executive (1992) *Manual Handling: Guidance on Regulations.* HMSO, London.
9 Health and Safety Commission (1992) *Guidance on Manual Handling of Loads in the Health Services.* HMSO, London.
10 CSP Professional Affairs Department (1996, 1997, 1996) No. PA 8 (November 1996) *Patient Handling Training.* No. PA 9 (April 1997) *Training for Manual Handling of Loads*; No. PA 35 (August 1996) *Treatment Involving Manual Handling.* CSP, London.
11 CSP Professional Affairs Department (1997) No. PA 41 (August 1997) *Joint Statement on Manual Handling CSP, RCN, COT.*
12 *Colclough* v. *Staffordshire County Council* June 30 1994, reported in *Current Law* No. 208 October 1994.

13 CSP Professional Affairs Department (1996) (November 1996) No. PA 8 *Patient Handling Training.* CSP, London.

14 CSP Professional Affairs Department (1997) No. PA 9 (April 1997) *Manual Handling of Inanimate Loads Training.* CSP, London.

15 CSP Professional Affairs Department (1995) No. PA 35 (August 1996) *Treatment Involving Manual Handling.* CSP, London.

16 Fazel, E. (1997) Handling of Extremely Heavy Patients. *National Back Exchange Journal* 2 April 1997, 9, 13–6.

17 *Bowfield* v. *South Sefton (Merseyside) Health Authority* (CA) 20 March 1991, Lexis Transcript.

18 *Beer* v. *London Borough of Waltham* (QBD) 16 December 1987, Lexis Transcript.

19 CSP (1995) No. PA 4 (January 1995), *Equipment Safety and Product Liability.* CSP, London.

20 Health and Safety Executive (1993) *A step by step guide to COSHH assessment* HMSO, London.

21 *R.* v. *Lincolnshire (Kesteven) Justices, ex parte Connor* (QBD) [1983] 1 All ER 901.

22 Blom-Cooper, L., Hally, H. & Murphy, E. (1995) *The Falling Shadow – One patient's mental health care 1978–1993,* Duckworth, London. (Report of an Inquiry into the death of an Occupational therapist at Edith Morgan Unit, Torbay 1995).

23 CSP Industrial Relations Department (1996) Health and Safety Briefing Pack No. 2 (September 1996) *Violence at Work.* CSP, London.

24 *South Bedfordshire Health Authority* v. *Lyle* (QBD) 12 October 1984, Lexis Transcript.

25 Geddes, W. & Pepper, M. (1994) Violence – You Don't Have To Be A Victim *In Touch* Autumn 1994, 73, 28–9.

26 Mora, K. (1994) Guidelines for Physiotherapists on Problems of violence and working alone. *Physiotherapists* **80**, 4, 236–8 and Mora, K. (1994) Harassment in the workplace. *Physiotherapy* **80**, 4. 239–43.

27 Health and Safety Commission (1997) *Violence and Aggression to Staff in Health Services.* HSE Books, London.

28 Alexandra Frean 'Funds for nurses who prosecute violent patients' *The Times,* 1 October 1998.

29 Harris, C. (ed) (1996) *Stress Check* published by *Therapy Weekly.*

30 CSP Industrial Relations Department (July 1997) *Briefing paper for safety representatives on stress.* CSP, London.

31 *Walker* v. *Northumberland County Council* (QBD) Times Law Report, 24 November 1994.

32 CSP Industrial Relations Department (1997) Health and Safety Briefing Pack No. 5 (July 1997) *Bullying At Work.* CSP, London.

33 Victoria Fletcher 'Teacher "bullied by staff" wins £100 000' *The Times,* 17 July 1998.

34 Barker, K.L. (1995) Repetitive Strain Injury: a review of the legal issues. *Physiotherapy* **81**, 2 103–6.

35 *Mughal* v. *Reuters Ltd* [1993] IRLR 571.

36 *Bettany* v. *Royal Doulton UK Ltd* reported in Health and Safety Information Bulletin (1994) Unidentifiable ULD/RSI can be occupationally caused HSIB (219) 20.

37 Jones, T. (1994) Strain gains. *Law Society Gazette* **91**, 30, 20–1.

38 Alexandra Frean 'Bank workers win claim for RSI' *The Times,* 23 May 1998.

39 *Pickford* v. *Imperial Chemical Industries Plc* (HL) The Times Law Report, 30 June 1998.

40 Roberts, S. (1996) It's good to talk – providing it doesn't affect your health *In Touch* Winter Issue 1996/7, 82, 27.

41 Smith, A. (1996) Upper Limb Disorders – Time to relax? *Physiotherapy* **82**, 1, 31–8.

42 Boyling, J. (1998) Repetitive Strain Injury – Moving ahead. *Physiotherapy* **84**, 3, 107–8.

43 Health and Safety Executive (1998) *Developing an Occupational Health Strategy for Britain*. HSE Books, London.

Chapter 12
Record Keeping

Record keeping is considered in this section because the standard of record keeping is most likely to come to the fore when litigation commences, a prosecution is initiated or a complaint is made. However it should not be ignored that the principal purpose of record keeping is to ensure the quality of care provided for the patient, to facilitate communication between professionals and maintain a record of the diagnosis, treatment and future plans for the patient. A good standard for documentation would be that if any health professional were to be called away in an emergency, his or her colleagues would be able to provide continuity of care on the basis of full comprehensive clear records. This chapter looks at the following issues:

- Principles of record keeping and standards of practice
- Transmitting records
- Storage of records and safe keeping
- Destruction of records
- Ownership and control of records
- Computerised records
- Litigation

Reference should also be made to Chapter 13 on giving evidence in court and statement writing, to Chapter 8 on confidentiality and to Chapter 9 on access by the patient and others to personal and health records.

Principles of record keeping and standards of practice

Standards

The CSP *Rules of Professional Conduct* set out the duty to ensure high standards of records keeping are maintained.

Rule 2 on the relationship with patients states that[1]:

'One of the rights every patient expects is that their medical records are full, clear and held securely. The duty of the physiotherapist, as part of their scope of practice and to comply with the patient's right, is to ensure that a full physiotherapeutic record is maintained. Details of what is required for that record is contained within the "Record Keeping Pack",[2] available from the Professional Affairs Department.'

Complementary to the *Rules*, the CSP has issued guidance on the general principles to be followed in record keeping[3], highlighting the following key features, that records should be:

- accurate,
- contemporaneous,
- legible,

- presentable,
- signed,
- dated.

There is also a guidance on computer generated records.

It should be clear from the Chapter 10 on negligence and Chapter 13 on evidence that the documentation can play a significant part in any court hearing and it is essential therefore that clear principles on the content, style, clarity, comprehensiveness and accuracy of records should be followed. Many civil cases may be contested several years after the events to which they relate and the records made at the time are therefore extremely important. Some of the basic principles are shown in Figure 12.1, taken from the NHS Training Directorate booklet *Just for the Record*.[4]

Figure 12.1 Principles of clinical record keeping.

Documents related to the central care plan should:

(1) assess and identify a patient's or client's problems/needs;
(2) plan the expected outcome and the treatment/interventions/care required to achieve it;
(3) put the planned treatment/interventions/care into practice; and
(4) evaluate the actual outcome with the expected outcomes, changing care or treatment where required.

Guidelines on actual recording

Figure 12.2 sets out some of the basic points to remember in writing the actual records.

Figure 12.2 Principles to follow in record keeping.

(1) Records should be made as soon as possible after the events which are recorded
(2) They should be accurate, comprehensive and clear
(3) They should be written legibly and be jargon-free
(4) They should avoid opinion and record the facts of what is observed
(5) They should be signed and dated by the maker
(6) They should not include abbreviations
(7) They should not be altered, unless the changes are made so that the original entry is clearly crossed out, but still readable
(8) Any change should be signed and dated

Recording non-events and 'no change'

■ What if there is no change in the care of the patient?

Physiotherapists often ask about what should be recorded when there is no change in the patient's condition and they simply continue the usual treatment. Many may write 'as above' to indicate that treatment has continued to plan. Is this sufficient? It is important that it is clear from the records what interaction there has been between patient and physiotherapist, what questions asked and what replies given and whether or not there are any changes in the patient's condition or the treatment plan. If the physiotherapist is able to follow the SOAP system of record keeping each time she sees the patient, then if the records are ever subject to scrutiny in a court case, the physiotherapist should be able to give a full explanation of the nature of her contact with the patient. It is important that a record should be made each time the physiotherapist sees the patient.

SOAP stands for 'subjective', 'objective', 'assessment', and 'plan' and covers:

- how patients are feeling,
- what they say about themselves,
- the objective examination by the physiotherapist,
- her assessment following that assessment and whether she intends to continue or to change the treatment plan.

Often there may be no change in any of these dimensions, but it is essential that the physiotherapist records the date when she saw the patient and that there was no change. Increasingly there is a tendency to interpret an absence of a record as meaning that there was no activity or interaction: 'If it's not written down, it didn't happen.' This is not in fact an inexorable rule of the courts, but clearly a witness is in a much stronger position in giving evidence if there is a comprehensive record.

Situation: No record

A baby in neonatal care suffered scarring and a foot drop possibly as the result of an intravenous drip tissuing. The parents sued the Trust and there was no record that the drip site was regularly inspected by nurses. A physiotherapist who was involved in the chest treatment and movement of the baby gave evidence that she saw no evidence that the vein had tissued, but she had not recorded that fact.

Because of the absence of recorded information it will be difficult for the staff in this case to show that appropriate care was taken of the child and that the intravenous drip was regularly inspected. In such a case the times on which the patient was seen and by whom could be very important.

The recording of the date of a treatment session may be extremely important if the patient is alleging that 'The physiotherapist only saw me twice', when the records of the physiotherapist may show far more frequent contact.

Illegibility

Several court cases have arisen as a result of illegible handwriting.

Case: *Prendergast* v. *Sam & Dee Ltd*

> The doctor prescribed amoxil (an antibiotic) for the patient which, because of bad handwriting, was misread as daonil (a drug used by diabetics) by the pharmacist. As a consequence of the wrong medication the patient suffered from severe hypoglycaemia and brain damage from oxygen shortage in the blood. The doctor was held 25% to blame and the pharmacist 75%. The latter should have been alerted to the misreading because of the dosage and the fact that the patient paid for the prescription.

More recently, in a coroner's inquest relating to the death of a woman following a routine hysterectomy, evidence was given that the junior doctor misread the consultant's prescription of 3 mg of diamorphine to be given by epidural as 30 mg[6].

Abbreviations

It is preferable if the use of abbreviations can be avoided. However realistically abbreviations and symbols can save time, but precautions must be taken to prevent mistakes. There are advantages in each NHS Trust or organisation agreeing a list of approved abbreviations with one specific meaning which can be used in that unit. A printed list of these abbreviations would then be provided in each set of records and accompany the records if they were sent to outside agencies. It could be made a disciplinary offence if abbreviations not on the approved list were used or if they were used for a different meaning. In this way the following ambiguities could be avoided:

PID   Pelvic Inflammatory Disease or Prolapsed Intervertebral Disc?

Pt.   Patient or Physiotherapist or Part Time?

CP   cerebral palsy or chartered physiotherapist?

BID   Brought in Dead or Twice?

NAD   Nothing Abnormal Discovered or Not A Drop (of urine)?

MS   Multiple Sclerosis or Mitral Stenosis?

NFR   Not For Resuscitation or Neurophysiological Facilitation of Respiration?

and so on.

All that has been said about abbreviations also applies to the use of symbols and signs and other hieroglyphics. Their use can certainly assist record keeping, especially in spinal care, but there must be a clearly approved list available for both patients and health professionals to access.

Reference should also be made to the publications of the NHS Training Authority on standards for record keeping[7]. The UKCC guidelines, *Standards for Records and Record Keeping*[8] are also of value to all health professionals.

Changing records

Records should not be altered. If the writer discovers that the wrong information was recorded, it would be possible to put a line through that information and initial this and then write the correct information. Any attempt to cover what was previously written by correction fluid or heavy blocking out will arouse suspicions. What was erroneously recorded should still be legible.

It was reported in the *Times* newspaper[9] that a casualty nurse who told the parents of a sick baby that he probably had a sniffle they should take him to the family doctor altered the notes when the baby died one hour later. She changed the words 'extremely pale' to 'quite pale' and added a pulse reading, although she had not taken his pulse. Even though an independent inquiry found that her actions probably had no bearing on the child's outcome, she faced internal disciplinary proceedings at which she was dismissed and such circumstances could also lead to professional conduct proceedings with the possibility of her being struck off the register of the UKCC.

Transmitting records

The Consumers Association in its *Health Which* April 1998 noted that in the chains of walk-in surgeries opening in stations and shopping centres GPs are failing to keep records and are not passing on relevant information to the patient's local GP[10]. Passing client information from one health professional to another who needs to know it is not a breach of confidentiality (see Chapter 8) and, indeed, failure to ensure that relevant information is passed on can amount to a negligent breach of the duty of care with foreseeable harm as a result (see Chapter 10).

If personal information is to be communicated by fax machines it is essential that care must be taken to preserve the confidentiality of the information, and that steps are taken to ensure that a designated person is appointed to receive it and that they do so straight away. In 1997 it was reported that a girl died after a fax error at hospital[11]. She suffered from giant cell hepatitis and had fallen ill on a visit to Middlesborough. Her records were faxed from her hospital in Crawley. Unfortunately they were sent to a fax machine in a locked room to which no one had access over the weekend. Doctors, unaware of her medical history, gave her an overdose of drugs.

Storage of records and safe-keeping

Records should be kept so that they are easily accessible to those who require to access them but at the same time with efficient controls to prevent unauthorised access and disclosure. The Audit Commission in its report on hospital records[12] considered that patients were being put at risk because their medical records are kept in a mess and sometimes lost. Failure to find records led to consultations being cancelled and to operations being postponed. It recommended that hospitals set up one main records library with good security.

■ What if records are lost by the physiotherapist?

It may be that the physiotherapist has records in her car, which is stolen, or they are lost between hospital departments. Clearly the failure to take reasonable care of records would be a disciplinable offence. Once the records are lost there is little which can be done to retrieve them although it may be possible to create a new patient file if parallel records are held by other departments. However such duplicate record keeping is not necessarily good practice (see below).

As a general rule records should not be left in a car. Even if the physiotherapist is visiting several patients in the community it is better for her to take all the records into each home (in a brief case so that there is no breach of confidentiality) rather than risk them being stolen in the car.

Destruction of records

Where litigation is being contemplated, reference should be made to the time limits within which action can be brought which are discussed in Chapter 10, bearing in mind the extended limitation periods that apply to children and those with a mental disability. In such circumstances, where there is a possibility of litigation, it would be extremely unwise to destroy any records.

In other circumstances records could be destroyed according to the advice given by the Department of Health[13] unless the records are so old as to amount to historical documents when the Public Records Act 1958 comes into play and legal advice should be taken.

Even though any critical time limits have been passed, most departments would prefer to transpose records onto microfilm rather than destroy them completely. However this is expensive and time consuming and might not always be justifiable. If a decision is taken that records can be destroyed it is important to prevent any breach of confidentiality during the destruction process.

Situation: Destruction on request

A physiotherapist is treating a patient who is suffering from mental illness. In one session she became very aggressive and this was noted by the physiotherapist in the records. The next session she was very apologetic and asked if the physiotherapist would delete the record of her outburst since it was so uncharacteristic and she was extremely contrite. What is the legal situation?

The physiotherapist should be very clear that the records cannot be changed. There is a statutory process by which a patient can request under the Data Protection Act 1984 and the Access to Health Records Act 1990 that records be amended if they are incorrect (see Chapter 9), but this does not apply here. Even though requested by the patient, deletion of the record would be a breach of professional practice. In July 1998 a GP who allowed a patient to destroy part of her records was found guilty of serious professional misconduct by the GMC[14]. He had allowed the patient, who was involved in acrimonious property dispute with her children, to remove a letter in which she was described as 'bad tempered' and another document referring to her drinking.

Ownership and control of records

Ownership

NHS records are owned by the Secretary of State and responsibility is delegated to the statutory health authorities. This also applies to the NHS records kept by general practitioners as part of their terms of service. Since April 1996 health authorities have been responsible for arranging the transfer of the records to a new GP where patients have indicated their wish to transfer and for collecting the records from the GP when a patient has died.

For NHS Trusts the ultimate decision on disclosure to others rests with the chief executive officer of the health authority or Trust. Thus statutes such as the Data Protection Act 1984 and Access to Health Records Act 1990 give to the holder of the records the ultimate decision making on whether access should be permitted. The holder should however consult the health professional who cared for the patient (see Chapter 9).

Records relating to private practice are owned by the health professional who made them. It can be agreed between the private practitioner and the patient before assessment and treatment commences as to what access is to be arranged and whether there should be patient held records. The patient receiving private care has the same statutory rights of access as the NHS patient (see Chapter 9).

Unified systems of record keeping

The development of a unified system of record keeping is on the agenda of many NHS trusts and community units. The aim is that all members of the multi-disciplinary team keep their patient records in the same patient folder to ensure that maximum co-operation and multi-disciplinary planning in the care of the patient takes place.

This development is to be applauded, but some physiotherapists may fear the loss of control over the records. They may also be tempted to provide an additional set of records in case the main set goes missing. The danger of this cautionary practice is that neither set may be complete or it may be assumed that there is only one set and that the fact that there are other records is not known.

The guidance provided by the CSP[15] suggests that if multi-disciplinary records comply with all the requirements stated in the guidance, including details of physiotherapy treatment, then that multi-disciplinary record will suffice as a physiotherapy record. If, however, such detail is not possible, then arrangements may need to be made to hold physiotherapy specific records that complete and complement the multi-disciplinary record. This situation arose when integrated care pathways (ICP) were applied to orthopaedic care by Pam Poole and Sue Johnson[16]. Physiotherapists found that they were keeping two sets of records. This is discussed in Chapter 20.

There is also a problem if the records kept by one discipline apparently contradict the records kept by another. Should this be the situation, the physiotherapist should not amend her records unless she knows them to be wrong. As always, any changes should be made so that the original writing is retained (i.e. correction fluid should not be used nor the original words blocked out) and any changes should be signed and dated.

Health and social services records

Difficulties have arisen over attempts to set up a unified record system which covers both health and social services records, since different statutes apply to the two in relation to access. Such differences are not insurmountable but any joint sharing of records should ensure that there are adequate controls over storage, access, confidentiality, and standards.

Client held records

Many different professionals are increasingly allowing clients to hold their own records. There are considerable therapeutic advantages in physiotherapy practice if clients are encouraged to keep their own records and so become responsible and involved in their progress.

There are some fears associated with the patient acting as custodian of the records. Fears, however, that records could be lost if the health professional ceases to be in control of the care of the records are generally unfounded. The evidence from ante-natal care with mothers holding their own records seems to indicate that they are less likely to go missing. Nevertheless such fears could lead to the setting up of a second system of record keeping at a central point. The dangers of this dual system have been considered above, that neither set might be complete and there might be inconsistencies.

There is also the fear that if records in the custody of the client go missing and litigation is commenced then the professionals will be at a disadvantage in defending themselves. The burden is, however, on the plaintiff to establish negligence on a balance of probabilities and this may be difficult to do if the documentation is missing and it is the plaintiff who is responsible for that loss.

Legal effect of lost records

If records have been deliberately destroyed and are not therefore available as evidence in court, there is a presumption summarised in the Latin tag *omnia praesumuntur contra spoliatorem*, i.e. there is a presumption against those who caused the loss[17]. Where the records are lost accidentally then the judge can determine in the light of other evidence available any inferences which are appropriate.

Computerised records

Some Trusts have made considerable progress with the computerisation of patient data and record keeping, but in other areas records are still kept in completely manual form. The Secretary of State for Health Frank Dobson announced on 24 September 1998 that there would be £1 billion investment to put all medical files on computer[18]. The initiative will take place over seven years and will enable records to be available for access on a 24 hour basis across the country and also permit patients access in their own homes. The initiative will link in an NHS website and an expansion of NHS Direct which offers the public a 24 hour telephone advice service on non-urgent health matters. £40 million is to be spent connecting GPs to the NHS Net.

Whilst the computer will avoid problems of illegibility, considerable care will still have to be taken. In August 1998 it was reported[19] that a student suffering from meningitis may have died as a result of her name being wrongly spelt on a computer. The omission of the letter 'p' in her surname, Simpkin, meant that her records could not be accessed and an inquiry found that she might have lived if vital results of blood tests, entered into the computerised records under the wrong name, had been seen by staff.

Litigation

It will be apparent from Chapter 10 on accountability and the discussion on the extended times within which an action can be brought that in many cases witnesses would be unable to remember any details of the events in issue and, in giving evidence, will be completely dependent on the records that were kept at the time. There is considerable value in staff who have been involved in litigation, disciplinary proceedings and other hearings sharing the lessons which they have learnt with their colleagues and illustrating the significant role which documentation played in their giving evidence. This topic is further discussed in Chapter 13.

Records of fact and hearsay

It is important to distinguish between what the patient says caused an injury, what symptoms the patient complains about and what the physiotherapist personally observes. Records should clearly identify where it is the patient who is providing information since this is hearsay. It does not, of course, follow that what the patient is reported as saying is factually correct. The patient may be proved wrong or, indeed, change his story. For example in one case[20] the records showed that the patient said he had had a running accident, but this was denied by the patient in court.

This does not mean that the physiotherapist should not take full notes of what the patient says as well as her own observations. In another case[21], the judge criticised the paucity of notes made by the physiotherapists, but these criticisms did not, fortunately, affect the outcome of the case.

This topic is further discussed in Chapter 13.

Legal status of records and evidential value of records

When does a record become a legal record is a question often asked; and the answer is that any record, any information however recorded, can be ordered to be produced in a court of law if it is relevant to an issue which arises in the court proceedings and if it is not privileged from disclosure. (Reference should be made to Chapter 8 on confidentiality and the powers and limitations of the court in requiring the production of witnesses and documents.)

It does *not* follow that what is contained in any records is necessarily accurate or true. It is possible for a completely fictitious account to be recorded. If, for example, the casualty nurse referred to above had not immediately written up her notes so that rather than adding to the record she had put down a totally fictitious pulse rate and written 'quite pale' in the first instance, the deception would possibly not have been discovered and the false record taken at its face value on an initial enquiry into the baby's death. Therefore, in determining the weight to be attached to the records and to determine the evidential value, the judge would listen to the makers of the records being cross-examined and in the light of that oral evidence determine how much value could be placed upon the written records.

Conclusions

The importance of high standards of record keeping cannot be over emphasised as part of the professional duty of care to the patient. If this duty is met, then the records should also provide essential evidence in the event of litigation or other court hearing or inquiry. Regular audit is essential to ensure that high standards are maintained.

 ## Questions and exercises _____

1   With some colleagues carry out an audit of the standards of record keeping amongst yourselves. Imagine that you were having to answer questions on the records in ten years time. How robust would the records be in protecting your practice?
2   What abbreviations do you consider could be usefully used in record keeping by physiotherapists? What steps would you take to ensure that there was no confusion arising from their use?
3   Consider ways in which the keeping of physiotherapy records could be made more efficient.

References

1   Chartered Society of Physiotherapy (January 1996) *Rules of Professional Conduct,* page 12. CSP, London.
2   CSP Professional Affairs Department (no date) *CSP Record Keeping Pack.* CSP, London.
3   CSP Professional Affairs (1994) No. PA 20 (November 1994) *General Principles of Record Keeping.* CSP, London.
4   NHS Training Directorate (1994) *Just for the Record: A guide to record keeping for health care professionals.* NHS Training Directorate, Bristol.
5   *Prendergast* v. *Sam & Dee Ltd* [1989] 1 Med LR 36.
6   Dominic Kennedy 'Hospital blamed in report on overdose death' *The Times,* 3 July 1996.
7   NHS Training Directorate (1994) *Just for the Record: A guide to record keeping for health care professionals* NHS Training Directorate, Bristol *and* NHS Training Directorate (1992) *Keeping the record straight.* NHS Training Directorate, Bristol.
8   UKCC (1993) *Standards for Records and Record Keeping* UKCC, London.
9   Paul Wilkinson 'Notes on dead baby altered by nurse' *The Times,* 7 November 1995.
10   Ian Murray 'Walk-in surgeries fail to keep records' *The Times,* 7 April 1998.
11   News item *The Times,* 16 December 1997.
12   Audit Commission (1995) *Setting the Records Straight: A Study of Hospital Medical Records* HMSO, London.
13   Department of Health (1989) Circular HC(89)20.

14   Peter Forster 'GP allowed patient to tamper with records' *The Times*, 7 July 1998.
15   CSP Professional Affairs Department (1994) No. PA 20 (November 1994) *General Principles of Record Keeping* CSP, London.
16   Poole, P. & Johnson, S. (1996) Integrated Care Pathways: An Orthopaedic experience. *Physiotherapy* **82**, 1, 28–30.
17   *Malhotra* v. *Dhawan* [1997] 8 Med LR 319.
18   Mark Henderson '£1bn scheme will put all medical files on computer' *The Times*, 25 September 1998.
19   Helen Johnstone 'Spelling mistake may have cost student her life' *The Times*, 28 August 1998.
20   *Peters* v. *Robinson* 27 January 1997, Lexis transcript.
21   *Jago* v. *Torbay Health Authority* (CA) 23 May 1994, Lexis transcript.

Chapter 13
Giving Evidence in Court

The increase in litigation where patients are seeking compensation for harm which has occurred makes it more likely that the physiotherapist may be called to give evidence in court on the alleged facts giving rise to the claim. In addition many physiotherapists (especially those in private practice) are developing their role as expert witnesses. This chapter covers both aspects and also looks at some of the rules of evidence and the terminology which is likely to be encountered. The following topics will be covered:

- Statement making
- Witness of fact
- Report writing
- Expert witness
- In court
- The future
- Conclusion

Statement making

Witnesses can refer to any contemporaneous records and statements in giving evidence and therefore, since it takes many years for some court hearings to take place, it is vital that comprehensive clear records have been kept and that statements are made at the earliest opportunity. If a physiotherapist is asked to prepare a statement she should ensure that she obtains advice from a senior colleague and, if possible, a lawyer. Many NHS Trusts now have solicitors who would provide assistance in the making of any statement. Her statement should be made with reference to the records which she has kept and the principles discussed in the previous chapter.

The statement should contain the elements shown in Figure 13.1.

***Figure 13.1*   Elements to include in a statement.**

- Full name, position, grade and location of maker
- Date and time the statement was made
- Date and time of the incident
- Full names of any persons involved e.g. patient, visitor, other staff
- A full and detailed description of the events which occurred
- Signature
- (Any supporting statements or documents should be attached)

The statement writer should ensure that the statement is:

- accurate
- factual
- concise
- relevant
- clear
- legible (usually typed)

Hearsay, i.e. repeating what another person has said, should be avoided. Other people could be asked to provide their own statements if they have relevant information relating to the subject. The statement maker should read it through, checking on its overall impact and whether all the relevant facts are included. A copy should be kept. Advice should be sought on its clarity and comprehensiveness and it should not be signed unless the maker is completely satisfied that it records an accurate, clear account of what took place. Many years later the statement could be used in evidence in court and it is an easy point for cross-examination (see below) if the witness is contradicting in court what she put in her statement.

Witness of fact

Any one who can give evidence on a matter relevant to an issue before the court can be summoned to appear. The only grounds for refusing to attend and give evidence are if the evidence is protected against disclosure in court by legal professional privilege or if, on grounds of national security or other public interest, a minister of state has signed a public interest immunity certificate that the information should not be disclosed. (Legal professional privilege and public interest immunity are considered in Chapter 8 on confidentiality.)

Giving evidence: the witness of fact

As a witness of fact the physiotherapist may be required to give direct evidence over a matter with which she has been involved. In giving evidence she should ensure that she keeps to the facts and does not offer an opinion. In some cases she may be asked to pronounce upon the prognosis of the client: she should not magnify the extent of the disability and the poor prognosis in order to obtain more compensation for the client. The practitioner has to ensure that her professional standards are maintained and she tells the court honestly the nature of the prognosis as she sees it. She may need guidance and training in how to withstand cross-examination. It is vital that she does not give facts which are outside her knowledge. Thus which ever party calls her as witness, she should not alter the facts or emphasis to support that party but should give her evidence according to professional standards of integrity. This is the best protection against hostile cross-examination (see below).

Physiotherapists who have not had any court experience may be surprised at the minutiae of detail which are considered in any court hearing. For example in one case[1] a physiotherapist and her senior manager were asked whether there were any steps under the traction couch as alleged by the plaintiff. In another case[2] a physiotherapist was required to give evidence of fact in a claim brought by a rugby football player against the club. He was the only person to have witnessed the accident and his failure to see any direct contact between the plaintiff's leg and a concrete post was a material fact in the judge finding against the plaintiff.

Cases other than negligence

Evidence from witnesses of fact could also be given at criminal court hearings and at civil proceedings for cases other than negligence. Thus in an action for 'passing off' the plaintiff company claimed that the defendant was marketing cushions for use in wheelchairs as though they were manufactured by the plaintiffs, a well-known producer of such cushions[3]. Evidence was given by physiotherapists that these cushions were invariably bought at the instance of and fitted by health care professionals who would not be deceived by any passing off claim. The plaintiffs therefore lost the case. A physiotherapist also gave evidence in a libel action brought by John Williams, the Welsh Rugby player[4].

Missing witnesses

Difficulties of course arise when a physiotherapist required to give evidence in court cannot be traced. Thus in a case heard in 1998[5] one of the problems was that

> 'the physiotherapist who had treated the plaintiff and whose evidence might have been relevant to the allegations of contributory negligence, had disappeared without trace at an early stage'.

If a witness is untraceable it may be possible for any statement prepared at the time to be placed before the court (although, of course, less weight will be given to it than would be the case if the witness were available to be cross-examined upon it).

Key points for witness of fact

Preparation

- Ensure that the records are available. Identify with stickers significant entries, but do not mark or staple or pin anything to the records. Read them through so that you are familiar with them.
- Try to obtain assistance from a lawyer or senior manager in preparation for

the court hearing, so that you are prepared for giving evidence in chief and answering questions under cross-examination.

- Try to visit the court in advance to familiarise yourself with its location, car-parking, toilet facilities etc.

At the court before the hearing

- Be prepared for a long wait and take work to do or something to occupy yourself with.
- Dress appropriately and comfortably but not too casually.
- Try to relax.

Giving evidence

- Keep calm.
- Give answers clearly and without exaggeration.
- Tell the truth.
- Do not feel that you are there to represent only one side; you must answer the questions honestly even though it might put the side cross-examining you in a good light.
- Take time over your answers and do not make up replies if you are unable to answer the question raised.
- Do not answer back or allow yourself to be flustered during the cross-examination.
- If you do not understand any legal jargon which is used, ask for an explanation.
- Keep to the facts and do not express an opinion.
- Ask for time to refer to the records if this is necessary.

Report writing

Expert witnesses will normally be asked to prepare a report by a solicitor representing one of the parties to the case. This report is vital since, if it is unfavourable to the party seeking it, the outcome may be that the case is settled or even withdrawn. On the other hand, if a party proceeds on the basis of a report that paints too rosy a picture of the case and where the expert witness fails to justify it under cross-examination, that party could lose the case or be awarded less compensation than had previously been offered in settlement and be heavily penalised in having to pay the other side's legal costs as well as their own.

Principles to be followed in report writing

- Identify the purpose of the report (likely readership and the kind of language which can be used) and therefore the appropriate style to be used.
- Identify the main areas to be included.
- Decide the order to be followed: sometimes chronological order is appropriate, at other times subject order may be preferable.
- Identify the different kinds of information used in the report and state the source of the material, e.g.

- ○ hearsay evidence
- ○ factual evidence observed or heard by the author of the report
- ○ evidence of opinion of another person
- ○ statements by others
- ○ similar fact evidence.
- Sign and date it but only after reading it through and being 100% satisfied with it.

Common mistakes in report writing

- Lack of clarity
- Too complex a style for reader
- Use of inappropriate jargon
- Use of misleading abbreviations
  - ○ Inconsistency
  - ○ Ambiguities
- Inaccuracies
  - ○ Lack of dates within the report
  - ○ Wrong names included
- Failure to follow a logical order
  - ○ Confusing account
  - ○ Mix of evidence and sources
  - ○ Opinion without facts
- Failure to cite facts to support statements
- Failure to give conclusions
- Failure to base conclusions on the evidence
- Lack of signature and/or date
- Failure to ask someone else to read it through.

Good report writing

For most purposes the style likely to be of greatest use is one of simplicity – with short sentences, clear paragraphing and sub-paragraphing, and avoidance of jargon and meaningless clichés. The report should begin with the statement as to its purpose, the person(s) to whom it is addressed, and the name and status of the writer. If it is confidential this should be highlighted at the beginning. Other documents which are relevant should be carefully referenced.

The CSP advice

Advice is given by the Professional Affairs Department of the CSP on reports for legal purposes[6]. This sets out a list of the routine requests from solicitors to physiotherapists and suggests that any report should follow the model of:

- history
- examination
- prognosis
- conclusion.

The CSP suggests that the points set out in Figure 13.2 should be remembered in report preparation.

Figure 13.2   CSP advice on report preparation.

- do not give an opinion on the cause of an injury, unless the physiotherapist was an eye witness
- distinguish between facts and opinions
- avoid abbreviations which may be misleading
- use a formal style and avoid 'purple prose'
- phrase the prognosis carefully and leave room for a re-statement at a later date
- be specific about suitability for work, describing the specific activities rather than a role
- sign the report as a Chartered Physiotherapist.

Advice on writing case reports is also given by an American author Irene McEwen[7].

■ How binding is a report written by a CP?

Every care must be taken to ensure that a report is written carefully. A person who has relied upon the accuracy of a negligently written report to his detriment would have a prima facie case against the writer of the report. Where a report has been written by an expert witness for a party to litigation, then the expert witness would be cross-examined on that report and any inadequacies, ambiguities and other weaknesses brought out. At this stage it is extremely embarrassing for the expert to wish to change the report, unless of course other evidence emerges which was not available at the time the report was written.

Expert witness

The skills of physiotherapists in assessment mean that their evidence is relevant in a wide variety of court and tribunal hearings as expert witnesses. An expert witness is invited to give evidence of opinion on any issue which is subject to dispute. It might be what would be the appropriate standards of care which would have been expected according to the Bolam test (see Chapter 10). It may be an opinion on the prognosis of the patient or the costs required to support a disabled patient, where the amount of compensation is disputed.

Reports and privilege

At present where an expert has prepared a report for a solicitor in anticipation or in the course of litigation, that report and any correspondence connected with it are protected by legal professional privilege and it cannot be ordered to be disclosed in court or the expert compelled to appear by the other side. However once the report is disclosed to the court it loses its professional privilege although this continues to attach to any correspondence between the parties which has not been disclosed. For example an expert may prepare a report on request but in the covering letter advise the solicitor that his client is likely to lose the case. Even if the solicitors do decide to disclose the report, the letter remains privileged.

Impartiality and professional integrity

An expert witness should not change her views according to the side which calls her. She may be asked to edit her report to make it more favourable to the side asking for her opinion. She should only agree to any amendments if she is satisfied that the changed report accurately represents her opinion and she is able to support it under cross-examination by oral evidence in court.

One useful rule for the practitioner to follow is to give an honest reasoned opinion whichever side calls her. She must not be partisan, nor should she exaggerate or belittle the amount of compensation. If she always gives an honest and professional view, she will be respected by the solicitors who will know that they will be able to trust her to withstand cross-examination as an expert witness and will know her to be reliable. She will not see the court battle personally as involving her and thus, whichever side wins, she will be able to feel that she has given an honest report to the court. A carefully prepared report, well substantiated, can reduce the length of a court hearing and enable many matters to be agreed by the parties, thus avoiding court time.

Duty of expert witness to the court

In a reported case[8] the court held that the expert witness had a responsibility to approach the task of giving evidence seriously and an expert should not be surprised if the court expressed strong disapproval if that was not done. In this case the expert in his report had stated that 'as far as I am aware no other previous seal manufacturer had used such a system'. In fact it became apparent not only that that system was used by others in the trade, but that the witness neither knew what systems were used by such others nor had made any effort to find out. More recently the House of Lords in the *Bolitho* case[9] has emphasised that expert witnesses must be able to show that the body of opinion which they are supporting has a logical basis (see Chapter 10).

The lesson from this is that an expert must not express an opinion unless it is clearly based on fact and where possible on established authorities or research.

A further lesson is that the expert should know and keep within her field of competence.

Case: *Miles* v. *Cain*[10]

Mrs Penelope Robinson, from the professional affairs department at the Chartered Society of Physiotherapy, gave evidence about the treatments provided and the extent to which the removal of clothes would have been necessitated.

In this case where the plaintiff was suing an unregistered physiotherapist for assault.

The judge commented:

'I accept her evidence. She was obviously being truthful and trying to help the court.'

Conflicting expert evidence

What is the situation if there is a clash between the evidence given by different expert witnesses, who both purport to speak on behalf of a body of competent professional opinion. This was the situation which arose in the *Maynard* case[11] which is mentioned in Chapter 10. The House of Lords held that where both sides were supported by equally competent professional opinion, then the plaintiff had not established the case.

Clearly there are advantages for experts to agree on the basic principles. Thus in one case[12] physiotherapy witnesses from the opposing sides, described by the judge as 'two impressive physiotherapists', agreed on the proposals for physiotherapy that the plaintiff would require in the future. In contrast in a case in 1995[13] the two expert physiotherapists disagreed over the approach (the extent to which a physiotherapist was required rather than others providing physiotherapy under guidance) and also over the extent to which existing physiotherapy treatment was sufficient for the child's needs.

The judge does not have to accept the evidence of any expert. Thus in *Miles* v. *Cain* described above (where an unregistered physiotherapist was sued for assault by a patient) two psychiatrists gave expert evidence as to whether the girl was telling the truth or not about the alleged trauma. The judge stated that the doctor for the plaintiff was

'unimpressive because I do not think he has sufficiently studied his brief . . . In my judgment it would be unsafe to utilise Dr Connell's views in formulating a judgment on the main issue as to whether the plaintiff is a liar or is fantasising.'

Of the other expert psychiatrist, the judge said 'I reject Dr Silverman also, distinguished though he is'.

It is essential that any expert opinion can be substantiated by the facts. In the light of the House of Lords ruling in the *Bolitho* case (see above and Chapter 10) judges are likely to look even more critically at the opinion of experts to ensure that it logically follows from the facts.

Lord Woolf's proposals to streamline expert evidence are discussed below.

Opinions on quantum

As well as being required to give evidence on how the standards of care which were provided matched up with the reasonable standard which could have been expected, experts may also be required to give evidence on quantum, i.e. the amount of compensation which the plaintiff is seeking. The expert must have clear factual evidence as to how she arrives at her estimate of needs of the patient and the cost of meeting these. For example in one case[14] a physiotherapist, Allison Sterling, was called to give evidence on the mobility problems of a client and stated that she had observed the patient using a walking frame, but 'when she pulls herself to her feet using the frame she is at risk of toppling backwards or sideways unless the frame is positioned in exactly the right position or if she fails to pull up strongly enough.'

The judge decided in the light of this and other evidence that an electric wheelchair was required for outdoor use and included the cost of such a chair in the compensation awarded.

Exaggerated claims

Some physiotherapists find that clients place considerable pressure upon them to make assessments in their favour since a considerable sum of compensation may be dependent upon the outcome.

Situation: Exaggerated claims

A physiotherapist was asked to assess a client for the purposes of quantifying the compensation payable in a road traffic case. The physiotherapist formed the view that the client was exaggerating his symptoms and that he in fact had far greater movement than he was admitting to. She noticed in particular that he was able to bend down and pick up his tea cup and saucer from the floor as they spoke. She included this fact in her report and received an extremely abusive reply from the client contradicting her.

In such a situation the physiotherapist has a professional responsibility to undertake an honest and thorough assessment and should not omit aspects of her findings even though these might be unwelcome to the client. It might help if she points out at the time some of those features which she observes which the client might later disagree with. The client might not be aware that her observations of his mobility are of greater importance than what he himself says about it, particularly where the client appears to be exaggerating his symptoms.

CSP guidelines

The CSP has laid down guidelines and criteria for the role of expert witness and has suggested that an expert, representing the profession by giving evidence as an expert, should:

- have been working within the specialty concerned for five years
- should be a Senior I or higher
- should have credibility with peers
- should have published something
- should have carried out a research project.

The CSP has a list of expert witnesses for each specialty and geographical area.

Points to remember

The expert witness:

- Does not take sides
- Outlines his/her professional credentials (status, experience, appointments and academic qualifications)

- Gives a professional, not personal, opinion
- Understands on what issues and topics he or she has expertise
- Provides a logical report (see above)
- Always supports opinion with fact
- Avoids confusing technical language and jargon
- Avoids being verbose
- Gives concrete understandable examples and uses everyday analogies
- Keeps facts and opinions relevant to the issues before the court
- Ensures that he or she understands the purposes of the proceedings
- Dates and signs the report.

Dos and don'ts of the expert witness

- Do find out where the court is and turn up
- Do make sure that the case has not been adjourned before travelling
- Do not stand on your dignity
- Do be acquainted with court procedure and the role of the judge, jury and counsel
- Do know how to address the judge and others
- Do dress appropriately
- Do not get emotional or forget what to say
- Do know your report and the facts contained in it
- Do not deviate from the report or introduce new material
- Do believe what you have written and what you are saying
- Do be dispassionate about the outcome
- Do not take an adversarial stance
- Do prepare for cross-examination
- Do remain calm under cross-examination
- Do not exaggerate
- Do keep to the facts
- Do not try to hasten the case along
- Do not try to be humorous.

Importance of records and other documentary evidence

Inevitably the value of a physiotherapist as a witness will depend significantly upon the clarity and comprehensiveness of any records which she kept and/or any statement she prepared at the time. Documentary evidence may include reports from pathology, X-rays, and any other relevant information, in whatever form it is held. All this information would have been disclosed to the other side during the process known as 'discovery of documents'. It is important that this discovery has been carried out properly. In one case[15] Frank Cunningham brought a case against North Manchester HA alleging lack of care by medical staff as a result of which he lost his leg, following a motorcycle accident. A retrial was ordered when it was discovered that the plaintiff's expert had only had access to miniaturised copies of the original X-rays and arteriograms, whereas the defendants' experts had seen the originals. Mr Cunningham subsequently accepted an offer of £325 000. He was a litigant in person.

In court

Cross-examination

This is the term applied to the opportunity of the one side, **A**, to question the witnesses called by the other side, **B** (and *vice versa*). In the adversarial system (see Chapter 2) which is the basis of English court procedure each witness of fact or expert witness is subjected to detailed questioning on the oral evidence they have just given by the lawyers acting on behalf of the opposing side. Through this process, if the legal representatives are competent and the case adequately prepared so the barrister knows what questions to ask, it is usually possible for the true facts of a matter to be brought out before the court for the judge or jury to decide.

This is particularly important if plaintiffs are bringing false or exaggerated claims. In *Jago* v. *Torbay Health Authority*[16] the judge ruled against the plaintiff (who was claiming compensation on the grounds that physiotherapy had been negligently undertaken), finding that he was guilty of self-deception, dishonesty and an element of fraud in what he said he could do and what he actually could do (neighbours had given evidence about his standing on a ladder and cutting a hedge). Both the plaintiff and the neighbours would have been subject to cross-examination and from this the judge could decide who to believe.

It is for this reason that appeal courts almost never overturn the findings of fact made by first instance judges, since they are the ones who have had the benefit of assessing the demeanour of witnesses when giving evidence and under cross-examination which the appeal court has not.

There are two distinct objectives in cross-examination. The one is to discredit the witness or show that his or her evidence is irrelevant to the point being established. The other is to use this witness to strengthen the case of one's own side.

In pursuing the first aim, the cross-examiner will attempt to:

* undermine the confidence of the witness;
* show up inconsistencies and/or ambiguities in the evidence;
* show how the evidence being given is contradicted by other witnesses;
* show how the witness is unreliable and/or unintelligent.

In pursuing the second aim, the cross-examiner will attempt to ensure that the witness (for side **A**):

* gives evidence helpful to side **B**;
* praises side **B**;
* corroborates evidence being given by side **B**.

Attempts may also be made to use the witness to testify on professional/expert matters and express opinions useful to the other side.

Preparation and an unshakeable conviction in the accuracy of your evidence is essential to be able to handle cross-examination and most physiotherapists would now be able to obtain expert advice from the solicitors acting for their NHS Trust before attending court on behalf of the employer.

Procedure

The stages which are followed in criminal courts and civil courts are shown in Chapter 2 on the legal system. Lord Woolf is currently reviewing the system for obtaining compensation in civil litigation and his recommendations are discussed in Chapter 10. His recommendations on the use of expert witnesses are considered below.

Rules of evidence

This is a complex area and the rules depend upon the nature of the court hearing. For example hearsay evidence (where a witness gives evidence about what was reported to him or her by an eye witness and of which he or she has no direct evidence) may be acceptable in some hearings, e.g. social security tribunals but not acceptable in civil or criminal hearings except in very specific circumstances.

Some of the issues which are covered by the rules include:

- rules on relevance, admissibility and hearsay
- weight of evidence
- burden of proof
- degrees (standard) of proof
- presumptions
- judicial notice
- competence of witness
- compellability of witness
- corroboration
- doctrine of privilege (see Chapter 8)

It is not possible in a work of this kind to give full details of the significance of the rules of evidence on the above topics and reference must be made to one of the specialist books listed for further reading.

The future

Following an interim report and a consultation paper[17], Lord Woolf published a final report, *Access to Justice*, in July 1996[18]. This is discussed in Chapter 10. One of the consultation papers related to the use of expert evidence. Lord Woolf considered that the uncontrolled adversarial nature of the present system of civil litigation was the main cause of excessive cost, delay and complexity. He therefore recommended a new system in which the courts would have an active role in case management, including control over the use of expert evidence. He recommended a fast track for cases below a certain financial limit where experts would normally be jointly appointed by the parties and would not be required to give oral evidence in court. Cases above this limit would be allocated to a multi-track, in which the court would have wide powers to define the scope of expert evidence and prescribe the way in which experts should be used in particular cases.

His proposals include the following:

- appointment of court experts and expert assessors;
- a clearer role for experts and guidance which emphasises their independence and their duty to the courts;
- appropriate choice and use of experts; and
- better arrangements for expert evidence at trial.

In his final report, *Access to Justice*, Lord Woolf stated that as a general principle single experts should be used. However, for medical negligence cases he had been advised by the Medical Negligence Working Group that there was no scope for the joint appointment of liability experts, except perhaps in the smallest and most straightforward cases. Lord Woolf regretted the polarisation of experts which so frequently took place and suggested that if joint instruction of experts was impossible, then it must be a prime objective to identify areas of agreement and disagreement between the experts as early as possible in the case.

In 1998 the Secretary of State for Health wrote to a wide range of organisations to invite their views on how to stop unnecessary litigation. The responses are to be used to formulate a strategy to tackle the increasing number of cases being brought against the NHS and the huge cost of meeting medical negligence claims[19].

Conclusion

There are considerable fears about giving evidence in court and it is vital that any witness, whether expert or witness of fact, should be properly prepared for the occasion. Even though they are not on trial themselves, their professional standing and integrity is being put to the test and it is therefore essential, that they follow the highest standard of professional practice.

 Questions and exercises _____

1 You have been asked to appear as a witness in a case. Draw up a list of your fears and try to work out ways in which these fears could be resolved.
2 Try to attend a court hearing and analyse the way in which it operates, the procedure followed and the actions of judge, jury (if present), barristers, solicitors, court clerk, court usher, witness, and any other person taking part in the court proceedings.
3 Prepare a protocol for the preparation of a report as an expert witness.

References

1 *McMenamin* v. *Lambeth Southwark and Lewisham Area Health Authority* (QBD) 28 October 1982, Lexis transcript.
2 *Simms* v. *Leigh Rugby Football Club Ltd* [1969] 2 All ER 923.
3 *Hodgkinson and Corby Ltd and Another* v. *Wards Mobility Services Ltd* [1994] 1 WLR 1564.
4 *Williams* v. *Reason and others* [1988] 1 WLR 96.

5   *Berry* v. *Calderdale Health Authority* (CA) 16 February 1998, Lexis transcript.
6   CSP Professional Affairs Department (1994) No. PA 1 (November 1994) *Reports for Legal Purpose*. CSP, London.
7   McEwen, I. (1996) *Writing Case Reports: A How-to Manual for Clinicians* published by the American Physical Therapy Association, Virginia USA (reviewed by Anne Parry in *Physiotherapy* **84**, 3, 150).
8   *Autospin (Oil Seals) Ltd* v. *Beehive Spinning (A firm)* The Times Law Report, 9 August 1995.
9   *Bolitho* v. *City and Hackney Health Authority* [1997] 3 WLR 1151; [1997] 4 All ER 771.
10 *Miles* v. *Cain* 25 November 1988, Lexis transcript.
11 *Maynard* v. *West Midlands Regional Health Authority* [1985] 1 All ER 635.
12 *Simpson* v. *South East Hampshire Health Authority* (QBD) 16 July 1997, Lexis transcript.
13 *Stephens* v. *Doncaster Health Authority* (QBD) 16 June 1995, Lexis transcript.
14 *Havenhand* v. *Jeffrey* (QBD) 6 December 1996, Lexis transcript.
15 *Cunningham* v. *North Manchester Health Authority* (CA) [1997] 8 Med LR 135.
16 *Jago* v. *Torbay Health Authority* (CA) 23 May 1994, Lexis transcript.
17 Lord Woolf (June 1995 and January 1996) *Access to Civil Justice Inquiry Interim Report* and *Consultation Paper* HMSO, London.
18 Lord Woolf (July 1996) *Access to Justice Final Report* HMSO, London.
19 Ian Murray 'NHS faces £2.3bn bill for negligence payouts' *The Times* 21 July 1998.

Chapter 14
Handling Complaints

An efficient system for hearing representations from the client about the services is one of the main ways in which the government saw the enforcement of the statutory duties under the community care legislation. In addition the Hospital Complaints Act 1985 sought to ensure that in each hospital there was an effective procedure for dealing with complaints by patients and their representatives. The recommendations of the Wilson Committee for dealing with hospital and primary care complaints were implemented in 1996 with the establishment of the complaints procedure which is discussed below. There are no plans at present to review the complaints procedures for Local Authorities or to integrate them within the health service system implemented post Wilson.

This chapter covers the following topics:

- Complaints relating to hospital and community health services
- The 1996 complaints procedure
- Complaints relating to local authority community services
- Complaints and the private sector
- The role of the Ombudsmen
- Other quality assurance methods
- Future developments

Complaints relating to hospital and community health services

There is a statutory duty under the Hospital Complaints Act 1985 for each health authority to establish a complaints procedure. Guidance requires authorities to establish a procedure in relation to community health services as well.

In addition, as part of the Patient's Charter initiative, local charters covering the handling of complaints are also required of providers. Such requirements may be included in the NHS agreement between health authority purchasers and providers.

The CSP has issued guidance on the NHS complaints procedure[1]. It gives the background to the new procedure, sets out the key policy objectives of the Department of Health, and looks at the main features of the new regulations. The CSP itself welcomes the new procedures and states its intention to monitor them.

Following the review committee chaired by Professor Alan Wilson into the handling of hospital complaints a consultation document was published[2]. The Department of Health accepted the principal recommendations of the Wilson Report and has published guidance for its implementation by NHS Trusts and health service authorities.

Wilson Report

The system for dealing with complaints relating to health services was seen to be confusing, bureaucratic, slow and inefficient. The report reviewed the current situation and set objectives for any effective complaints system. The principles it identified are set out in Figure 14.1.

Figure 14.1 **Principles of an effective complaints system.**

(1) Responsiveness
(2) Quality enhancement
(3) Cost effectiveness
(4) Accessibility
(5) Impartiality
(6) Simplicity
(7) Speed
(8) Confidentiality
(9) Accountability.

The report recommended that these principles should be incorporated into an NHS complaints system.

The areas covered by its recommendations are shown in Figure 14.2.

Figure 14.2 **Recommendations of the Wilson report on the review of complaints procedures.**

(1) There should be a common system for all NHS complaints
(2) The complaints procedure should not be concerned with disciplining staff
(3) Staff should be empowered to deal with complaints informally
(4) There should be training of staff
(5) Support should be provided for complainants and respondents
(6) The degree of investigation should relate to the complainant's required degree of response
(7) Conciliation should be made more widely available
(8) Time limits should be set
(9) Deadlines should be set for:
    (a) the acknowledging of complaints (two working days)
    (b) the response to the complaint (three weeks)
    (c) further action and response (two weeks)
(10) Confidentiality should be preserved and complaints filed separately
(11) There should be a system for recording and monitoring
(12) Impartial lay people should take part in the system

Continued

Figure 14.2 **Continued.**

(13) Key aspects of the system should be set by the Department of Health but detailed implementation and operation should be left to individual organisations

(14) Threefold procedures:
stage 1 – immediate first line response
stage 2 – investigation/conciliation
stage 3 – action by FHSA (now HA) officer or chief executive officer for Trusts. A panel should be set up to consider those complaints which cannot be resolved in the earlier stages.

(15) There should be training in communication skills

(16) Oral and written complaints should be treated with the same sensitive treatment

(17) Community service staff should have particular training in responding to complaints

(18) Purchasers should specify complaints requirements in their contracts with non-NHS providers

(19) Complaints about policy decisions should be referred to the Health Service Commissioner if they cannot be resolved locally by the purchasers

(20) Where more than one organisation is involved it should be the organisation which receives the complaint which makes sure that a full response is sent

(21) Community care – there should be close liaison with local authorities and the Government should consider further integration of NHS and local authority complaints procedures

(22) Stage 2 procedures – there should be a screening officer

(23) The jurisdiction of the HSC should be extended to GPs and the operation of the FHSA service committees

(24) Recommendations on implementation.

The 1996 complaints procedure

This came into effect on 1 April 1996 and implements the majority of recommendations contained in the Wilson Report. Three stages are recognised.

First stage – local resolution

The complaint should be dealt with speedily and often an oral response will suffice. Where investigation or conciliation is required an initial response should be made within two working days and a final response within four weeks. Chief executives should personally approve and sign the response to all formal complaints. In family health services, practices will be expected and encouraged to set up their own practice based complaints procedure.

Second stage – independent review

Consideration of an application for independent review
If complainants remain dissatisfied after the first stage, they can apply for further consideration by an independent panel. This request will be considered by a non-

executive director of the Trust or health authority to which the complaint was made. This non-executive director will be known as 'the convenor' and will have the decision as to whether the complaint should be referred to an independent review panel. The circumstances in which it is not recommended that there should be an independent review are shown in Figure 14.3.

Figure 14.3 **Situations where there will be no independent review.**

- Where legal proceedings have commenced or there is an explicit indication by the complainant of the intention to make a legal claim against:
  ○ a Trust or health service authority; or
  ○ one of their employees;
  ○ or against a family health services practitioner.

- It is considered that the Trust/health authority has already taken all practicable action and therefore establishing a panel would add no further value to the process. However, consideration of the cost of instituting an independent review is not an appropriate reason for refusing to proceed.

- Further action as part of local resolution is still believed to be appropriate and practicable – for example conciliation – so that referral back to the chief executive is considered preferable to instituting the independent review process.

Where the convenor refuses to refer the complaint for independent review, the complainant must be informed of his right to complain to the Ombudsman.

Independent review panels

All panels have an independent lay chairman. The convenor, who may or may not be the same one who referred the case, (i.e. a non-executive director of the Trust or health authority) is also a member.

- For non-clinical complaints, the panel comprises a non-executive director of the relevant health authority or, where appropriate, a GP fundholder.
- For family health service complaints, the panel comprises, the convening health authority non-executive director and an independent lay person.
- For clinical complaints, the panel is advised by two independent clinical assessors following advice from the relevant professional bodies.

The panel is established as a committee of the Trust/health authority and the assessors are appointed by the Trust/health authority to advise the panel.

Third stage – Health Service Commissioner (HSC) (Ombudsman)

The final option for unresolved complaints will be recourse to the Ombudsman. Legislation which came into force on 1 April 1996 widened his jurisdiction to cover complaints relating to the exercise of clinical judgement and those about family practitioners. Disciplinary matters, however, are still not included in his jurisdiction. (The role of the HSC is considered in more detail below.)

Time limits

The time limit for making a complaint is six months from the event giving rise to the complaint; or six months from the complainant becoming aware of the cause for complaint up to a maximum of one year after the cause for complaint arose. There is a discretion to extend this time limit where it would be unreasonable in the circumstances of a particular case for the complaint to have been made earlier and where it is still possible to investigate the facts of the case.

Complaints within the family health services

As can be seen, these are brought within the common complaints system. Disciplinary procedures are kept separate from the complaints system.

Complaints and Community Health Councils

Community Health Councils have a significant role to play in both the representation of their community at large and also in facilitating any complaint by an individual. Patient leaflets and notices should contain the name of the CHC secretary and the address of the CHC.

Complaints and litigation

Case: *R v. Canterbury and Thanet DHA and another, ex parte F and W*[3]

> Complaints were made under the previous hospital complaints procedure by eight families that a doctor employed by the first defendants and seconded to the second defendants diagnosed sexual abuse when it should not have been so diagnosed and delayed in telling the parents of the diagnosis. A legal aid certificate was obtained by one of the complainants. The doctor withdrew her co-operation in view of the possibility of legal proceedings. The defendants subsequently considered that an inquiry was inappropriate. The complainants applied for judicial review contending *inter alia* that there was a duty to review their complaints.

The court held that the complaints procedure was not appropriate where litigation was likely because:

- the purpose of the inquiry was either to obtain a second opinion and a change of diagnosis or to enable the health authority to change its procedures in the light of matters brought to its attention during the investigation; and
- the procedure depends on the co-operation of the doctor concerned which obviously would not be forthcoming if legal proceedings were likely.

The issues raised in the above case will not be resolved by the implementation of the Wilson Report. To require a complainant to agree not to bring legal proceedings whatever the outcome of the investigation would appear to be unjust and may mean that some complainants may not make use of the complaints system. Thus the possibility of resolving the issues without recourse to litigation will be lost.

Complaints relating to local authority community services

The requirement that a complaints procedure should be established stems from section 7B of the Local Authorities Social Services Act 1970 (as inserted by section 5 of the National Health Service and Community Care Act 1990). This enables the Secretary of State to require local authorities to establish a procedure for considering any representations (including complaints) which are made to them by a qualifying individual, or anyone acting on his behalf, in relation to the discharge of, or any failure to discharge, any of their social services functions in respect of that individual.

A qualifying individual is one entitled to the provision of services by the LA and whose need for those services is known to the LA. Directions have been issued by the Secretary of State in 1990 for complaints procedures and they cover

- representations and their consideration;
- the monitoring of the operation of the procedures; and
- other general aspects.

Policy guidance was issued in *Caring for People: Community Care in the next decade and beyond*, pages 59–72[4]. This covers the objectives of social services departments' (SSDs') complaints procedures and the need to ensure that the procedure is developed after consultation. It defines the essential requirements of a complaints procedure and these are shown in Figure 14.4.

***Figure 14.4*   Requirements of a complaints procedure.**

(1) An officer should be designated to co-ordinate the consideration of complaints.

(2) Key stages should be identified together with staff responsibilities.

(3) Members and staff of the authority should be familiar with the arrangements, responsibilities and key stages.

(4) Every registered complaint should be considered and responded to within 28 days of receipt and, if this is not possible, an explanation should be given with a full response within three months.

(5) The authority should respond to the complainant and advise on further options for the complainant.

(6) The review panel should meet within 28 days of the complainant's request.

(7) The review panel's decision to be recorded within 24 hours of the completion of their deliberations and sent formally to the authority, the complainant and anybody acting on his behalf.

(8) The authority should decide on its action with regard to the review panel's recommendation within 28 days of the receipt of the recommendation, with appropriate notification to specified persons.

(9) The authority should keep a record of all complaints received and the outcome in each case, and identify separately those cases where the time limits imposed by the directions have been breached.

Policy guidance also covers the following matters:

- the operation of the procedure in terms of staffing
- the form of complaint
- the response to complaints
- the review stage
- monitoring
- publicity
- support for complainants
- assessment decisions
- special cases
- voluntary and private sector provision
- nursing homes
- collaborative assessments
- elected members
- the role of the Mental Health Act Commission
- the Children Act 1989
- the Disabled Persons (Services, Consultation and Representation) Act 1986
- training.

An Annex gives details of the setting up and role of the Review panels.

Complaints and the private sector

Individual hospitals and private practitioners can set up their own complaints procedures. There would be advantages, however, in their following the same principles as those accepted for the public sector. There would in particular be benefit to them in ensuring that at some stage in the procedure the complainant would be able to secure the assistance of an independent person or review panel. It may be that those working in independent practice could provide a panel from which independent persons could be chosen to investigate or mediate a complaint.

The role of the Ombudsmen

If a complainant is not satisfied with the response of the authority to a complaint, he can apply to the Ombudsman for further investigation: the Health Service Commissioner (HSC) in respect of complaints about the NHS and the Local Authority Commissioner in respect of complaints about local authority services. In April 1996 the jurisdiction of the HSC was extended to include the investigation of matters concerned with the exercise of clinical judgment and also complaints about family practitioner services.

The HSC has a duty to prepare a report which is submitted to Parliament under section 14(4) of the Health Service Commissioners Act 1993. The Select Committee of the House of Commons has the power to investigate further any complaint reported by the HSC, if necessary summoning witnesses to London for questioning. The HSC is completely independent of the NHS and the Government and has the jurisdiction to investigate complaints against any part of the NHS about:

- a failure in service;
- a failure to purchase or provide any service an individual is entitled to receive; or
- maladministration (administrative affairs).

Other quality assurance methods

Individuals who have complaints about the services provided in the NHS do not have any contractual right to bring an action before the court for breach of contract. If harm has been suffered as a result of a failure or omission, they may have a successful claim in the law of negligence (see Chapter 10) or if a service has not been provided they may in exceptional circumstances be able to bring a case of breach of statutory duty for failure to provide that service (see Chapter 6). Otherwise they must rely upon the complaints procedures.

There are, however many other mechanisms to ensure the maintenance of high standards of health care although these cannot be directly implemented by the patient. The Labour Government's White Paper put forward a strategy for improving quality assurance and its mechanisms.

These mechanisms include a National Institute of Clinical Effectiveness (NICE), a Commission for Health Improvement (CHIMP) and a framework for national standards. The establishment of Clinical Governance whereby chief executives and Trust Boards will be held accountable for the clinical performance of their organisations will provide more evidence to the patient about the standards of care locally.

The CSP has provided an information paper on *Quality Assurance in Health Care*[5] explaining the terminology used by providing a glossary and giving other sources of information. Reference should also be made to a package produced by the University of Dundee[6].

Physiotherapists will be expected to take part in quality assurance and audit initiatives as part of their routine work in ensuring standards are set and maintained. The CSP gives advice on conducting a survey as part of Quality Assurance[7]. It emphasises the importance of clear preparation for the survey and points to consider in designing a questionnaire.

Future developments

There is no clear evidence as yet as to whether the new complaints system implemented on 1 April 1996 has succeeded in following the principles set out in Figure 14.1. Monitoring is through the Patient's Charter standards and it is likely that league tables will be published. It is however dangerous to assume that an absence of complaints is indicative of a satisfactory service, or that many complaints show that an organisation is worse than one with fewer complaints. The reasons why people do not complain even when there is a perceived reason to complain are many and it could be that the organisation with no complaints is so appalling that patients consider that complaining would be a waste of time. Any league tables should highlight the speed and efficiency with which complaints are handled.

It is in the interests of all health professionals to ensure that any complaints by parents and children relating to the provision of health services are resolved as speedily as possible informally without requiring the complainant to make use of the formal procedure. Physiotherapists should have the confidence to realise

- that complaints can be a useful way of monitoring and improving the services to clients,
- that it takes courage to make a complaint, especially where the client suffers from a chronic condition, and
- that improvements can be made if clients are prepared to discuss with the health professionals ways in which the services could be enhanced.

Every complaint should be dealt with objectively and no assumptions made about the genuineness or grounds for the complaint until it has been effectively and thoroughly investigated. Complaints should be seen as only a small part of the quality assurance mechanisms in every organisation.

Questions and exercises

1 Draw a diagram showing how a complaint by a client of physiotherapy services would be processed.
2 A client tells you that he is not happy with the care provided by another health professional. What action do you take and what advice do you give?
3 In what way could the handling of informal complaints be improved?

References

1 CSP Professional Affairs Department (1997) No. PA 34 (August 1997) *New NHS Complaints Procedure* CSP, London.
2 DoH (1994) *Being Heard. The Report of a review committee on NHS complaints procedures.* Department of Health, London. (The Wilson Report).
3 *R* v. *Canterbury and Thanet District Health Authority and South East Thames Regional Health Authority, ex parte F and W* (QBD) [1994] 5 Med LR 132.
4 DoH (1990) *Policy guidance Caring for People: Community Care in the next decade and beyond* HMSO, London.
5 CSP Professional Affairs Department (1994) No. PA 14 (November 1994) *Quality Assurance in Health Care.* CSP, London.
6 Postgraduate School of Ninewells Hospital and Medical School (1995) *Moving to Adult: An education package for various health professionals including physiotherapists.* University of Dundee, Dundee.
7 CSP Professional Affairs Department (1991) No. PA 15 (March 1991) *Quality Assurance – Conducting a Consumer Satisfaction Survey* CSP, London.

Chapter 15
Equipment Issues

Physiotherapists use equipment in the treatment of patients and may also be involved in work relating to the assessment for, provision of, installation of and maintenance of equipment. A useful encyclopedia covering the choice and different laws covering specific items of equipment is *Equipment for disability* compiled by Michael Manelstam[1].

No easy line can be drawn between the role of the occupational therapist and that of the physiotherapist in relation to the ordering, supply and maintenance of equipment. Different authorities and NHS Trusts have worked in different ways and often these differences are historical rather than planned. What is essential is that there is clarity and consensus between the different professional groups in each area as to who is responsible for what.

This chapter covers the following topics:

- Legal rights against the supplier
- The Consumer Protection Act 1987
- Medical Devices Agency and warnings
- Maintenance of equipment
- Exemption from liability and written instructions
- Equipment as a resource
- Choice of equipment and instruction by physiotherapists
- Conclusions

Legal rights against supplier

Common law action in negligence

The law of negligence enables an action to be brought against the manufacture of a defective product if harm has been caused to a consumer or third person. This principle was established in the leading case of *Donoghue* v. *Stevenson*[2]. This form of action is discussed in detail in Chapter 10 on negligence. It should be noted that, in order to succeed, the plaintiff must establish:

- that there was a duty of care;
- that there has been a breach of this duty of care; and
- that as a reasonably foreseeable result of that breach of duty
- harm has been caused.

Contractual action against supplier

The supplier is under a contractual duty to provide goods in accordance with the contract terms. In addition, where the purchaser is a private individual purchasing from a person in course of business, he or she can rely on the legal rights given under the Sales of Goods and Services legislation, which, by implying certain terms (e.g. that the goods are fit for the purpose for which they are sold) into such a contract, provides additional protection over and above that contained in the contract documents.

Where the purchaser is a large consortium or organisation in its own right, the fact that it could threaten to remove the contract to other suppliers may assist both in enabling the purchaser to have terms that give it protection written into the contract at the outset and in enforcing the performance of the contract terms without any recourse to legal action.

The Consumer Protection Act 1987

The parts of the Act are set out in Figure 15.1.

Figure 15.1   **Consumer Protection Act 1987.**

Part I   Product Liability
Part II   Consumer Safety
Part III   Misleading Price Indications
Part IV   Enforcement of Parts II and III
Part V   Miscellaneous and Supplemental.

Part I on product liability covers the sections shown in Figure 15.2.

Figure 15.2   **Product liability under the Consumer Protection Act 1987.**

Section 1   Purpose and construction of Part I
Section 2   Liability for defective products
Section 3   Meaning of defect
Section 4   Defences
Section 5   Damage giving rise to liability
Section 6   Application of certain enactments
Section 7   Prohibition on exclusions from liability
Section 8   Power to modify Part I
Section 9   Applications of Part I to the Crown.

The provisions of this Act are discussed in this chapter but reference should be made to other legal rights of action in Chapter 11 on health and safety.

Basis of the Act

The Consumer Protection Act 1987 enables a claim to be brought where harm has occurred as a result of a defect in a product. It was enacted as a result of the European Community Directive No. 85/374/EEC. It is a form of strict liability in that negligence by the supplier or manufacture does not have to be established. The plaintiff will, however, have to show that there was a defect. The supplier can rely upon a defence colloquially known as 'state of the art' i.e. that the state of scientific and technical knowledge at the time the goods were supplied was not such that the producer should have discovered the defect (see below).

A product is defined as meaning any goods or electricity and includes a product which is comprised in another product, whether by virtue of being a component part or raw material or otherwise.

Who is liable under the Consumer Protection Act?

The producer

Section 2(1) states that 'where any damage is caused wholly or partly by a defect in a product, every person to whom section (2) below applies shall be liable for the damage.'
Section 2(2) includes the following as being liable:

- the producer of the product;
- any person who by putting his name on the product or using a trade mark or other distinguishing mark, has held himself out to be the producer of the product; and
- any person who has imported the product into the EC in the course of business.

The supplier

In addition to producers or original importers as set out under section 2(2), section 2(3) provides that any person who has supplied the product to the person who suffered the damage or to any other person shall be liable for the damage, if:

- the person who suffered the damage requests the supplier to identify one or more of the persons who were producers (as set out above);
- that request is made within a reasonable period after the damage occurs and at a time when it is not reasonably practicable for the person making the request to identify all those persons; and
- the supplier fails, within a reasonable period after receiving the request, either to comply with the request or to identify the person who supplied the product to him.

This provision makes it is essential for the physiotherapist to keep records of the manufacturer/supplier of any goods (including both equipment and drugs) which she provides for the client. In the absence of her being able to cite the name and address of the manufacturer or the company that supplied the goods to her, she may become the supplier of the goods for the purposes of the Act and therefore have to defend any action alleging that there was a defect in the goods which caused harm. Harm includes both personal injury and death and loss or damage of property.

Where a social services authority or health service body supplies equipment for use in the community then that body can become the supplier for the purposes of the Consumer Protection Act. If harm results from a defect in the equipment the appropriate supplier must provide the client with the name and address of the firm from which the equipment was obtained otherwise it will become itself liable for the defects. Records of the sources of equipment are therefore essential in order that clients can be given this information.

What is meant by a defect?

This is defined in the Act as set out in Figure 15.3.

Figure 15.3 **Definition of defect: Consumer Protection Act 1987
– section 3.**

(1) Subject to the following provisions of this section, there is a defect in a product for the purposes of [Part 1 of the Act] if the safety of the product is not such as persons generally are entitled to expect; and for those purposes 'safety', in relation to a product, shall include safety with respect to products comprised in that product and safety in the context of risks of damage to property, as well as in the context of risks of death or personal injury.

(2) In determining ... what persons generally are entitled to expect in relation to a product all the circumstances shall be taken into account, including—
(a)   the manner in which, and purposes for which, the product has been marketed, its get-up, the use of any mark in relation to the product and any instructions for, or warnings with respect to, doing or refraining from doing anything with or in relation to the product;
(b)   what might reasonably be expected to be done with or in relation to the product; and
(c)   the time when the product was supplied by its producer to another.

Defences

Certain defences are available under section 4 and are shown in Figure 15.4.

Figure 15.4　**Defences under the Consumer Protection Act 1987 – section 4(1).**

(a)　that the defect is attributable to compliance with any requirement imposed by or under any enactment or with any Community obligation; or

(b)　that the person proceeded against did not at any time supply the product to another; or

(c)　that the following conditions are satisfied, that is to say—
  (i)　that the only supply of the product to another by the person proceeded against was otherwise than in the course of a business of that person's; and
  (ii)　that section 2(2) above [that the person is the producer or importer] does not apply to that person or applies to him by virtue only of things done otherwise than with a view to profit; or

(d)　that the defect did not exist in the product at the relevant time; or

(e)　that the state of scientific and technical knowledge at the relevant time was not such that a producer of products of the same description as the product in question might be expected to have discovered the defect if it had existed in his products while they were under his control; or

(f)　that the defect—
  (i)　constituted a defect in a product ('the subsequent product') in which the product in question had been comprised; and
  (ii)　was wholly attributable to the design of the subsequent product or to compliance by the producer of the product in question with instructions given by the producer of the subsequent product.

What damage must the plaintiff establish?

Compensation is payable for death, personal injury or any loss of or damage to any property (including land) (section 5(1)). The loss or damage shall be regarded as having occurred at the earliest time at which a person with an interest in the property had knowledge of the material facts about the loss or damage (section 5(5)). Knowledge is further defined in subsections 5(6) and (7).

There have been few examples of actions being brought under the Consumer Protection Act 1987 in health care cases and only a handful of cases brought under it have been reported. One reported in March 1993[3] led to Simon Garratt being awarded £1400 against the manufacturers of a pair of surgical scissors which broke during an operation on his knee, with the blade being left embedded. A second operation was required to remove it. Had he relied upon the law of negligence to obtain compensation he would have had to show that the manufacturers were in breach of the duty of care which they owed to him. Under the Consumer Protection Act 1987 he had to show the harm, the defect and the fact that it was produced by the defendant.

National Consumer Council Report

A report by the National Consumer Council[4] in November 1995 recommended that consumers should be assisted in using their rights under this Act. Specific recommendations of the Report are shown in Figure 15.5.

***Figure 15.5*   Recommendations of the National Consumer Council on product liability.**

(1) Department of Trade and Industry should review its collection of home accident statistics to alert those responsible to dangerous products on the market.

(2) The Act should be amended so that compensation can be claimed for damage costing less than £275 caused by unsafe goods.

(3) The Act should be altered:
    (a) to reverse the burden of proof in cases where a product has failed and it appears self-evident from the failure that it must have been unsafe; and
    (b) (where there has been a failure to warn in pharmaceutical or medical cases) to provide a rebuttable presumption that the consumer would not have consented to the treatment if the warning had been given.

(4) The development risk defence should be amended to bring the legislation in line with the European Directive.

(5) Local authorities should be given a statutory duty, properly funded, to give advice and assistance to consumers.

(6) Criminal courts should be required to consider compensation in all cases of prosecutions under safety legislation.

(7) Manufacturers should improve recall procedures for unsafe goods.

(8) Manufacturers should produce new instructions to alert buyers to the possible dangers of injuries caused by particular goods.

(9) A new procedure should be introduced for class actions which would allow a single claim for compensation by all those injured by a particular product.

(10) The Lord Chancellor's Department and the Office of Fair Trading should explore how to raise the profile of the Act.

(11) The Department of Trade and Industry or the Lord Chancellor's Department should look at consumer protection legislation to develop a strategy to make sure that it can be used effectively for the purposes for which it was introduced.

Since the client is not an employee, she cannot use the provisions of the Employer's Liability (Defective Equipment) Act 1969 (see Chapter 11).

CSP Guidance on Consumer Protection

Professional Affairs paper No. 4 gives guidance on equipment safety and product liability[5]. It emphasises the importance of:

● record keeping
● procedure sheets
● equipment inventory
● the labelling of equipment
● clear procedures covering loan and issue of equipment
● procedures for the servicing of equipment.

Defining responsibility

It is essential when equipment is first supplied that the responsibility for it and the rights of action, if any defect be discovered, should be clearly defined. This is discussed below.

Situation: Dangerous nebuliser

An NHS Trust has nebulisers which are used for patients suffering from chronic chest conditions and are given out by the physiotherapists to patients for home use. Unfortunately the patient suffered a severe electric shock when using the nebuliser and is seeking compensation from the NHS Trust.

In this situation the possible defendants are:

- The NHS Trust if its employees failed to purchase safe equipment or if its employees fitted the equipment negligently.
- The suppliers or manufacturers if there was a defect in the nebuliser. They could be liable under the Consumer Protection Act 1987. However if it were to be shown that the reuse of the nebuliser and its maintenance was at fault, then they might be able to show that because of this intervention the NHS Trust had become the supplier of the equipment.
- Any person who tampered with the nebuliser.

The causes for the nebuliser causing an electric shock would have to be investigated in order to establish responsibility.

Medical Devices Agency and warnings

The Medical Devices Agency (MDA) was established to promote the safe and effective use of devices. In particular its role is to ensure that whenever a medical device is used it is:

- suitable for its intended purpose;
- properly understood by the professional user; and
- maintained in a safe and reliable condition.

Guidance has been issued by the CSP on the role of the Medical Devices Agency[6]. This is a government appointed body which has an advisory role in drafting regulations and issues publications on specific matters, 'device bulletins' (DBs) and 'safety notices' (SNs).

What is a medical device?

Annex B to safety notice 9801[7] gives examples of medical devices. It covers the following:

- equipment used in the diagnosis or treatment of disease, monitoring of patients (e.g. syringes and needles, dressings, catheters, beds, mattresses and covers, physiotherapy equipment)
- equipment used in life support (e.g. ventilators, defribilators)
- *in vitro* diagnostic medical devices and accessories (e.g. blood gas analysers) (Regulations are to come into force in 2000 on *in vitro* diagnostic devices.)
- equipment used in the care of disabled people (e.g. orthotic and prosthetic appliances, wheelchairs and special support seating, patient hoists, walking aids, pressure sore prevention equipment)
- aids to daily living (e.g. hearing aids, commodes, urine drainage systems,

domiciliary oxygen therapy systems, incontinence pads, prescribable foot-wear)

- equipment used by ambulance services – but not the vehicles themselves (e.g. stretchers and trolleys, resuscitators)

Other examples of medical devices include condoms, contact lenses and care products and inter-uterine devices.

Essential requirements

Regulations[8] require that from 14 June 1998 all medical devices placed on the market (and made available for use or distribution even if no charge is made) must conform to 'the essential requirements' including safety as required by law, and bear a CE marking as a sign of that conformity. Although most of the obligations contained in the Regulations fall on manufacturers, purchasers who are positioned further down the supply chain may also be liable – for example, for supplying equipment which does not bear a CE marking or which carries a marking liable to mislead people[9]. This marking is the requirement of the EC Directive on medical devices[10]. The manufacturer who can demonstrate conformity with the regulations is entitled to apply the CE marking to a medical device.

The essential requirements include the general principles that:

- A device must not harm patients or users, and any risks must be outweighed by benefits.
- Design and construction must be inherently safe and, if there are residual risks, users must be informed about them.
- Devices must perform as claimed and not fail due to the stresses of normal use.
- Transport and storage must not have adverse effects.

Essential requirements also include prerequisites in relation to

- the design and construction
- infection and microbial contamination
- mechanical construction
- measuring devices
- exposure to radiation
- built-in computer systems
- electrical and electronic design
- mechanical design
- delivery of fluids to a patient
- the function of controls and indicators.

Excepted devices

Exceptions to these regulations include the following:

- *In vitro* diagnostic devices to be covered by a separate directive (still being prepared)

- active implants (covered by the Active Implantable Medical Devices Regulations[11])
- devices made specially for the individual patient ('custom made')
- devices undergoing clinical investigation
- devices made by the organisation ('legal entity') using them.

Implementation of the regulations

In January 1998 the MDA issued a device bulletin[12] giving guidance to organisations on implementing the regulations. The Bulletin covers the sections shown in Figure 15.6.

Figure 15.6 **Device bulletin of the MDA January 1998.**

- Strategies for deploying, monitoring, and controlling devices
- Purchasing medical products
- When a device is delivered
- Prescription of devices
- Record keeping
- Maintenance and repair
- Training
- Community issues

The MDA has powers under the Consumer Protection Act 1987 to issue warnings or remove devices from the market.

Devices are divided into three classes according to possible hazards, class 2 being further subdivided. Thus:

Class 1   – low risk, e.g. a bandage
Class 2a – medium risk, e.g. a simple breast pump
Class 2b – medium risk, e.g. a ventilator
Class 3   – high risk, e.g. an intraortic balloon.

Any warning about equipment issued by the Medical Devices Agency should be acted upon immediately. Notices from the Agency are sent to Regional General Managers, chief executives of health authorities and NHS Trusts, directors of social services, managers of independent health care units and rehabilitation service managers. Failure to ensure that these notices are obtained and acted upon could be used as evidence of failure to provide a reasonable standard of care.

For example safety notice SN 9707 May 1997 drew attention to Arjo shower trolleys and the risk of side rail failure due to corrosion. It advised that the welding on the side rail hinges should be inspected and replacements obtained from the manufacturer if necessary. Were harm to occur as a result of such a failure which should have been remedied by the physiotherapist her employer might be sued for its vicarious liability for her negligence.

An example specific to physiotherapy that would now be the subject of a DB is the Directorate warning issued in 1988 by the Canadian Environmental Health about Interferential Therapy Equipment. It recommended that the output of such equipment should be limited to 50 mA owing to the possibility of causing cardiac fibrillation if the current was applied across the chest. This warning was endorsed by the CSP in February 1995. On the other hand Wendy Emberson[13] suggests that the use of Interferential Therapy in the treatment of asthma, in particular, is not dangerous and indeed should be supported by research within a professional that has all the knowledge and understanding of electrotherapeutic treatments. She asserts that

> 'the warning has served to prevent the necessary research and development of a technique that has been clinically demonstrated to have possible benefits for at least the asthmatic patient.'

Adverse Incident Reporting procedures

In 1998 the MDA issued a safety notice[14] requiring healthcare managers, healthcare and social care professionals and other users of medical devices to establish systems to encourage the prompt reporting of adverse incidents relating to medical devices to the MDA. The procedures should be regularly reviewed, updated as necessary, and should ensure that adverse incident reports are submitted to MDA in accordance with the notice.

What is an adverse incident?
The safety notice defines this as

> 'an event which gives rise to, or has the potential to produce, unexpected or unwanted effects involving the safety of patients, users or other persons.'

Such incidents may be caused by shortcomings in:

- the device itself
- instructions for use, servicing and maintenance
- locally initiated modifications or adjustments
- user practices including
  - training
  - management procedures
  - the environment in which it is used or stored or
  - incorrect prescription.

The incident is 'adverse' where it has led to or could have led to the following:

- death
- life threatening illness or injury
- deterioration in health
- temporary or permanent impairment of a body function or damage to a body structure
- the necessity for medical or surgical intervention to prevent permanent impairment of a body function or permanent damage to a body structure
- unreliable test results leading to inappropriate diagnosis or therapy.

Minor faults or discrepancies should also be reported to the MDA.

Liaison officers

The safety notice suggests that organisations should appoint a liaison officer who would have the necessary authority to:

- ensure that procedures are in place for the reporting of adverse incidents involving medical devices to the MDA;
- act as the point of receipt for MDA publications;
- ensure dissemination within their own organisation of MDA publications; and
- act as the contact point between MDA and their organisation.

Medical devices and the community

The MDA device bulletin published in January 1998[15] gives specific guidance on equipment used in the community. It suggests that the delivery and collection of equipment procedures should include checks that:

- the correct equipment has been delivered in good order;
- the end-user has received training or
- the end-user has been told not to use the device until trained; and
- the delivery and collection process does not risk cross-contamination.

The guidance emphasises that good device management is the same for hospitals and the community. It covers in particular:

- delivery and commissioning of loan equipment;
- collection of equipment when no longer needed;
- checking and testing returned equipment;
- adaptation of equipment;
- insurance; and
- device safety for medical and dental surgeries.

Specific guidance on sterilizers, dental X-ray equipment and resuscitators is also provided. For the latter it suggests that the best practice is for the equipment to be checked daily including the pressure in the oxygen cylinder, whether the bag is working, that any drugs are still in date, and that any sterile materials are in date and the packaging is undamaged.

Maintenance of equipment

It follows that as a result of the regulations relating to medical devices there should be clear procedures over the maintenance and servicing of any equipment. Often when equipment is installed or handed out for use at home, there is no clarity over who has the responsibility for ensuring that the equipment is regularly checked and, if necessary, serviced or maintained. It is essential that there should be procedures to determine this responsibility when the equipment is first supplied. Some equipment must by law be regularly serviced: for example lifts. When this equipment is installed, an agreement for the future inspection and servicing of the lift should be arranged.

Responsibility for the maintenance would normally reside with the owner of the equipment. If the NHS Trust or the social services authority remains the owner and the equipment is merely loaned to the client then the Trust/authority should set up an appropriate system for inspection and maintenance. This system should also take into account the avoidance of cross-infection.

MDA guidance

The MDA guidance[16] suggests the use of a computer system to identify equipment in terms of:

- whether it is simple
- whether it requires:
  - assembly
  - fixing
  - that a prescribing professional be present
  - special instructions for the end-user
- the time and personnel needed to ensure successful and safe delivery, installation and end-user training.

Client owned equipment

Where the equipment is transferred into the ownership of the client or clients purchase it themselves, then the client would usually be the one responsible for inspection and maintenance. However the authority would have a responsibility to ensure that all the necessary information was passed on to the client. Account would also have to be taken of the physical and mental capacity of the client to undertake this responsibility. Since the NHS is based on the principle that services are supplied free at the point of delivery, unless there is specific statutory provision (as there is in the case of prescriptions), it would be unlawful for an NHS Trust to supply equipment on loan to a patient and then expect the patient to arrange to pay the maintenance costs. For example nebulisers provided by an NHS physiotherapy department must be serviced and maintained by the NHS.

Once the responsibility for ensuring inspection and maintenance is defined, then should harm result from a failure to inspect and/or maintain, liability should be clear.

Failure to ensure that the equipment is in working order could lead to litigation if harm occurs to a patient.

Inventory

Each physiotherapy department should ensure that they keep a list of equipment which is given out for use in the community and that information is kept on the dates for servicing. There should also be a regular review to ensure that the equipment is still in use or whether it should be recalled. The inventory should have details of:

- nature of the equipment
- date issued
- name of patient

- name of physiotherapist
- item/s issued
- manufacturer/model/number
- labelling of equipment
- date of service.

Situation: Old equipment

A physiotherapist obtained from a client's home equipment used in treating enuresis. Unknown to her this was a very old model. She reissued it without ensuring that it was checked by the electrical maintenance department and was horrified to hear that a child had been burnt as the result of a fault in the equipment.

In the above situation there has been clear negligence by the physiotherapist in reissuing the equipment. She should have ensured that it was checked over before the equipment was passed to another client. Her employer would be vicariously liable for her negligence.

Ultrasound units

The responsibility for ensuring that equipment is regularly maintained and checked should be clearly defined.

For example Stephen Pye[17] discusses the calibration and performance of ultrasound physiotherapy machines with reference to current national and international standards, current practices and published surveys of machine performance. He concludes that 'gross faults – resulting in either immediate injury or totally ineffective treatment – can be present in new, factory-checked machines'. He emphasises that all machines require a vigorous programme of testing and calibration in order to deliver outputs within 20% or 30% of that indicated by the front panel. The records of the tests are essential to prove that the physiotherapist has taken all reasonable care to ensure that the machines are safe and effective. He spells out some important recommendations both for the individual practitioner and for the physiotherapist educators.

The output of an ultrasound unit must be checked on a weekly basis to see that it is working and giving the correct output. Other tests would measure the treatment time, the treatment frequency, and pulse timing. In addition every year there should be a check on a precision measurement device that is traceable to nationally recognised standards.

A one day forum was held in July 1997 to review the current situation on calibration[18]. There was a general consensus that one of the contributing factors to why poor calibration status of physiotherapy equipment had lasted so long was

'a lack of awareness and training at physiotherapist level. It was also generally agreed that physiotherapists have an absolutely key role to play in ensuring that the equipment bought from manufacturers is calibrated using International Specification Standards and is fit for its purpose.'

Adaptation of equipment

If equipment is modified for the specific uses of the client, every care should be taken to ensure that it remains safe. The following situation is taken from the Bulletin issued by the MDA in January 1998.

Situation: Adapting a wheelchair

> A physiotherapist inadvertently destabilised a wheelchair by changing the frame structure to accommodate a reclined backrest angle without considering stability effects, or consulting the manufacturer.
>
> In so doing, she would have affected the safety properties of the wheelchair, and thus probably invalidated the CE marking which the manufacturer placed on the wheelchair as a sign that it conformed to the essential requirement of the Medical Devices Regulations 1994 (see above).

As a result of the physiotherapist's adaptation, her employers may also have become in law liable as a supplier under the Consumer Protection Act 1987 and subject to a claim should any harm befall the patient or another person.

Maintenance of hospital equipment

There is a danger that, in these days of increasing pressure on resources, some of the equipment used within physiotherapy departments is not systematically serviced and maintained and unacceptable risks are taken.

Situation: On the blink

> A physiotherapist was aware that an alarm clock was not completely reliable. She had applied for a replacement but in its absence continued to make use of the old one. She set up a patient for ultra violet treatment setting the alarm. She was then called by an assistant to help with another patient. She forgot about the first patient. When she remembered, she discovered that the alarm had not sounded and the patient had probably suffered serious harm.

One cannot imagine any possible defence being offered in the above situation. There is clearly negligence on the part of the physiotherapist and her employer will be vicariously liable for the harm.

Exemption from liability and written instructions

Effect of exemption notices

Some authorities use a form which is signed by the client to exempt themselves from liability should harm occur. An example of such a form is shown in Figure 15.7.

Figure 15.7   **Example of notice attempting to exempt from liability.**

I ... acknowledge that the following equipment has been provided to me by the ...
NHS Trust

(1) ...
(2) ...
(3) ...

and I agree to be responsible for the installation and maintenance of this equipment
and not to hold the ... NHS Trust liable for any loss, harm or injury caused by the said
equipment.

Signature:

Witness:

Date:

The notice in Figure 15.7 would *not* be effective in removing liability from the
NHS Trust or Social Services Department if one of their staff had been negligent
in carrying out their duties and responsibilities. This is because the provisions of
the Unfair Contract Terms Act prohibit evasion of liability for negligence if
personal injury or death occurs as a result. If there has been negligence then the
notice will be of no effect (see Chapter 10).

Sometimes, however, the notice is not to exempt from liability but to instruct
the client on the use of the equipment and to ensure the client will be safe. To
provide this kind of written instruction may well be a duty. However any attempt
to use it as an exemption notice will not be effective if personal injury occurs.

An exemption notice may, however, be effective if loss or damage to property
occurs (see Chapter 10).

An example of a disclaimer is discussed by Porter and James[19] in an article on
an assessment for bathing by occupational therapists. A bath clinic was set up
and its use and value monitored. A responsibility disclaimer clause was
investigated with the legal adviser for the county council. He recommended that,
following correct instruction in the fitting and use of the equipment, this clause
would absolve the OT of any responsibility should the client not follow the
instruction correctly. Consequently, this was included in the instruction sheet for
fitting and use of the equipment given to all those issued with the traditional bath
board and seats. This did not absolve the OT of the responsibility for giving
correct professional instruction on the use and fitting of equipment and still
required that she was confident of the client's/carer's competence to follow these
instructions prior to the issue of the equipment.

The limitations of the disclaimer notice must be noted. It cannot relieve the
physiotherapist if she has been at fault. However, if she has taken all reasonable
care, it could act as a reminder to the client that the advice must be followed and
that failure to follow the advice will absolve the physiotherapist and her
employer from liability for any harm that follows in consequence. The notice is
not so much a disclaimer as a reminder of the effects of contributory negligence
(see glossary and Chapter 10).

Use of specialist equipment by a non-client

The same principles apply if it is feared that the equipment would be used by someone other than the client.

Situation: Loaning out equipment by the client

> Walking aids were provided for the client who allowed a friend to use them. The friend suffered harm whilst using these aids when they broke under her weight. Is the physiotherapist liable?

If written instructions had been given when the equipment was delivered that the equipment should not be used by anyone else, then the NHS Trust should not be liable for that other person's harm, if the equipment was safe for the client. Again the written instructions act not as a disclaimer, but as information about the correct use of the equipment. If the physiotherapist has given all the necessary information and instruction according to the Bolam test, neither she nor her employer should be found liable in negligence.

Failure by the client to follow instructions

The same principles would apply where the client fails to follow instructions: the physiotherapist should not be regarded as negligent if she has used all reasonable care in instructing the client and warning of the dangers of ignoring this advice. However the physiotherapist must take account of any disabilities of the client in giving this advice and in some situations would have to explain to a carer how the equipment should be used. Physiotherapists may say that they have no time to put instructions to the client or carer in writing but if this could be done it could prevent a lot of wasted time, make the instructions clearer for client and carer and also give them a document to which they could refer. In addition, of course, in the event of any dispute over what instructions were given, the physiotherapist could refer to the document.

Equipment as a resource

Determining priorities

Given the limitation on resources it is inevitable that there is often a waiting list for equipment for home use. Even if the equipment is available there might still be a delay in arranging installation. This is a major concern to those who have recommended equipment since there may be liability if harm should occur whilst the client is waiting for the equipment.

However the determination of priorities is part of the duty of care owed by the professional to the client. If a professional fails to assess the urgency of a client's need for equipment and harm befalls the client, then there is likely to be an investigation as to the priority which had been attached to that client's needs in comparison with the needs of others.

In the case of *Deacon* v. *McVicar*[20] the judge ordered the disclosure of the records of the other patients on the ward at the same time as the plaintiff patient in order to assess whether sufficient regard had been given to the needs of the plaintiff patient in comparison with the needs of the other patients on the ward at the same time. This is an unusual step but it indicates that the determination of priorities is a legal duty and can be evidenced from the records.

Client demands

■ When can a physiotherapist refuse to supply equipment or equipment of the patient's choice?

Often there may be no clinical need for the patient to have specific equipment, or equipment of the standard insisted upon by the patient. For example the patient may request a more sophisticated walking aid (such as a shop trolley). The physiotherapist has to be responsible in the allocation of resources and providing a more sophisticated item for one patient may mean that the resources are not available for others. Similar problems arise with temporary residents, are they entitled to receive the equipment necessary for their short stay? The answer depends on all the circumstances. If the equipment is available and the duration short, then it might be reasonable to provide a temporary resident with the equipment. However the costly installation of equipment may not be justified.

Some equipment is lent for the short term, but thereafter patients are expected to purchase it themselves (for example TNS machines).

If the equipment is properly described as medical equipment, provided under the NHS, then there will probably be a duty to provide this both in the short term and the long term since facilities under the NHS are free at the point of delivery, unless there is statutory provision for charging (e.g. prescriptions).

Where decisions have to be made over the priority in the allocation of equipment the physiotherapist should ensure that reasonable defensible decisions are made and are clearly recorded.

Refusal of patient to return equipment

Where property is loaned to a patient there is a duty upon the patient or carer to return the equipment when there is no longer a medical need, e.g. after the death of the patient. It should be made clear when the equipment is initially supplied that it is only on loan, that it must be returned on any request by the hospital and that good care must be taken of it. This should also be put in writing. If the patient refuses to return the equipment legal proceedings could in theory be taken, although in practice the cost of such a step is unlikely to be justified. If possible the equipment should be labelled as hospital equipment and speedy collection of the equipment when it is no longer needed should prevent it being passed on to friends, jumble sales or to a charity. Co-operation with district nursing services over what equipment has been supplied and the duty to retrieve it following a death should make it easier to recover the equipment. It may be worthwhile to have an amnesty day every so often, when the local residents are invited to return property to the hospital on a 'no questions asked' basis.

Responsibility for damage to the equipment

Who is responsible if equipment is loaned to a patient and is damaged? Normally, if there is no evidence of deliberate damage, the hospital would not pursue any claim against the patient. If however the equipment is deliberately broken or misused, or even damaged through carelessness, the NHS Trust as the owner of the equipment has a theoretical legal right against the bailee (see glossary) of the equipment since it was loaned on the understanding that care would be taken. However again it is unlikely that any hospital would wish to pursue this legal right except in extreme circumstances.

Insurance cover

At the same time that responsibility for the inspection and servicing of the equipment is decided, the liability for providing insurance cover should be agreed where this is deemed necessary. It may be that the NHS Trust or local authority has its own group policy for insurance cover which can be used to protect an individual client. It may be that the client is covered by his or her own house or personal insurance cover. The physiotherapist should ensure that this question is raised and answered. The MDA Bulletin points out that

> 'Equipment loaned by the NHS or social services departments normally remains the property of those statutory services and users cannot be required to insure it. However where end-users are using equipment in public places (e.g. powered wheelchairs) it may be advisable for them to consider third party insurance against personal liability in case of accident.'[21]

A survey carried out by the NHS executive between January and April 1998 concluded that over £55 million a year is being spent on commercial insurance premiums by NHS Trusts. The Government intends to set up a risk pooling scheme for non-clinical liabilities under Section 21 of the NHS and Community Care Act 1990. The NHS Litigation Authority, which manages the Clinical Negligence Scheme for Trusts, has been asked to consider how and over what timescale they might adapt their operations to include a new scheme for non-clinical risks.

Choice of equipment and instruction by physiotherapists

The physiotherapist has to make a determination of the nature of the equipment required by the client, the supplier and any other features in relation to the individual circumstances and physical and mental capabilities of the client. The individual circumstances will also require consideration of the carers and their capacities. Alternatives other than the provision of equipment are also important. For example it may be that there is a danger in the client making use of the equipment on his/her own and additional visits by community staff are necessary instead.

Even simple equipment such as a walking or support stick has to be prescribed and chosen with full professional judgement. For example Chris Wilkin[22] in a challenging article takes the topic of the issuing of sticks and walking frames to show changes in practice from the traditional model of issuing aids based on the patient's medical condition – axillary crutches for a fractured femur or pelvis, elbow crutches for fractured tibia and fibula etc. – to a wider approach. He suggests that other factors are now taken into account in determining the suitability of an aid. He recommends that, instead of considering only the patient's condition, the patient's needs should also be considered. These include:

- the need to maintain normal reciprocal movement
- for the equipment to fit into the patient's home
- for the carers and other members of the household to find it acceptable
- to remove stress from an unstable area
- to relieve pain
- to compensate for decreased balance
- to change the position of the centre of gravity of the patient in relation to the base of support
- to cope with emergency situations, either real or perceived.

His paper poses a dilemma in terms of how the Bolam test would apply, especially when he writes

'If you can follow the logic of this paper but just cannot bring yourself to issue an aid which now somehow feels "wrong" you are, I suggest, probably being influenced by a traditional mode of thinking.'

It is important in such a case for a physiotherapist to ensure that the records show the reason for the non-traditional choice of aids, since it is likely that if litigation were to be brought several years later, when the memory of the reasons for the choice has gone, it may still seem a 'wrong' decision and therefore appear indefensible when in fact it was fully justified.

Failures by the physiotherapist in selecting equipment which no reasonable therapist would have selected for a specific client, could lead to liability if harm is incurred. In addition the physiotherapist must be aware of the cost implications of the equipment which she is recommending and have access to a value for money audit which is kept up to date. The Disability Equipment Assessment Centre at Southampton provides such a service of equipment evaluation[23].

Situation: Choice of walking frame

A physiotherapist recommends that a disabled person should be supplied with a particular walking frame. However she failed to take into account the nature of the flooring in the house. The patient slips whilst using the frame at home. Who is responsible for the accident?

If the patient can show that any reasonable physiotherapist would not have provided that particular type of frame, then there is evidence of negligence by the physiotherapist. It may be however that the accident was not caused by the type of frame but there were inherent defects within the frame, in which case the patient may have a case under the Consumer Protection Act 1987.

Wheelchairs

The announcement by John Bowis, a junior health minister, in February 1996[24] that severely disabled persons are to be offered powered wheelchairs on the National Health Service under a £50 million scheme emphasises the need for training within the NHS in the selection and use of such equipment. The scheme started in April 1996. It was accompanied by a voucher system which gives wheelchair users more choice and financial help from the NHS if they choose to buy from the private sector. The money is to be phased over four years. (It should be noted that there can be dangers in using wheelchairs in vans and other transport – see Chapter 16.)

Many items of equipment will require instruction from the physiotherapist before the patient is able to use it safely. The physiotherapist should provide a reasonable standard of care in giving this instruction, where possible providing a written leaflet for the patient. (Reference should be made to Chapter 27 on the liability which can arise from instructing others. See also Chapter 10 on negligence)

Refusal by client to use hoist

It may be that a hoist has been provided to reduce the risk in manual handling, but the client or carer refuses to use it. The physiotherapist can show them the reasons why a hoist is advisable and give them clear instructions in its use, but cannot prevent their ignoring such advice and instructions when they are on their own. The Trust would not be liable for any harm which client or carer thereby incurs. However the client could not refuse to use a hoist if health care support workers or other health professionals were in attendance. Their health and safety should not be endangered by the refusal of the client and the client might have to be warned that it may not be possible to provide the service required if the health and safety of employees is put at risk.

Rehabilitation Supplies and Services Association (RSSA)

This is a trade association for manufacturers, distributors and maintainers of 'active' (electrical and mechanical) rehabilitation equipment[25]. It was formed in response to the needs of the Organisation of Chartered Physiotherapists in Private Practice (OCPPP) which wished to compile a list of 'approved suppliers' for its accredited members. It sets basic minimum operating standards to which its members have to work in order to remain in the association. There are three categories of membership: sales, manufacture and service.

If a complaint is alleged against an RSSA member it can be made to the RSSA which will consider the complaint, offering an independent point of view and the chance to mediate a satisfactory conclusion. If the complaint is upheld and the RSSA member fails to meet its obligations then it risks being removed from the register of members.

Keeping up to date

All specialisms throughout the wide scope of physiotherapy practice are required by their professional rules of conduct and by the duty of care which they owe to their clients in the law of negligence to ensure that they keep up to date in relation to the developments within equipment and technology. The following are a few examples of recent developments.

Chatham and others used an incremental test of respiratory endurance (the TIRE) as a method of fixed load respiratory muscle training in normal volunteers. He concluded that this method increased the strength and endurance of respiratory muscles[26].

Keeping up to date with high technology developments in medicine can be demanding and highly specialised. Thus Fiona Makin[27] discusses the use of a vented electric left ventricular assist device as an alternative to conventional cardiac transplantation. She emphasises that:

'It is vital that physiotherapists working in this specialty remain critical, yet constructive, regarding new technological advances, in order that future patients receive effective and well-researched rehabilitation, which offers them maximal physical and psychological support to return to daily life.'

Electromyography (EMG) biofeedback units are reviewed by Lee Herrington[28]. These units are used in treating certain musculoskeletal conditions. He shows the common faults in EMG interpretation and emphasises that:

'It has to be used with care, because of the limitations of the equipment itself and the potential errors when interpreting the true meaning of the level of EMG activity displayed. The actual signal produced can be used only to demonstrate the time of activation and in the grossest form the amount of EMG activity of a given muscle. It cannot be used for direct between-muscle comparison or in any way to describe the amount of force being generated.'

Clearly any physiotherapist who was to use this equipment would be judged according to the Bolam test in drawing any conclusions from its results.

Professional warnings

Physiotherapists have a professional duty to be aware of any information which can affect their safe practice. For example the CSP has issued guidance on burns and interferential therapy[29] It warns physiotherapists of the danger of the possibility of an insulating layer of debris forming between the metal connection and the rubber electrode where the connection between the lead and electrode is metal. The result could be the reduction in the size of the electrode and an increase in the current density which could cause a burn.

The physiotherapist must be alert to any warnings issued by the Medical Devices Agency and must in turn ensure that she completes the appropriate forms to feed back any dangers or hazards which come to her attention.

Conclusions

Liability for the supply of equipment which causes harm, has been clarified over recent years and the work of the Medical Devices Agency makes clear the legal responsibilities of the physiotherapist. To keep up to date with technical developments in equipment is becoming a heavy burden for physiotherapists, but specialisation and clear allocation of responsibilities should ensure that the physiotherapist is supported in keeping up to date within her own specialist area and that the client is safe.

 Questions and exercises

1 Review the procedure you follow in choosing equipment for a client.
2 Draw up a leaflet to give to the client about the supply of equipment in the home and which covers instruction on use, maintenance, insurance and any other aspects you consider necessary.
3 A client is considering bringing a claim against manufacturers because of faulty equipment. What advice could you give her about her rights?

References

1 Disabled Living Foundation (1993) *Equipment for disability.* Manelstam, M. (compiler) 3rd edn. Jessica Kingsley Publishers Ltd, London.
2 *Donoghue* v. *Stevenson* [1932] AC 562.
3 Dimond, B.C. (1993) Protecting the consumer. *Nursing Standard* **7**, 24, 18–19.
4 National Consumer Council (1995) *Unsafe Products: How the Consumer Protection Act works for consumers.* National Consumer Council.
5 CSP Professional Affairs Department (1996) No. PA 4 *Equipment Safety & Product Liability.* CSP, London.
6 CSP Professional Affairs Department (1997) No. PA 33 (July 1997) *Medical Devices Agency.* CSP, London.
7 Medical Devices Agency (January 1998) SN 9801 *Reporting Adverse Incidents Relating to Medical Devices.* MDA, London.
8 Medical Devices Regulations 1994 SI No. 3017 of 1994 (came into force 1 January 1995; mandatory from 14 June 1998) Directive 93/42/EEC.
9 Medical Devices Agency (January 1998) DB 9801 *Medical Device and Equipment Management for Hospital and Community-based Organisations.* MDA, London.
10 Directive 93/42/EEC (concerning medical devices).
11 Directive 90/385/EEC (came into force 1 January 1993 and is mandatory from 1 January 1995).
12 Medical Devices Agency (January 1998) DB 9801 *Medical Device and Equipment Management for Hospital and Community-based Organisations.* MDA, London.
13 Emberson, W. (1996) Asthma and Interferential Therapy (IFT). *In Touch* Spring Issue 1996, 79, 2–8.
14 Medical Devices Agency (January 1998) SN 9801 *Reporting Adverse Incidents Relating to Medical Devices.* MDA, London.
15 Medical Devices Agency (January 1998) DB 9801 *Medical Device and Equipment Management for Hospital and Community-based Organisations* MDA, London.
16 Medical Devices Agency (January 1998) DB 9801 *Medical Device and Equipment Management for Hospital and Community-Based Organisations.* MDA, London.

17 Pye, S.D. (1996) Ultrasound Therapy Equipment – Does it Perform? *Physiotherapy* **82**, 1, 39–44.

18 Zequiri, B. (1997) Calibration and Safety of Physiotherapy Ultrasound Equipment. *Physiotherapy* **83**, 10, 559–60.

19 Porter, J. & James, F. (1991) To Bath or Not to Bath? A joint initiative to resolve the problem of increasing demand for bath assessments; Parts 1 and 2. *British Journal of Occupational Therapy* **54**, 3 & 4, 92–4 & 135–8.

20 *Deacon* v. *McVicar and Another* (QBD) 7 January 1984, Lexis transcript.

21 Medical Devices Agency (January 1998) DB 9801 *Medical Device and Equipment Management for Hospital and Community-based Organisations*. MDA, London; *see also* HSG(96)34 *Powered indoor/outdoor Wheelchairs for severely disabled people.*

22 Wilkin, C. (1996) Pragmatics in the Issuing of Sticks and Frames. *Physiotherapy* **82**, 5, 331.

23 *For example see* Pain, H., Ballinger, C. Gore, S. & McLellan, D.L. (1994) An Evaluation of Kettle Tippers. *British Journal of Occupational Therapy* **57**, 1, 5–8.

24 News Report *The Times*, 24 February 1996.

25 See *In Touch* Winter 1996/7, 82, 29.

26 Chatham, K. *et al.* (1996) Fixed load incremental respiratory muscle training: a pilot study. *Physiotherapy* **82**, 7, 422–426.

27 Makin, F. (1996) The vented electric left ventricular assist device: an alternative to cardiac transplantation *Physiotherapy* **82**, 5, 295–8.

28 Herrington, L. (1996) EMG Biofeedback: What can it actually show? *Physiotherapy* **82**, 10, 581–3.

29 CSP Professional Affairs Department (January 1995) No. PA 22 *Burns and Interferential Therapy*. CSP, London.

Chapter 16
Transport Issues

Since many physiotherapists are required to drive a car as part of their duties and many legal problems can arise, devoting an entire chapter to this topic is justified. Issues relating to driving by disabled persons will also be considered. Concerns centre on the following areas:

- What is permitted in the course of employment
- Transporting other people and equipment
- Insurance issues
- Crown cars and lease cars
- Employer's responsibilities on transport and insurance
- Tax situation and private mileage
- Driving by disabled people

What is permitted in the course of employment

In Chapter 10 on negligence it was noted that an employer is only vicariously liable for the acts of the employee if the employee was acting in the course of employment. Many community professionals transport others as part of their work – clients, carers, colleagues and others.

Where this is clearly indicated in the job description then the employer would have to accept that it is vicariously liable for any harm caused by the employee whilst driving in the course of employment. The employee, if driving her own car, would have to ensure that all the necessary measures in terms of appropriate insurance cover have been taken.

Acting in the course of employment would cover all those journeys between the hospital, social services and clients homes, but it would not cover the physiotherapist deviating from the route and going to a supermarket to do her shopping. This would be described in legal terms as 'a frolic of her own' and the employer is not vicariously liable for any harm that occurs during such a ride.

Giving lifts

It may be however that an employee is forbidden to give lifts to others and yet disobeys these instructions.

Situation: Giving lifts

A physiotherapist is aware that she is not permitted within her job description to give lifts to others. She visits an isolated cottage where the General Practitioner has called and left a prescription which the client has not been able to take to a chemist. She realises that the client has no transport and offers to take a carer to the chemist's shop and return with the medication. On the return journey she is involved in an accident. Her insurance company claims that it should not be liable for the injury to the passenger since she had not notified it that she took passengers as part of her job. Her employers claim that she was not acting in course of employment since she was forbidden to transport persons other than clients and she was employed as an physiotherapist not a chauffeur.

The fact that she was forbidden to take passengers will not necessarily take her actions outside the definition of 'in the course of employment' (see Chapter 10). However she is likely to face disciplinary proceedings. In contrast if she picked up hitch hikers this would be unlikely to come within the course of employment. The employer would probably not be liable for any harm caused to the hitch-hikers.

It is of great benefit if employer and employee spell out exactly what use can be made of an employee's car for work purposes to prevent a dispute arising at a later time. It is also essential to clarify the use for insurance purposes (see below).

Any person injured in a road accident where the driver does not have insurance cover or cannot be traced may be able to recover compensation from the Motors Insurers' Bureau.

Transporting other people and equipment

People

Even where the employer expressly agrees that the physiotherapist can use her car for transporting clients, legal issues can arise if the client is injured or causes an accident.

■   What if the passenger becomes disturbed?

Situation: Disturbed passenger

A physiotherapist arranges to take an elderly mentally infirm patient to visit a leisure centre. On the journey the client becomes very disturbed and tries to get out of the car and succeeds in opening the back door and falls out. Is the physiotherapist liable?

This situation is of concern to many community physiotherapists. If the incident is reasonably foreseeable then it could be argued that the physiotherapist should have taken the precaution of arranging 'child locks' on the car so that this could not occur. Alternatively the precautions may have involved taking an assistant with her. Her duty of care to the client would require her to take reasonable precautions against events which are reasonably foreseeable. Before embarking on the journey she should have made an assessment as to whether the client would be safe in the car and whether or not an assistant should have sat with the client. In making this decision she should be aware that she is responsible for taking precautions to meet all reasonably foreseeable risks of harm to the client or to others.

■ What if the community professional took passengers on the basis that they were taken at their own risk?

Such an arrangement is prohibited under road traffic legislation and such a device could not be used to exempt the driver from liability for the passenger's safety.

Any notice purporting to exclude liability for death or personal injury arising from negligence is invalid (see Figure 10.1 for the provisions of the Unfair Contract Terms Act 1977). However with mentally competent adults there may be contributory negligence (see Chapter 10) if they do not take all reasonable steps to ensure their own safety, such as using seat belts provided.

Case: *Eastman* v. *S.W. Thames Regional Health Authority*[1]

Damages were awarded against the health authority in respect of injuries which the plaintiff sustained when travelling in an ambulance without a seat belt. Although the ambulance driver was acquitted of all blame for the accident it was held by the Court that a duty of care was owed to advise passengers to wear a seat belt. The defendants appealed to the Court of Appeal.

The appeal was allowed. It was held that adult passengers possessed of their faculties should not need telling what to do. The ambulance attendant was under no obligation to point out the existence of seat belts and a notice recommending their use. It should be noted that this case refers to the duty of care to adults possessed of their faculties. Where a health professional is transporting a client in her own car and the client is frail or mentally incompetent the courts would probably accept that a duty of care was owed to ensure that the client was reasonably safe. This might in exceptional circumstances require child proof locks or a person in attendance.

■ What if a passenger causes damage to the physiotherapist's car?

It depends upon the circumstances as to whether there is likely to be any liability on the part of the employer. It would have to be established that the employer was aware that harm could occur and failed to take reasonable precautions against that harm arising. If such fault could not be found, then the employer would not be liable, and the physiotherapist would be responsible for paying for the damage to be rectified.

■ What if a client carried in the car is suffering from an infectious disease which another patient picks up whilst being transported in the same vehicle?

There would be a duty upon the physiotherapist, if she is aware that she is carrying in her car a person suffering from an infectious disease, to ensure that after this use the car is cleaned and disinfected to prevent any cross-infection. If she fails to do this to a reasonable standard then she and her employer could be liable. Similar provisions apply to any equipment which she is removing from a client's home: she would have a responsibility to ensure that the equipment and her car was thoroughly cleaned to prevent the risk of cross-infection.

Equipment

It is also important that the physiotherapist is clear on her duties in relation to the transporting of equipment. To ensure that the client obtains equipment without delay she may be inclined to decide to take equipment herself rather than wait for a van to be provided by her employers. She should take special precautions to ensure that her visibility in the car is not impaired and that she does not suffer injury from manually handling equipment on her own. Should such injury occur, and she attempts to bring a claim, she may be met with the defence of contributory negligence (see glossary) – that it was her own responsibility.

If the equipment is stolen her insurance company may not be prepared to pay compensation for the loss unless there is an express term covering such liability and the physiotherapist had made it clear in her application for insurance cover that the carrying of equipment for work purposes was part of her agreed activities. (See below on concerns about wheelchairs being used in vehicles when they are not designed for that purpose.)

Insurance issues

Absolute disclosure is required in any insurance contract and therefore, if there is any likelihood that the employee will require to use the car during work, this and the reasons should be disclosed. Should the driver not inform the insurers of a significant fact, this could invalidate the cover even though that particular omission had no relevance to the claim in question. An interesting recent development has been the suggestion that if a driver uses his car for car boot sales without the consent of the insurance company this could invalidate his car insurance. This highlights the importance of ensuring that an insurance company is given full details of every use made of the car.

Crown cars and lease cars

Insurance and road tax

Crown cars
Where the employee has the use of a crown car insurance is normally provided through the employer and the crown is exempt from the provisions of the road traffic legislation requiring payment of road tax.

Lease cars
Usually the company providing the car would ensure that the appropriate insurance cover is taken out. However this is not always so and the driver must check that she has the correct insurance cover.

Servicing

With both crown and lease cars there may be service agreements, which enable the user to have the car serviced at regular intervals as part of the agreement. The responsibility would be upon the user to ensure that the car was regularly maintained and also to ensure that any faults were reported and rectified. Should an accident occur because the user has failed to take action to remedy a defect, the user could face disciplinary proceedings from the employer and in some cases also face criminal prosecution herself.

Permitted use

The definition of the permitted use of the crown car or lease car should also cover the use of the car outside the catchment area of the Trust, e.g. if the physiotherapist were to attend a conference or course. It should be made absolutely clear whether or not this is a permissible use of the car.

■ What if a physiotherapist is required to have a car for work but is unable to afford to get the car repaired or to pay for its MOT?

If it is a requirement of the post that the physiotherapist uses her own car in the course of employment, then failure to have a car in working order could mean that the physiotherapist is unable to perform her job. This may justify dismissal or transfer to another post where driving a car is not necessary. It may be however that she is able to use a crown car or have one on lease. It depends upon local arrangements within the Trust or other employer.

Employer's responsibilities on transport and insurance

■ What duties does an employer have in relation to transport by employee?

The following case illustrates the question.

Case: *Reid* v. *Rush and Tompkins Group plc*[2]

> The plaintiff suffered severe injuries whilst driving the defendant's Land Rover in Ethiopia in the course of his employment by the defendant. It collided with a lorry. The accident had been caused solely by the negligence of the lorry driver who could not be traced. The plaintiff contended that the defendant was in breach of its duty of care as employer in failing either to insure him so as to provide suitable benefits in the event of injury resulting from third party negligence or to advise him to obtain such insurance for himself; and that had he been so advised he would have obtained personal accident cover. The basis for these arguments was that there was an implied term in the contract of employment requiring such insurance cover or advice, or that there was a duty of care owed in the law of negligence by the employer to the employee; or that the employer had a duty of care because of the special relationship which existed between them.

None of these arguments succeeded. The Court of Appeal held that there was no duty on the employer to take all reasonable steps to protect the employee's economic welfare whilst acting in the course of employment even if loss was foreseeable. The Court of Appeal cited the case of *Edwards* v. *West Hertford-shire Hospital Management Committee*[3] in support of this decision. The duty of the employer was limited to the protection of the employee against physical harm or injury.

If therefore the employer fails to warn employees to take out insurance cover, that is the responsibility of the employee even if the car is used solely for work purposes. Where the employer assists the employee in the purchase of the car or provides the transport, the respective duties of employer and employee in relation to the transport should be made clear at the outset to prevent any misunderstanding or omissions.

Paying fines and fees

- If the physiotherapist incurs a parking fine when visiting a patient in the community, is she liable to pay that fine?

- Does it make any difference if she was driving a crown car?

The answer is that the employee would be personally responsible for the fine since she has broken the law by parking in a prohibited area. The fact that she was parking as part of her duties would be irrelevant since the commission of a criminal offence would normally not be regarded as being in the course of employment. Similarly if she was in a hospital car, it would still be her personal responsibility.

Where parking fees are charged on a hospital site it is entirely a matter of discussion between employees and employers over the fees charged and the sanctions which can be used if an employee ignores the parking conditions. Employers may find however that the fact that certain staff are extremely difficult to recruit may influence the terms and conditions of service, and this may include offering more favourable parking terms to attract and retain staff.

If an employee refuses to use her car unless the employer is prepared to pay parking fines or parking fees, and if driving a car is a requirement of her contract of employment, then the dismissal of that employee may be reasonable and fair.

Tax situation and private mileage

It is impossible in a work of this kind to cover the details of the law relating to the taxation of the benefit obtained from the use of cars provided by employers and the way in which private mileage is treated by the Inland Revenue. However it is important that those employees who have the use of a car provided by the employer should keep accurate records of their use of the car for private purposes, as well as their use of the car for work. Records should be made as soon as possible after the journey.

Physiotherapists in private practice will also need to keep comprehensive records of all costs associated with the car in calculating their profit and income tax.

Driving by disabled people

Under the Road Traffic Acts it is an offence for an individual to drive a car if they are suffering from a physical or mental defect which impairs their driving safely. Physiotherapists may be confronted with patients very anxious to drive when it is medically contra-indicated.

Situation: Insisting on driving

> A physiotherapist is treating a patient who has suffered a stroke. Movement on the left side is restricted but the patient is anxious to drive since he acts as the sole carer for his wife who has motor neurone disease. The physiotherapist suspects that he is driving contrary to clinical advice. What is the legal position of the physiotherapist?

This is not an uncommon situation since the inability to drive can be seen as a considerable hardship for many people who have suffered neurological damage or physical injuries. Many patients may therefore be tempted to commence driving before they are physically or mentally fit to do so. The physiotherapist can advise such patients that they are committing a criminal offence. In serious cases where the physiotherapist considers that there is a grave danger of serious harm to other people, it would probably be an exception to her duty of confidentiality to advise the DVLA or others of the dangers (see Chapter 8 on confidentiality). However it would be preferable to attempt to persuade the driver to cease to drive or to notify the DVLA himself and show him any appropriate literature.

Wheelchairs

An information sheet has been issued by the Joint Committee on Mobility for Disabled People[4] stating that manufacturers are becoming increasingly worried that their products are being used as vehicle seats when they were never designed for such purposes. The Department of Transport is working with wheelchair manufacturers and restraint manufacturers in order to improve the situation in the future.

Disabled parking and badges

The scheme

Physiotherapists may be involved in the assessment of the eligibility of a disabled person to have a badge which will entitle her to park in parking bays designated for the disabled. Each local authority has a duty to implement the provisions of the Chronically Sick and Disabled Persons Act 1970 and assist in travelling arrangements for disabled persons.

The Department of Transport has devised a scheme known as the Orange Badge scheme which provides parking concessions for the disabled. The scheme is implemented by social services departments and operates through out England, Scotland and Wales except for Central London, road systems near some airports such as Heathrow, private roads and certain town centres where access is prohibited or limited to vehicles with special permits. Central London has an independent concessionary scheme operated by the City of London, the City of Westminster, the Royal Borough of Kensington and Chelsea, and part of the London Borough of Camden.

The concessions

The Orange Badge scheme allows a holder to park free of charge and without time limit at parking meters, without a time limit at other places where non-holders' time is limited, and up to three hours on single or double yellow lines. The orange badge must be displayed. Some routes are designated as 'red routes' and these are subject to special controls on stopping, loading and unloading, but some concessions may be made for orange badge holders. There is a list of places where an orange badge holder cannot park which includes on a zebra or pelican crossing, where there are double white lines in the centre of the road, and similar places of danger.

Entitlement

Where a person is entitled to the mobility element of the disability living allowance a parking permit would normally be issued without further assessment. Other claimants may be required to produce medical evidence from their own doctor or to be assessed by the local authority.

If the disabled person is refused a permit, there should be in place an appeal mechanism. A physiotherapist who has carried out the assessment should be prepared to justify both her findings and her conclusions and she should follow the guidance given in Chapter 13 on report writing and giving evidence.

It should be noted that entitlement to receive an orange badge does not necessarily mean that the disabled person is fit to drive and any change in the physical or mental condition of the driver which impairs driving ability should be reported to the Driver and Vehicle Licensing Agency (see list of addresses).

Conclusion

Whether a physiotherapist is provided with a car from her employer or a lease car, or whether uses her own transport, it is essential that she makes enquiries relating to any conditions laid down in relation to insurance cover and the exact terms on which she is allowed to use the car in connection with work. She should also be aware of any regulations which affect the rights of a disabled person in relation to transport.

 ## Questions and exercises _____

1   Whilst giving a lift to a carer, contrary to the instructions of your employer, you are involved in an accident which leads to the carer being injured. What is the situation in law?
2   Draw up a procedure which can cover the use of crown, lease or employee-owned cars.
3   Advise a client on how to obtain a parking permit for disabled persons.

References

1 *Eastman* v. *S.W. Thames Regional Health Authority* (CA) The Times Law Report, 22 July 1991.
2 *Reid* v. *Rush and Tompkins Group plc* (CA) The Times Law Report, 11 April 1989.
3 *Edwards* v. *West Hertfordshire Hospital Management Committee* [1957] 1 WLR 1415.
4 Joint Committee on Mobility for Disabled People (1997) Travelling in Vehicles while in a Wheelchair. *Physiotherapy* **83**, 6, 305.

Section D
Management Areas

Chapter 17
Employment and the Statutory Organisation of the NHS

This chapter sets out the basic principles of employment law and how they relate to the physiotherapist. It also considers the statutory organisation of the NHS and the physiotherapist as manager. Those in private practice should refer to Chapter 19. However the private practitioner may also be an employer of others in which case she should be aware of the principles of employment law in relation to those whom she employs.

The topics to be covered include:

- The employment contract
- Protection against unfair dismissal
- Employee protection and health and safety
- Local bargaining
- Rights of the pregnant employee
- Rights in relation to sickness
- Protection against discrimination
- Trade unions
- Whistle blowing
- Future changes in employment law
- Statutory framework of the NHS
- The White Paper on the new NHS
- The physiotherapist as manager
- Conclusions

The employment contract

Formation of the contract

As soon as an unconditional offer of employment (by the employer) or to be employed (by the employee) has been accepted by the other party, a contract of employment comes into existence. This may be at the interview or it may be by letter from the prospective employee accepting an offer of a post. The contract may be subject to conditions, e.g. receipt of satisfactory references or a satisfactory medical examination. If these prove not to be satisfactory, then the contract will either not come into existence, or cease to exist.

Even though the contract has been agreed, the employee may not actually start working for several weeks. If the employee were to do anything incompatible with the contract prior to starting work, e.g. accepting a job from another employer, she would be in breach of the original contract. The remedies for breach of contract are, however, unlikely to be pursued by the aggrieved employer (see below).

Effect of the contract

As a result of the contract of employment both employer and employee have duties and rights. These duties and rights arise from:

- express terms, either agreed by the parties individually or resulting from collective bargaining procedures;
- implied terms; and
- terms set by statute.

Express terms

Some duties arise by express agreement between the parties. These would include the basic terms of the contract – title of the post, starting date, salary, holidays, sickness, pensions, etc. Some of these terms may have already been part of collective bargaining within the work place. Thus health service employees may have agreed terms nationally through the Whitley Council bargaining procedures (unless their Trust has negotiated contractual terms with its own employees) and if it is agreed that an employee is to commence at a specific level then all the other terms and the General Conditions of Service will flow from that. The national conditions set through the Whitley Council mechanisms or the Government's review body are gradually being replaced by local collective bargaining (see below).

The employee might also agree specific terms with the employer when commencing: e.g. that a previously booked holiday can be taken or that she can start the day an hour later than usual because of child commitments. Such terms are enforceable, but written evidence of the agreement that the term is part of the contract of employment would be of considerable assistance to an employee who claimed that these terms were not being upheld.

Implied terms

The law implies into a contract of employment certain terms which are binding upon both parties even though such terms were never expressly raised by the parties. Figure 17.1 lists the terms which would be implied by law as obligations upon the employer and Figure 17.2 lists the terms which would be implied by law as obligations upon the employee.

Figure 17.1 **Implied terms binding upon the employer.**

- A duty to take reasonable care for the health and safety of the employee, including the duty to ensure that the premises, plant and equipment are safe, that there is a safe system of work and that fellow staff are competent.
- A duty to co-operate with the employee to enable him to fulfil his contract of employment.
- An obligation to pay the employee.

Figure 17.2 **Implied terms binding upon the employee.**

- A duty to obey the reasonable instructions of the employer.
- A duty to act with reasonable regard to health and safety.
- A duty to co-operate with the employer, including the duty to account for profits, to disclose misdeeds and not to compete with the employer.
- A duty to maintain the confidentiality of information learnt during employment.

The basic principle is that where express terms cover the issue terms will not have to be implied. Thus a contract would normally state the pay to be given to the employee. However where this is not done, the court would imply that there is a duty for the employer to pay the employee a reasonable amount. Alternatively where very little has been agreed the court might hold that in the absence of agreement over significant terms there is no binding contract, i.e. the contract is void for uncertainty. The employee would be entitled to receive payment for any work performed, on a quasi contractual basis.

In the case of a junior hospital doctor it was argued that there was an implied term that an employer would take care of its employees and not ask them to work an excessive amount of overtime[1]. In this case the junior doctor became ill as a result of the excessive amount of overtime he was asked to work.

Statutory rights

The employer does not have complete discretion over what terms it can negotiate with the employee. Acts of Parliament require the employer to recognise certain rights, known as statutory rights, to which the employee is entitled. The employer could offer terms which improve upon these rights, but not reduce them. Certain qualifying conditions stipulate which employees are entitled to benefit from these statutory rights. Many rely upon a specified length of continuous service (see below).

Figure 17.3 sets out the principle rights given by statute.

Figure 17.3 **Statutory rights (Employment Rights Act 1996).**

- Written statement of particulars
- Itemised statement of pay
- Time off provisions:
  - to take part in trade union (TU) duties and training
  - to take part in TU activities
  - to look for job or undergo training if made redundant
  - to attend ante-natal clinics
  - to act as JP and certain public service duties
- Provisions relating to pregnancy and maternity (including pay)
- Sickness pay

Continued

Figure 17.3   Continued.

- Health and safety rights
- Rights relating to TU membership and activities
- Bank holidays
- Guarantee payments
- Redundancy payment
- Medical suspension payment

Employment protection legislation required different lengths of continuous service as a condition of being eligible for these statutory rights, with part timers having to serve for a longer period of time. However this has been held to be discriminatory since more women are likely to be part timers and an increasing number of statutory rights have no continuous service as a prerequisite (see below).

The minimum wage and the Working Time Directives

The National Minimum Wages Act 1998 aims to combat poverty pay. Subject to certain exceptions the national minimum wage will apply at the same rate to all workers, regardless of the sector in which they work. The Act creates a framework for the minimum wage to be implemented and enforced, but the details are contained in regulations issued by the Secretary of State. The Act refers to workers, including agency workers and homeworkers, and creates the Low Pay Commission which works with the Secretary of State in creating the minimum wage and advising on policy matters.

The Working Time Regulations 1998 SI 1998 1833 (in force from 1 October 1998) implement the Council Directive 93/104 ([1992] OJL307/18) concerning certain aspects of the organisation of working time and provisions concerning working time in Council Directive 94/33 ([1994] OJL 216/12) on the protection of young people at work. Obligations are imposed on employers concerning:

- the maximum average weekly working time of workers,
- the average normal hours of night workers,
- the provision of health assessments for night workers,
- rest breaks to be given to workers engaged in certain times of work, and
- keeping records of workers' hours of work.

Performance of the contract

Both parties under the contract of employment have a duty to fulfil the express, implied and the statutory requirements in the contract of employment. Failure by the employee to fulfil her contractual requirements could result in her facing disciplinary proceedings. Failure by the employer to fulfil its contractual obligations could result in the employee claiming that she has been constructively dismissed (see glossary) by the employer, i.e. the employer has shown an intention of no longer abiding by the contract of employment and this therefore gives the employee the right either to see the contract as ended by this breach of contract or of treating the contract as continuing but being able to claim damages or compensation for this breach of contract. Rights in connection with constructive dismissal are considered below.

It is a basic principle of contract law that one party to a contract cannot unilaterally change the terms of the contract without the consent of the other person. Thus an employer who required an employee to work in a different capacity or in a different location could be seen as being in breach of the contract of employment if the capacity and the location were express terms in that contract.

Termination of the contract

A contract of employment can come to an end in the following ways:

- Performance
- Expiry of a fixed term contract
- Giving notice
- Breach of contract by one or other party
- Frustration.

Performance
A contract which specifies that a stated service is to be provided will come to an end when those services have been given. Thus a physiotherapist in private practice might agree that she will attend for ten sessions. On the completion of those ten sessions the contract, unless renewed, will come to an end.

Fixed term contract
A fixed term contract will come to an end at the passing of the specified time unless the contract is renewed.

Notice
Under the employment protection legislation the employee is entitled to a minimum length of notice terminating the job. The period depends upon the length of continuous service. However there will usually be agreed in the contract of employments notice provisions which are in excess of the statutory requirements. Such terms will require the employer to give the employee notice of an intention to end the contract and vice versa. Where the employer dismisses an employee without regard to the length of notice this constitutes a wrongful dismissal and damages calculated at the rate of pay for the proper notice period are due. However the employee might also have a case for unfair dismissal if there are not adequate grounds for ending the contract or if the employer has acted unreasonably in treating certain grounds as justifying dismissal and further compensation will be due (see below).

Breach of contract
By the employer   If the employer is in fundamental breach of the contract of employment, the employee might see herself as being constructively dismissed and bring an application for unfair dismissal (see below).

By the employee   Where an employee is in breach of contract the employer can, if the circumstances justify, see the contract of employment as at an end and dismiss the employee. The employee does however have the right to claim that the dismissal is unfair if the circumstances do not justify such action (see below).

Frustration

Where an event occurs which was not in the contemplation of the parties at the time the contract was agreed and this makes the performance of the contract impossible, then the contract will end by law without any requirement for the employer to terminate it. Each case depends on its own facts and the following events have been seen as frustrating and therefore bringing to an end a contract of employment – death, imprisonment and blindness (in a pilot). (The law of contract is further considered in Chapter 19 in relation to the private practitioner.)

Protection against unfair dismissal

One of the most important statutory rights has been the right not to be unfairly dismissed. This is given to those employees who have worked continuously for the same employer for 2 years for at least 16 hours a week or for 5 years for at least 8 hours a week. This requirement of 2 years continuous service has recently been challenged and the Court of Appeal[2] has ruled that it is incompatible with the equal treatment enshrined in the Equal Treatment Directive of the European Community[3].

Case: *R v. Secretary of State for Employment ex parte Seymour-Smith & Another*; *Seymour-Smith and Perez*

> The facts of the case are that Ms Seymour-Smith was employed by a firm for 15 months when she was dismissed and Ms Perez was employed by a different firm for a similar period. Neither had the required two years continuous service to bring an application before the industrial tribunal for unfair dismissal. They therefore sought judicial review of the statutory instrument which had lengthened the qualifying time for such applications from one year to two years[4]. They claimed that the proportion of women who could comply with the two year qualifying period is considerably smaller than the proportion of men, so as to amount *prima facie* to a indirect discrimination against women and was therefore contrary to the EEC directive.

The decision of the Court of Appeal that the present law was incompatible with the EEC directive was taken by the Secretary of State to the House of Lords. The House of Lords[5] allowed the appeal of the Secretary of State and held that the EC Directive only affected the rights of the individual against the state and therefore an employee could not use the Directive on Equal Treatment to pursue an action for unfair dismissal. It would request a preliminary ruling of the European Court of Justice regarding the construction of the Treaty of Rome. The European Court of Justice ruled that it could be seen as discriminatory, but whether it was so on the facts should be determined by the national court[7]. The White Paper *Fairness at Work*[6] (see below) envisages that the qualifying period for bringing an unfair dismissal application should be reduced from two to one years of continuous service.

One possible step which is being taken by employers, which is not necessarily to the benefit of employees, is to take more employees on fixed term contracts, since the employment protection law permits an employer in such a contract to have a term whereby the employee agrees to waive the right to bring an application for unfair dismissal if the fixed term contract is not renewed.

Exceptions to the continuous service requirement

There are certain dismissal situations where no continuous service requirement exists:

- Dismissal in connection with TU activity and membership
- Dismissal in connection with pregnancy
- Dismissal in connection with discrimination
- Dismissal in connection with health and safety
- Dismissal for asserting a statutory right.

Application for unfair dismissal

If an allegation of unfair dismissal arises, and the employee has failed to win an internal appeal, an application to an industrial tribunal can be made. The time limit for making such an application is three months from the date of dismissal. If the setting up of the internal appeal is protracted the employee may need to protect her rights by applying to the industrial tribunal within the time limit and then asking for an adjournment pending the hearing of the internal appeal.

The Advisory, Conciliation and Arbitration Service (ACAS) will contact the employee in an attempt to conciliate between the parties, so that a hearing of the case is unnecessary. ACAS has a general duty of promoting the improvement of industrial relations. It can provide advice on employment legislation and industrial relations and can also assist in the settling of disputes. It has also published a *Code of Practice* on disciplinary practice and procedures in employment. Failure by any employer to follow the ACAS guidelines will not make the employer liable to proceedings but this evidence could be used against the employer in evidence before an industrial tribunal.

The employee must show that there has been a dismissal and not a resignation. A dismissal may be:

- an ending of the contract of employment by the employer;
- a constructive dismissal where the employee is able to regard the contract as ended by the employer's fundamental breach of contract; or
- the failure to renew a fixed term contract.

There is however the power for the employer to exclude from such a contract the employee's right to apply to an industrial tribunal if the fixed term is not renewed.

Once the employee has established the dismissal then the employer must defend the case.

Defence to an unfair dismissal application

The employer must show the reason for the dismissal and the fact that the reason is recognised in law as capable of being a reason for dismissal. He must also show that he acted reasonably in treating this statutory reason as justifying the dismissal. The statutory reasons that can render a dismissal fair are:

- conduct;
- capability;
- redundancy;
- going on strike;
- legal impossibility; or
- other substantial reason.

The factors which are taken into account in determining the reasonableness of the dismissal and the employer's action are:

- consistency;
- following the ACAS Code of Practice;
- clarity;
- hearing the employee's case;
- allowing the employee to be represented;
- giving a series of warnings; and
- making a fair investigation of the facts.

Case: *Watling* v. *Gloucestershire County Council*[8]

One of the conditions on which an occupational therapist was employed was that he would obtain permission to engage in any outside work and he would only see private clients in the evenings and at the weekend. In 1990 he was seen by an area manager seeing a private client during the normal working week. He was given a strong warning that when he saw his private clients for alternative therapy it was to be outside his normal working hours. In 1993 there was again evidence that he was seeing a patient in ordinary working hours and that he was calling up a private client during his working time.

A disciplinary hearing was held and he was found guilty of gross misconduct in two respects – firstly in seeing a private patient during working hours and secondly in ignoring the very clear and emphatic warning which he had been given. He was summarily dismissed for gross misconduct.

He failed in his application to the industrial tribunal which found the dismissal to have been fair and he also failed in his appeal to the Employment Appeal Tribunal (EAT). His defence that he was doing no more than taking an early lunch was rejected on the grounds that lunch hours are for lunch and not for seeing private patients. It was also alleged on his behalf that the management were aware that he was seeing private clients during the day and that the flexibility which he was permitted in the ordering of his work and the taking of his lunch break enabled him to see private clients. However the EAT was satisfied that the employers has conducted a reasonable and fair enquiry into what had happened and that the decision of the industrial tribunal was beyond any sensible criticism.

Employee protection and health and safety

The Trade Union Reform and Employment Rights Act 1993 (now consolidated in the Employment Rights Act 1996) has given to the employee considerable protection against dismissal where the employee is taking action on grounds of health and safety. There is no continuous service requirement placed upon the employee to obtain protection against dismissal or any other action short of dismissal. In Figure 17.4 is set out a summary of section 100 of the Employment Rights Act 1996.

***Figure 17.4* Employment Rights Act 1996 section 100(1).**

[Dismissal in health and safety cases is unfair in cases where]

(a) having been designated by the employer to carry out activities in connection with preventing or reducing risks to health and safety at work, the employee carried out (or proposed to carry out) any such activities,

(b) being a representative ... on matters of health and safety at work or member of a safety committee ... [he] performed (or proposed to perform) any functions as such...,

(c) being an employee [where there was no safety representative or committee or it was not reasonably practicable to use these means] he brought to his employer's attention, by reasonable means, circumstances connected with his work which he reasonably believed were harmful or potentially harmful to health or safety,

(d) in circumstances of danger which [he] reasonably believed to be serious and imminent and which he could not reasonably have been expected to avert, he left (or proposed to leave) or (while the danger persisted) refused to return to his place of work or any dangerous part of his place of work, or

(e) in circumstances of danger which he reasonably believed to be serious and imminent, he took (or proposed to take) appropriate steps to protect himself or other persons from the danger.

The criteria for judging the appropriateness of the employee's actions are 'all the circumstances including, in particular, his knowledge and the facilities and advice available to him at the time.' (section 100(2)).

A defence is available to the employer if the employee's actions were so negligent, that a reasonable employer might have dismissed him as the employer did (section 100(3)).

Interim relief is available where an application is made to a tribunal in the case of a complaint of unfair dismissal (section 128 of the Employment Rights Act 1996). The tribunal has the power to establish whether the employer is willing to reinstate the employee pending the determination of the complaint.

The provisions shown in Figure 17.4 should give the employee much greater protection when bringing issues of health and safety hazards to the attention of the employer so that she should not be victimised. (see also section on whistle blowing below).

Local bargaining

Most physiotherapists are employed by NHS Trusts, some by social services departments and a minority are employed in the private sector. Within the NHS the framework of collective bargaining under the Whitley Councils was gradually being dismantled as local bargaining replaced centrally negotiated terms and conditions. This may change with the government's overall review of the NHS but the physiotherapist needs to ensure that she understands the principles of contract law and employment law in order to make maximum use of the system of local bargaining.

The introduction of NHS Trusts has presented the health based physiotherapist with a very different environment to that which existed prior to the implementation of the 1990 Act. Under the internal market physiotherapists are having to show the value of physiotherapy treatment to their patients in order to ensure the contracts for purchasing physiotherapy services are in place. Even when the internal market is abolished, it will still be essential for the physiotherapist to convince those who arrange the budgets for long-term service agreements that physiotherapy service provides added value for patients (see below). The physiotherapist is still likely to face conflict over the number of recommended sessions for a patient. The budget holder may, for example, stipulate six as a norm, when the physiotherapist may consider that a far greater number is justified.

Rights of the pregnant employee

Statutory rights given to the pregnant employee are:

- time off to attend for ante-natal care;
- maternity leave;
- maternity pay;
- right to return after confinement; and
- protection against dismissal on grounds of pregnancy or childbirth

New provisions in relation to the statutory maternity pay were introduced in October 1994 which gives a universal statutory right of 14 weeks maternity leave during which the employee would be paid a standard rate of statutory maternity pay and a right to receive pay during suspension on grounds of pregnancy, of having recently given birth or of breastfeeding.

The above rights are those given by statute. Many employers however give far more generous benefits than those given as a statutory right. The employee cannot, however, have both. The Whitley Council conditions are in many ways superior to the statutory rights for those who have been in employment for more than two years. Any locally agreed conditions cannot, of course, be worse than those to which women are entitled by statutory right and these are subject to review under the Family Friendly Policies set out in the White Paper *Fairness at Work* (see below). The Employment Relations Bill 1999 increases lengths of maternity leave and introduces a right to parental leave and a right to time off for domestic incidents.

Rights in relation to sickness

Employees are entitled to receive statutory sick pay from their employer when they are sick. Those who are not in work or are self-employed may be able to claim state incapacity benefits instead. These include sickness benefit, invalidity benefit, and severe disablement allowance.

Statutory sick pay is payable for up to 28 weeks incapacity, with spells separated by a period of not more than eight weeks counting as one.

Many employees receive superior sickness benefits under their contracts of employment. In the NHS most employees with the necessary continuous service have, under Whitley Council conditions, sickness cover of six months full pay and six months half pay.

Protection against discrimination

Race and sex discrimination

The main legislation protecting persons against discrimination over race and sex is the Race Relations Act 1976, the Sex Discrimination Act 1975 and subsequent amendments. Also the Equal Pay Act 1970 implies an equality clause into any employment contract, that a woman employed on like work to a man is entitled to have similar terms and conditions.

The basic principles under the race and sex discrimination laws, and these apply both within and outside the employment field, are shown in Figures 17.5 and 17.6.

Figure 17.5 **Principles of protection against discrimination on grounds of race.**

Basic principle
Discrimination on grounds of colour, race, nationality or ethnic or national origin is unlawful.

Direct discrimination
This occurs where one person treats another less favourably on racial grounds than he would treat a person of another race.

Indirect discrimination
This exists when an employer applies a requirement or condition which, although applicable to all people, is such that the proportion of people of one race who can comply with it is smaller that the proportion in another, or where the employer cannot show that the requirement is justifiable on other than racial grounds and it is to the detriment of the complainant because she cannot comply with it.

It is also unlawful to victimise or segregate on grounds of race.

Exempt areas
- Genuine occupational grounds (e.g. the essential nature of the job requires a particular physique and authenticity (like playing the Moor in *Othello*))
- National security
- Charitable trusts

Continued

Figure 17.5   Continued.

Other provisions
It does not apply to immigration rules, or civil service regulations.

Enforcement
This is through an application to an industrial tribunal.

Assistance can be provided by the Commission on Racial Equality (CRE) which has a statutory duty to work towards the elimination of discrimination, to promote equality of opportunities and to keep the Race Relations Act under review. The CRE can itself take action in relation to advertisements which indicate an intention to discriminate. It has the power to seek an injunction to prevent discrimination on racial grounds.

Figure 17.6   Principles of protection from discrimination on grounds of sex.

Basic principle
To treat a person less favourably on the grounds of sex than a person of the other sex would be treated is unlawful. It is also unlawful for an employer to discriminate against a person on grounds of marital status.

Indirect discrimination
This occurs where an employer applies a requirement or condition which, even though it applies equally to all persons, is such that the proportion of people of one sex who can comply with it is considerably smaller that the proportion in the other and where the employer cannot show justification on other than sexual grounds and it is to the detriment of the complainant. It is also unlawful to victimise or segregate on grounds of sex.

Exempt areas
- Genuine occupational qualification
  - essential nature of the job requires a person of a different sex
  - authenticity, decency and privacy, personal services
  - work abroad which can only be done by a man
  - the job is one of two held by a married couple
- National security
- Work in private households
- Charitable trusts
- Ministers of religion
- Sports and sports facilities
- Police and police cadets (in respect of certain terms only)

Enforcement
This is through an application to the industrial tribunal

Like the CRE the Equal Opportunities Commission (EOC) has a duty to work towards the elimination of discrimination and in promoting the equality of opportunities. It keeps the Sex Discrimination Act under review and can bring action itself in the event of advertising which indicates an intention to discriminate unlawfully. It can also bring an action for an injunction to prevent a person discriminating unlawfully.

A test case[9] on the Equal Pay Act 1970 was brought by speech therapists who claimed that they were employed on work of equal value with male principal grade pharmacists and clinical psychologists employed in the NHS whose salaries exceeded theirs by about 60%. Part of the argument circulated around the nature of speech therapy and what was the relevant profession to it in comparative terms. The employers pointed out that speech therapists had been considered in the past to be a profession auxiliary to medicine, and were therefore grouped with almoners, chiropodists, dieticians, medical laboratory technicians, occupational therapists, physiotherapists and radiographers. In contrast clinical psychologists had been treated as comparable to scientists such as physicists and biologists. The Court of Appeal referred the case to the European Court of Justice[10]. This decided that the fact that differences in pay were mainly arrived at through collective bargaining is not sufficient objective justification for the difference in pay between the two jobs. It is for the national court to determine whether and to what extent the shortage of candidates for a job and the need to attract them by higher pay constitutes an objectively justified economic ground for the difference in pay between the jobs in question. The case is now awaiting a rehearing by the industrial tribunal to apply the European ruling.

Disability discrimination

There is a long history of attempts to persuade Parliament to legislate in protection of the rights of disabled persons. The Disability Discrimination Act was passed in 1995 and will when fully implemented give the disabled person certain rights in relation to employment, pensions and insurance, the provision of goods and services, access to premises, education and public transport. The main provisions of the Act are set out below in Figure 17.7.

Figure 17.7 **The Disability Discrimination Act 1995.**

Part I   Definitions of disability and disabled person.

Part II   Employment: discrimination by employers, enforcement provisions, discrimination by other persons, occupational pension schemes and insurance services.

Part III Discrimination in other areas: goods, facilities and services, premises, enforcement.

Part IV   Education.

Part V   Public transport: taxis, public services vehicles, rail vehicles.

Part VI   National Disability Council.

Part VII Supplemental: Codes of Practice, victimisation, help.

Part VIII Miscellaneous.

Implementation

The first rights under the Disability Discrimination Act 1995 Part III came into force 2 December 1996. The remaining provisions of Part III are to be implemented in two stages. From October 1999, service providers will have to take reasonable steps to change practices and procedure that make it unreasonably difficult for disabled people to use a service. From 2004 service providers must take reasonable steps to remove, alter or provide reasonable means of avoiding physical features that make it impossible for disabled people to use that service.

Definition of disability

The Disability Discrimination Act 1995 defines a person as having a disability if

'he has a physical or mental impairment which has a substantial and long-term adverse effect on his ability to carry out normal day-to day duties.'

Guidance may be issued by the Secretary of State about the matters which must be taken into account in the application of this definition.

Employment

In Part II, which covers discrimination in employment, it is made unlawful for an employer to discriminate against a disabled person (i.e. unjustifiably treat the disabled person less favourably) in arrangements for recruitment, and also in the terms of employment which are offered, including opportunities for promotion and training and other benefits. The disabled employee is also protected against dismissal or other detriment on the grounds of disability. Regulations are being made to cover these provisions and also to define further the duties of the employer in relation to physical arrangements. Small businesses are exempt from these provisions if the employer has fewer than 20 employees.

The disabled person has the right to apply to an Industrial Tribunal over any discrimination. There are also provisions covering discrimination in respect of contract workers and discrimination by TU organisations. Discrimination on the part of occupational pension schemes and insurance services is also made illegal.

Goods, services, education and transport

Part III covers discrimination in the provision of goods, facilities and services. It will be unlawful for a provider of services to discriminate against a disabled person by refusing to provide him with services, or in relation to the standard or terms of the service. There will be a duty on service providers to take such steps as are reasonable to make alterations to buildings and the approach or access, and to provide auxiliary aids, such as audio tapes or sign language. Regulations may be passed to determine what is reasonable and on the implementation of this duty.

In the provisions relating to discrimination in education, it will be a requirement for the annual report of each county, voluntary or grant-maintained school to include information on the arrangements for the admission of disabled pupils, the steps taken to prevent disabled pupils from being treated less favourably than other pupils and the facilities provided to assist access to the school by disabled pupils. Similar requirements are made in relation to further and higher education.

Taxi accessibility regulations are to be made to ensure that disabled persons and persons in wheelchairs can get into and out of taxis safely and also be carried in safety and in reasonable comfort. Taxi drivers will also have a duty to carry the guide dogs and hearing dogs of passengers without making an additional charge. Regulations may also be made relating to public service vehicles and the access and carriage of disabled persons and wheelchairs.

The National Disability Council (NDC)

Part VI establishes the NDC. This Council will, following consultation, advise the Secretary of State on relevant matters as requested, and prepare Codes of Practice. Unlike the EOC it will not have the power to take cases to an industrial tribunal.

In theory the framework is in place for a major revolution to take place in the lives of disabled persons. However in practice the value of the Act depends on the more detailed guidance and regulations being passed and the extent to which the government places its weight behind the legislation. Much too depends upon the NDC in advising the government and in highlighting unjustified discrimination.

In August 1998 it was stated that more than 1700 claims had been lodged with tribunals since the implementation of the Act in December 1996[11] and large awards are being made. Thus a shift chemist with poor eyesight who qualified as disabled argued that, when made redundant, he had been discriminated against because of his disability and was awarded £103 146 including £3500 for injury to feelings.

There has been much debate about the financial consequences of the implementation of the provisions. It has been estimated that the cost to employers of taking on disabled person will be £8 million and adapting buildings and improving access could cost between £380 million and £1.13 billion.

Rehabilitation of Offenders Act 1974

The aim of this Act is to prevent discrimination against those who have had criminal convictions. It works by regarding certain offences as 'spent' after a certain length of time. This means that the person does not have to disclose the offence and to dismiss an employee on grounds that he or she failed to disclose a spent offence is automatically unfair. However the Act does not apply to serious crimes and many occupations are excluded from its effects, including health service employment[12]. Under Schedule 1 to the Statutory Instrument detailing the exceptions all members of any profession coming under the aegis of the Professions Supplementary to Medicine Act 1960 are excepted from the provisions of the 1974 Act and no convictions considered spent. All convictions will remain on the record and have to be disclosed to prospective employers.

Trade unions

Industrial action

The protection and immunities which trade unions and their members enjoyed in the 1970s and 1980s have been eroded until they have very few rights in relation to protection as a result of industrial action. Industrial action itself is defined in narrow terms if it is to be construed as 'lawful'. Rules are laid down in relation to elections and the holding of secret ballots before a strike can commence. Secondary industrial action is prohibited, so that TUs are not immune from liability for the effects of any secondary action.

The individual citizen has been give a right to prevent disruption to his supply of any goods or services because of unlawful industrial action. If he can show that he has been or will be deprived of goods or services and that the industrial action is unlawful then he can apply to the court for an order to restrain the action. The establishment of a Commissioner for protection against unlawful industrial action enables legal advice and representation to be paid for, though the Commissioner will not itself bring proceedings on behalf of an individual.

Unlawful industrial action includes the following: that

- which constitutes a tort;
- which is not supported by ballot;
- of which proper notice is not given;
- which is not in furtherance of a trade dispute;
- which is secondary action;
- which promotes a closed shop;
- which is to support an employee dismissed whilst taking part in unofficial industrial action;
- which is unlawful picketing.

Members' rights

The law relating to the constitution, membership, elections, funds, accounts and other forms of control was consolidated in the Trade Union and Labour Relations (Consolidation) Act 1992. An employee's right to join an independent trade union and to take part in its lawful activities is protected so that dismissal in relation to such activities is automatically unfair without any continuous service requirement.

The office of the Commissioner for the Rights of Trade Union Members was established following the Employment Act 1988. His task is to assist TU members who have complaints against their TU. He can also give assistance in relation to the right to a ballot before industrial action and the right to inspect a union's accounting records, and also in relation to complaints about TU elections and the register of members. Since the Employment Act 1990 the Commissioner has the power to assist in proceedings arising from alleged breaches of the union rules such as appointment to office, disciplinary proceedings, and authorisation of industrial action. However under the Labour Government proposals the post of Commissioner for the Rights of Trade Union Members is to be abolished.

Whistle blowing

This is the term which refers to a person (usually an employee) who draws attention to concerns which have health and safety implications. Because of a fear that such persons, many of whom have a professional duty to draw attention to dangers and hazards, would be victimised as a result of their actions, the Department of Health issued a circular recommending that each Trust and authority should set up a procedure whereby an individual employee could raise these concerns with the management internally without being victimised and thus not needing to bring in the media or other external bodies.

In September 1997 Alan Milburn, a Health Minister ordered health chiefs to remove gagging clauses in NHS employment contracts[13] whilst at the same time indicating the government's support for the private member's bill that became the Public Disclosure Act (see below). He stated that:

> 'There have been a number of well-publicised cases where NHS staff have felt obliged to raise concerns about inadequacies in the provision of health care publicly. In doing so they have provided an important safeguard for the public.'

A letter was sent out from the Human Resources (personnel) section at the NHS Executive to chief executives in the health service emphasising that staff should be encouraged to report to managers where they have concerns, but that where this is not possible, staff should be allowed to speak to the media.

The Public Interest Disclosure Act 1998

The Public Interest Disclosure Act received the royal assent on 2 July 1998. The basic provisions of this Act are shown in Figure 17.8.

Figure 17.8 **Basic provisions of the Public Interest Disclosure Act 1998.**

Section 1	Protected disclosures
Section 2	Right not to suffer detriment
Section 3	Complaints to employment (industrial) tribunal
Section 4	Limit on amount of compensation
Section 5	Unfair dismissal
Section 6	Redundancy
Section 7	Exclusion of restrictions on right not to be unfairly dismissed
Section 8	Compensation for unfair dismissal
Section 9	Interim relief
Section 10	Crown employment
Section 11	National security
Section 12	Work outside Great Britain
Section 13	Police officers
Section 14	Remedy for infringement of rights
Section 15	Interpretative provisions of 1996 Act
Section 16	Dismissal of those taking part in unofficial industrial action
Section 17	Corresponding provisions for Northern Ireland
Section 18	Short title, interpretation, commencement and extent.

The explanatory memorandum envisages that the Act will protect workers who disclose information about certain types of matters from being dismissed or penalised by their employers as a result. The Act applies to disclosures relating to:

- crimes,
- breaches of a legal obligation,
- miscarriages of justice,
- dangers to health and safety, or
- dangers to the environment

and to the concealing of evidence relating to any of these.

To qualify for protection, the worker making the disclosure must be acting in good faith throughout and must have reasonable grounds for believing that the information disclosed indicates the existence of one of the above problems. Disclosures are protected if they are made to the employer or other person responsible for the matter; to a Minister of the Crown, in relation to certain public bodies, to a regulatory body designated for the purpose by order and for the purpose of seeking legal advice. The Act comes into force on days to be appointed by the Secretary of State.

The Clothier and Bullock reports

Following the offences by Beverly Allit, the Clothier Inquiry made several recommendations to detect the possibility of personal disorder in applicants for nursing posts. It suggested that there should be procedures for management referrals to Occupational Health and the criteria to trigger such referrals should be clarified. There would therefore be a duty on any employee who suspects that a colleague is acting suspiciously to advise the appropriate manager.

The Clothier recommendations were reinforced by an inquiry chaired by Richard Bullock following the case of Amanda Jenkinson, a Nottinghamshire nurse who was jailed for a harming a patient.

The Government have accepted the recommendations that all NHS staff will have a pre-employment health assessment. Information provided to Occupational Health staff will remain confidential unless disclosure is necessary because a member of staff is considered to be a danger to patients, other staff or themselves. In these circumstances there should be disclosure to the appropriate person or authority.

Grievance procedures

As stated above the Department of Health has recommended that each Trust should provide a procedure to ensure that an employee can raise any concerns to the awareness of senior management without suffering victimisation. The jurisdiction of the Health Service Commission does not extend to complaints and grievances of staff (see Chapter 14) but it may be that the Commission for Health Improvement set up under the White Paper proposals (see below) will be receptive to complaints from staff where these relate to deficiencies in the standards of care available to patients.

Future changes in employment law

At the time of writing there are major changes to take place in the law relating to employment including the following[14]:

- **Working Time Directive** – (see above)
- **Parental Leave Directive** – By 1999 working parents will have the right to a maximum of three months' parental leave after one year's service.
- **Part-time Work Directive** – This will eliminate discrimination against part-time workers.
- **Employment Rights (Dispute Resolution) Act 1998** – This promotes a new voluntary arbitration scheme to settle unfair dismissal claims.
- **White Paper *Fairness at Work*[15]** – This sets out proposals for major changes in employment law which are shown in Figure 17.9.

***Figure 17.9*   Fairness at Work: main proposals.**

Rights for individuals:
- national minimum wage;
- Public Interest Disclosure Act;
- Employment Rights (Dispute Resolution) Act;
- abolition of the cap on the compensation that industrial tribunals can award in unfair dismissal cases;
- a reduction from two years to one in the qualifying period for unfair dismissal claims;
- consultation on removal of waiver of unfair dismissal rights in fixed term and zero hours contracts.

Collective rights:
- implementation of European Works Council Directive;
- changes in legislation on representation and recognition of TUs;
- changes in law on industrial action ballots and notice;
- abolition of Commissioner for the Rights of Trade Union Members (CRTUM) and Commissioner for Protection Against Unlawful Industrial Action (CPAUIA).

Family Friendly policies:
- Working Time Directive;
- Young Workers Directive;
- Parental Leave Directive;
- extension of maternity leave to 18 weeks;
- reasonable time off for family emergencies;
- protection against dismissal in exercising rights to parental leave and time off for urgent family reasons.

Statutory framework of the NHS

Following the NHS and Community Care Act 1990 NHS Trusts were established with the intention that they should become the principal providers of NHS secondary and community health care. Purchasers were either GPs, who were approved as fundholders to hold a budget to purchase secondary and community health care services for their patients, or health authorities.

In April 1996 health authorities were reorganised: the former district health authorities (DHAs) and family health services authorities (FHSAs) were abolished and in their place were established new health authorities which have the responsibility of commissioning and, in conjunction with GP fundholders, purchasing services from providers, as well as carrying out the responsibilities in relation to the primary health care services formerly undertaken by FHSAs.

However, the underlying principles of the internal market created in the 1990 legislation remained unchanged by the 1996 Act and the purchase and provision of health care is agreed in NHS contracts. Other changes introduced by the 1990 Act relate to the functions of the LAs in community care provision and these are considered in Chapter 18.

The White Paper on the new NHS

The internal market had created a different context within which physiotherapists worked and presented them with new challenges. Once again change is imminent but the emphasis on value and standards will remain (see below). The White paper on the NHS[16] envisages that the internal market will be abolished, but proposes that long-term service level agreements covering at least three years for the provision of services should be in place. The significance of this change is yet to be seen.

The main features of the White Paper on the NHS are shown in Figure 17.10.

Figure 17.10   **Main features of the White Paper.**

- Abolition of the internal market and GP Fundholding
- Establishment of Primary care groups leading to primary care trusts
- Establishment of the National Council of Clinical Excellence
- Establishment of the Commission for Health Improvement
- Setting up of National Service Frameworks
- Introduction of NHS Direct
- Introduction of Clinical Governance

Standards and guidelines

Following implementation of the White Paper there will be greater emphasis on standard setting in the light of research findings on clinical effectiveness and excellence. Standard setting and monitoring will become an even more significant part of the physiotherapist's professional responsibilities. The CSP has provided information on clinical guidelines[17] and guidance on developing clinical protocols[18]. It is too early to assess the impact of the concept of clinical governance on the role of the individual physiotherapist but if chief executives of Trusts are, from April 1999, to be held clinically accountable for their Trusts it is likely that more specific clinical targets will be laid down for each department, including physiotherapy.

Legal standards in the duty of care are discussed in Chapter 10 on the law of negligence and the extent to which clinical guidelines, protocols, procedures and practices are enforceable through the courts is considered in that chapter and also covered in a fascinating work by Brian Hurwitz[19].

Selling physiotherapy

In 1995 the CSP issued an information pack for GPs on purchasing physiotherapy[20]. It covers the following areas:

- the aim of physiotherapy
- who should provide physiotherapy
- the development of Chartered Physiotherapists
- the contribution of physiotherapy to General Practice
- the effect on practice workload
- Who may benefit from physiotherapy
- the range of clinical and other services offered by chartered physiotherapists
- physiotherapy service provision
- management and organisational issues
- quality issues.

There is also a relevant pack provided by the Department of Health in 1996 on all the professions allied to medicine[21]. which includes examples of service level agreements.

Even when the internal market is abolished this guidance will still be of value since it is still essential that physiotherapists can justify their work to health commissioners and to local health groups or primary care trusts and the managers of NHS Trusts. They will need to show the value added that physiotherapy can bring to a clinical situation, thereby justifying the investment in care and treatment by the physiotherapist. Even though the internal market might not exist in name there will still be value in developing managed care schemes for physiotherapy services. The CSP has prepared guidance, *Patterns of Health Care Delivery: Managed Care*[22]. It advises its members to understand the economics of any given disease/disorder, to know the standards and guidelines governing delivery of health care and to understand care interventions and their interrelationships as part of the overall care process. It states:

> 'Physiotherapists need to carefully examine managed care and disease management schemes to ensure that they do not compromise their clinical autonomy in order to achieve short term cost benefits. Failure to preserve physiotherapists' clinical autonomy, perhaps swapping it for standardised, inflexible care packages in the name of cost control, may compromise patients' welfare.'

This advice will still be relevant following the abolition of the internal market.

Outcome measures

In this area the research on outcome measures is vital. Thus Rosemary Chesson and colleagues[23] surveyed the outcome measures used in therapy departments in Scotland. They found that the major influences on outcome measures were:

- clinical decision making
- purchaser/provider agreements/contracts
- cost/benefit analysis
- patients' expectations

- health service research
- needs assessment
- quality/audit
- service prioritisation and
- professional credibility/parity of esteem.

They found that there was greater use of outcome measures between their first survey and their second and that outcome measures were more commonly used in care of the elderly rather than any other specialty. Most respondents incorporated patients' views into their outcome measures, but only six were using systematic methods.

The CSP has provided guidance on outcome measures[24].

Physiotherapy as part of primary health care

Situation: Unmet need

A GP practice arranges for services from the physiotherapy department for the rehabilitation of a patient. Six sessions are agreed. At the end of this time, the physiotherapy department recommends that the patient should have a further six sessions, but the GP is not prepared for them to be funded. What is the situation?

After the reforms following the NHS and Community Care Act 1990 if the GP fundholder was not prepared to pay for services for his patient, there was little a provider could do other than to complain to the health authority which provided funds for the GP fundholder or to try and negotiate with the GP to persuade him to change his mind. As a result of the changes envisaged in the White Paper it is hoped that there will not be such disputes. This remains to be seen.

The White Paper envisages the ending of GP fundholding and its replacement by consortia of GP practices which, with local authorities and others, can develop primary health groups. Eventually these primary care groups could be given trust status. The possibility of enhancing the role of the physiotherapist in primary health care will become evident. Lessons of those already operating within GP fundholding are of value. For example Catherine Minns and Christine Bithell report on muscoskeletal physiotherapy with sessions held in GP fundholding practices[25]. Customers preferred the location but the physiotherapists interviewed stressed the importance of a health and safety policy, continuous professional development, management support and essential equipment at the GPFH site. There were also concerns that there was less control of their work than would have been the case in hospital based practice. These issues must be taken up in any development of physiotherapy as part of primary health care.

The physiotherapist as manager

Managing a department

Many physiotherapists may be concerned at how the law impinges upon their role as a manager of a service and most of the general chapters in this book will provide specific information for many of the issues which confront a manager.

They should of course also be able to look for assistance from solicitors to the Trust and personnel officers or health and safety and other specialists employed within the organisation.

Situation: Liability of a manager

A senior physiotherapist who had charge of a department discovered that, during her annual leave, a basic grade physiotherapist had used a defective alarm clock and as a consequence a patient was injured. Is the manager liable?

The principle of vicarious liability, which means that the employer is liable for the negligence of an employee whilst acting in the course of employment (see Chapter 10) does not apply to the relationship of senior to junior members of staff. Provided that work has been appropriately delegated and supervised, a senior is not liable for the negligence of a junior. In this situation the manager is not personally liable because the basic grade has acted negligently. However she may be liable on her own account. Was she aware that the alarm clock was defective? If so, she should have removed it from the work place for repair, so that it could not be used inadvertently. If there is evidence that she has failed to follow a reasonable standard of care in management issues such as these, then she would be personally and professionally liable.

It follows too that any field of management which is directly the responsibility of the physiotherapist could, if she had failed in fulfilling her duties, result in her liability. Thus failure in ensuring a safe system of work, failure to draw the attention of senior management to any inadequacies in resources (including staffing and equipment), or failure to establish an appropriate system for determining priorities, could all result in her personal liability, for which her employer will also be vicariously liable.

A manager will also have responsibilities for the health and safety of staff. She should be aware of any unreasonable stress being suffered by individual employees and should ensure that there is no bullying. It is also her responsibility that risk assessment is undertaken in the department. (See Chapter 11 for health and safety laws.)

Situation: Manager's responsibilities

A physiotherapist complains to the manager that she is receiving unwelcome attention from a patient. The manager tells her that this is an expected part of her work with patients and that she should try to ignore the problem. Unfortunately, the physiotherapist is assaulted by the patient when she is alone with him in the gymnasium. She suffers significant injuries.

An inquiry should be undertaken into this incident. It is clear from the few facts given here that the manager acted entirely inappropriately and failed to take the situation seriously. The employee might well have grounds for suing the employer for compensation for the injuries which she suffered, because of the failure of the manager to take reasonable precautions to ensure her safety.

Some of the main topics of concern for the physiotherapist manager are considered in *Management in Physiotherapy* edited by Robert Jones[27].

Managing a clinical interest or occupational group

Some physiotherapists may find that they are involved in running a clinical interest or occupational group. They may be unfamiliar with the administrative demands of such work and it is essential that they take advice on the responsibilities involved. It is hoped that such work is unlikely to lead to legal disputes, but clarity of role, responsibility and procedure is essential to prevent any possible arguments. The CSP has issued guidance[27] for its 31 clinical interests and occupational groups. This covers:

- The role of chairman, committee papers, agenda.
- The secretary's role, meetings, AGMs etc., agenda, minutes.
- The treasurer's role.
- The role of the research officer and public relations officer.
- Courses, conferences and study days.
- Links with CSP.

It describes how a clinical interest group can become recognised and provides a model constitution for clinical interest and occupational groups.

Conclusions

Over the next few years there will be significant changes in the laws relating to employment as workers' rights are expanded across the European Community and the Government's White Paper *Fairness at Work* is implemented. Major changes are also envisaged for the NHS following the White Paper on *The New NHS* published in 1997. The effects of clinical governance, the National Institute for Clinical Excellence and the Commission for Health Improvements are not yet known. The challenges for managers in keeping up to date and ensuring that procedures and practices are amended to take account of these major changes will be significant.

 Questions and exercises _____

1 Prepare a protocol for the preparation of local bargaining. What additional terms would you like to see included in local contracts of employment with physiotherapists?

2 Look at the letter setting out your contract conditions and identify the source of each term i.e. statutory, express as a result of personal agreement, express as a result of collective bargaining. What terms would be implied?

3 There are very few men who are employed as physiotherapists or physiotherapist assistants. What action do you consider your NHS Trust or social services employer could take to encourage the recruitment of more men, without breaking the law on sex discrimination?

4 Obtain sight of the NHS agreement or the long-term service specification which stipulates the terms on which physiotherapy services are provided. To

what extent do you consider that these terms meet the patient's needs and how can they be used as an instrument in quality assurance?

5 You have just been appointed as a senior manager within the physiotherapy department. How does the law impact upon your new responsibilities?

References

1 *Johnstone* v. *Bloomsbury Health Authority* [1991] ICR 269.

2 *R* v. *Secretary of State for Employment, ex parte Seymour-Smith and Perez* [1995] IRLR 464.

3 EEC Equal Treatment Driective 76/207 – Articles 1(1), 2(1) and 5(1), 1976.

4 HMSO (1985) Unfair Dismissal (Variation of Qualifying Period) Order 1985 SI 1985 782.

5 *R* v. *Secretary of State for Employment, ex parte Seymour-Smith* [1997] 1 WLR 473.

6 Department of Trade and Industry (1998) *White Paper: Fairness at Work* Stationery Office, London.

7 *R.* v. *Secretary of State for Employment ex parte Seymour-Smith & Another*, The Times European Law Report 25 February 1999.

8 *Watling* v. *Gloucestershire County Council* 1994 EAT/868/94, Lexis transcript.

9 *Enderby* v. *Frenchay Health Authority and the Secretary of State for Health* [1991] IRLR 44.

10 *Enderby* v. *Frenchay Health Authority and Health Secretary* (C-127/92) October 1993 (ECJ) [1994] Current Law 4813, [1994] 1 All ER 495.

11 Frances Gibb 'Putting the pain into being fired' *The Times* 11 August 1998.

12 HMSO (1975) *Rehabilitation of Offenders Act 1974 (Exceptions) Order 1975* SI No. 1023.

13 Jill Sherman 'Ungagged Whistle-blowers to get legal protection' *The Times* (page 1) 26 September 1997.

14 Edward Fennell 'Now for the summer of teasing changes' *The Times* (page 37) 14 July 1998.

15 Department of Trade and Industry (May 1998) *Fairness at Work*. Stationery Office, London.

16 DoH (1997) *The New NHS: Modern Dependable*. HMSO, London.

17 CSP Professional Affairs Department Information Paper No. 36 (no date) *Clinical guidelines: Reference list*. CSP, London.

18 CSP Professional Affairs Department (1995) *Protocols Pack: An introduction to developing clinical protocols for Chartered Physiotherapists*. CSP, London.

19 Hurwitz, B. (1998) *Clinical Guidelines and the Law*. Radcliffe Medical Press, Oxford.

20 CSP Professional Affairs Department (1995) *Purchasing Physiotherapy: Information for General Practitioners and Fundholding Practice Managers*. CSP, London and see *In Touch* Winter 1995, 74, 38–40.

21 *Getting Involved and Making a Difference: Purchasing and the Professions Allied to Medicine* published by Department of Health gives examples of service level agreements. 1996/7 no date given.

22 CSP Professional Affairs Department (1995) Information Paper No. 28 (August 1995) *Patterns of Health Care Delivery: Managed Care*. CSP, London.

23 Chesson, R., Macleod, M. & Massie, S. (1996) Outcome Measures Used in Therapy Departments in Scotland. *Physiotherapy* **82**, 12, 673–9.

24 CSP Professional Affairs Department (1995) *Outcomes Pack: An introduction to implementing outcomes of care for Chartered Physiotherapists*. CSP, London.

25 Minns, C. & Bithell, C. Muscoskeletal Physiotherapy in GP Fundholding Practices. *Physiotherapy* **84**, 2, 84–92.

26 Jones, R.J. (ed.) (1991) *Management in Physiotherapy*. Radcliffe Medical Press in conjunction with CSP, Oxford.

27 CSP Professional Affairs Department (1997) *Clinical interests and occupational groups*. CSP, London.

Chapter 18
Community Care

In the last chapter we looked at the legal issues which arise in relation to employment law and at the organisation of care within the NHS. In this chapter we look at the legal issues arising from physiotherapy practice in the community, whether the physiotherapist is working for health care trusts or (very infrequently) the social services. The community role of physiotherapists has increased enormously over the past decade and most trusts providing community services would now have physiotherapy services in the community. Since 1993 major changes have resulted from the community care legislation with which the community physiotherapist should be familiar. This chapter considers the effect of these developments upon the role of the physiotherapist and the legal issues which can arise in community care.

Topics considered are:

- The community physiotherapist
- Community care changes
- Assessments
- Community care plans
- Long-term care and NHS/social services responsibilities
- Residential and nursing home provision
- Inspection
- Legal concerns of the community physiotherapist
- Conclusions

Reference should be made to Chapter 15 for equipment issues, to Chapter 16 for transport issues, to Chapter 19 for private practice and to Chapters 20, 21, 22, 23 and 24 covering individual client groups.

The community physiotherapist

'A community physiotherapist needs to have an in depth understanding of the sociological, environment and economic factors that influence peoples lives and be able to adapt their intervention accordingly. The physiotherapist should have good working relationships with primary health care, local authority, voluntary and private sector personnel in their area.'

This is set out by the Association of Chartered Physiotherapists in the

Community which has produced *Standards of Good Practice* (1995) covering the following topics:

- The role of the community physiotherapist
- Resource management (Standard 1)
- Referrals (Standard 2)
- Professional matters (Standard 3)
- Management issues (Standard 4)
- Human resources (Standards 5, 6 and 7)
- The junior physiotherapist (Standard 8)
- The physiotherapist helper (Standard 9)
- Administrative support (Standard 10)
- Health promotion (Standard 11)
- Communication and team work (CSP Standards 1 to 6)
- Documentation (CSP Standards 8 to 10)
- Assessment/patient management (CSP Standard 11)
- Informed consent (CSP Standards 12 to 14)
- Health and safety (CSP Standard 20)
- Quality assurance (CSP Standards 21 to 25)

Multi-disciplinary work

The physiotherapist working in the community will probably find that she is working as part of a multi-disciplinary team, though the extent of team working varies considerably across the country. In mental health care community mental health teams are in some districts extremely sophisticated. The impact of the White Paper[1] which aims at enhancing primary health care and the development of local health groups should encourage more multi-disciplinary working for those suffering from physical disabilities.

The law does not recognise a concept of team liability[2]. If, therefore, a physiotherapist is given an instruction from the team that she finds unacceptable professionally, she would have a duty to inform the team of the reasons why the instruction clashed with her professional duties. To say in a civil action for compensation 'I was obeying the instructions of the team' would not constitute a valid defence.

If the physiotherapist is appointed a key worker it is essential that she stays within her sphere of competence, and that she obtains the appropriate training and supervision if she is asked to perform activities and take on responsibilities which would not normally be seen as those of a physiotherapist.

Research and development

Under the proposals of the White Paper on the NHS, the emphasis will be on research based practice. The physiotherapist will be expected to be aware of recent research findings on clinical effectiveness and will also be expected to take part in research projects herself. Research is carried out on all aspects of physiotherapy, including work in the community.

Joanna C. Seymour and Kathleen M. Kerr[3] describe a survey carried out to investigate community based physiotherapy in the Trent Region. They conclude that the services (in 1996) were still very much in a developmental stage. However on the positive side physiotherapists in the community service were

'experienced practitioners running an efficient service, and treating a wide range of conditions in patients of both sexes and a variety of ages. Resources in terms of equipment appeared to be adequate and access to assistants reasonable, although it seems that more efficient use could be made of this resource. There is sound support network, linked to a well-established service training programme.'

They also comment on negative issues and suggest the following areas for further investigation:

● caseload analysis,
● referral documentation,
● administrative support,
● use of assistants,
● provision of paediatric physiotherapy, and
● the potential for implementation of health education/health promotion strategies.

Cherry Land (also in 1996) conducted a survey on how community physiotherapists in Cornwall used their time[4]. Her conclusions were that two thirds of the time in an average week was spent on direct patient related activity. She emphasised that, when calculating activity levels for the purpose of contract setting, local data about time use needs to be used in conjunction with realistic estimates of 'on-duty hours' and 'patient input hours' which take account of annual leave, sick leave, study leave and the need to provide cover for absent colleagues. Action to maximise the efficiency of the service in question should also play a part; for example time can be wasted in the physiotherapist having to go back to referrers to obtain adequate clinical information.

Cherry Land warned of the danger of using the data recorded as the sole basis on which to calculate activity levels and this point was followed up by Janet Cross[5] with evidence of two audits of time spent by community physiotherapists based at the Radcliffe Infirmary Oxford. The results were very similar to Cornwall with the activities in descending order of time taken being:

● 'face to face'
● patient support
● travel
● administration
● study and teaching.

Such information is essential in showing the effect of having rotating staff and the need to train new staff to think in terms of community physiotherapy as a specialised service. It is also needed to establish norms of work patterns and to develop costings for the service.

Pauline Pope evaluated the management of the physical condition of people with chronic and severe neurological disabilities living in the community[6]. She extended the physiotherapy services offered at a day centre to include such a management programme encompassing the home environment. She concluded that physical management is not always possible, practicable or acceptable in patients' homes. Disabled people in the community need more rather than less regular access to specialist centres, particularly when physical management is not established at home. She also concluded that disabled people requiring specialist equipment are not best served by the current procurement system.

Community care changes

The Griffiths report

Debate on the value of developing community care goes back to the late 1950s and 1960s and progress was made to a limited extent in reducing the size of long-stay NHS institutions, both for the mentally disturbed and for the elderly. The greatest impetus to the more recent changes however was the report prepared by Sir Roy Griffiths.

In December 1986 the then Secretary of State, Norman Fowler, asked Sir Roy Griffiths, who had undertaken the report into hospital management, to undertake a review of community care policy. His terms of reference were as follows:

'To review the way in which public funds are used to support community care policy and to advise . . . on the options for action that would improve the use of these funds as a contribution to more effective community care.'

In addition he was instructed

'that the review should be brief and geared towards advice on action as was the review of management in the health service in 1983.'

The report was presented in February 1988. In his letter of response to the Government Sir Roy Griffiths made some radical suggestions which were initially not enthusiastically received. His main recommendations are summarised in Figure 18.1.

***Figure 18.1* Summary of Griffiths recommendations.**

- Strengthening and clarifying the role of central government.
- Clarifying the role of local social services authorities in assessing needs, developing local priorities and determining priorities.
- Transferring to local authorities the responsibility for funding residential and nursing home accommodation for those unable to pay.
- Enhancing the role of health authorities in the provision of medically required community health services and their role in the assessment of needs.

Basically the recommendations were for a radical change in the funding of accommodation in the community and greater emphasis on clear lines of managerial accountability. Provision in future had to be on the basis of an assessment of need and the development of local plans, drawn up by the local authorities in conjunction with health authorities and the voluntary sector.

White Paper

In November 1989 a White Paper was published, *Caring for People: Community Care in the next decade and beyond*[7]. Figure 18.2 sets out the key objectives of the White Paper's proposals.

Figure 18.2   Objectives of White Paper *Caring for People.*

(1)   To promote the development of domiciliary, day and respite services to enable people to live in their own homes wherever feasible and sensible.

(2)   To ensure that service providers make practical support for carers a high priority.

(3)   To make proper assessment of need and good care management the cornerstone of high quality care.

(4)   To promote the development of a flourishing independent sector alongside good quality public services.

(5)   To clarify the responsibilities of agencies and so make it easier to hold them to account for their performance.

(6)   To secure better value for taxpayers' money by introducing a new funding structure for social care.

The White Paper explained how these objectives would be met in practice and outlined the roles and responsibilities of the social services authorities and also those of the health services. Emphasis was placed upon quality control and achieving high standards of care, collaborative working and service for people with a mental illness. It also considered the issue of resources and the links with social security. Separate chapters cover Wales and Scotland.

The NHS and Community Care Act 1990

Many of the recommendations of the White Paper were incorporated in the NHS and Community Care Act 1990. The main provisions of this Act in relation to community are listed in Figure 18.3.

Figure 18.3   The community care provisions of the NHS and Community Care Act 1990.

Section 46(3): Statutory definition of community care

Sections 42 to 45: The provision of accommodation and welfare services, charges for accommodation and the recovery of charges provided by local authorities

Section 46: The provision of a community care plan by each local authority

Section 47: Assessment of needs for community care services

Section 48: Inspection of premises used for provision of community care services

Section 49: Transfer of staff from health service to local authorities

Section 50: Power of Secretary of State to give directions and instruct local authorities to set up complaints procedures

Section 51 to 58: Provisions for Scotland

It should be noted that Section 7 of the Local Government Social Services Act 1970 requires a local authority to act under the guidance of the Secretary of State in exercising its social services functions.

Community care services

Section 46(3) provides the first statutory definition of community care services and it is given in Figure 18.4.

***Figure 18.4* The NHS and Community Care Act 1990 – section 46(3).**

'Community care services' means services which a local authority may provide or arrange to be provided under any of the following provisions—

(a)   Part III of the National Assistance Act 1948 [provision of accommodation for those over 18 who need it because of age, illness disability or any other circumstances];

(b)   section 45 of the Health Services and Public Health Act 1968 [covers arrangements for promoting the welfare of 'old people'];

(c)   section 21 of and Schedule 8 to the National Health Service Act 1977 [the provision of services for the care of mothers and young children; prevention, care and after-care; home help and laundry facilities];

(d)   section 117 of the Mental Health Act 1983 [the duty of the health authority and local social services authority to provide, in co-operation with relevant voluntary agencies, after care services for any person who has been detained under specified sections of the Mental Health Act 1983].

Three main topics in the community care provisions will be considered in the first part of this chapter: the duty to assess, the duty to prepare community care plans, and the care management approach.

Assessments

Statutory provision

Section 47 of the NHS and Community Care Act 1990 places upon the local authority a duty to carry out an assessment for any individual who would appear to be eligible to have its services.

The assessment is of the 'needs' of the individual for these services and it is on the results of the assessment that the local authority decides whether those needs call for the provision of services. There are, however, emergency provisions in section 47(5) and (6) enabling urgent needs to be met temporarily without the formality of a prior assessment.

Disabled persons

There is a statutory requirement (section 47(2)) upon local authorities to proceed under the Disabled Persons (Services, Consultation and Representation) Act 1986 if, at any time during the assessment of needs, it appears that the client is a disabled person. They need not wait for a request from the client but must inform him that they will be doing so and inform him of his rights under the 1986 Act (see Chapter 20).

Section 47(7) states that the section is 'without prejudice' to section 3 of the Disabled Persons (Services, Consultation and Representation) Act 1986. This means that it does not affect the provisions of the 1986 Act which exist in parallel with the provisions for giving information under the 1990 Act. 'Disabled person' has the same meaning as that used in the 1986 Act.

Involvement of health and housing authorities

Under section 47(3)(a) the local authority must notify the relevant health authority if, at any time during the assessment, it appears that the person may need services provided under the National Health Service Act 1977.

Under section 47(3)(b) a similar provision exists if there is seen to be a need for the provision of any services which fall within the functions of a local housing authority.

In such circumstances the local authority has a duty not only to notify the health authority and/or housing authority but also to invite them to assist, to such extent as is reasonable in the circumstances, in the making of the assessment. In making a decision as to the provision of the services needed for the person in question, the local authority shall take into account any services which are likely to be made available for him by the health authority or housing authority.

Central government directions and guidance

The Secretary of State has the power to make directions relating to assessments (section 47(4)). Subject to this the local authority shall carry out the assessment in such manner and take such form as it considers appropriate.

Guidance has been issued to local and other authorities for use in carrying out the assessments, *Caring for People: Community Care in the next decade and beyond; Policy guidance*[8]. In addition the Social Services Inspectorate has prepared several handbooks on guidance in care management and assessment for managers and practitioners.

Entitlement to assessment

Entitlement is not defined in the section other than in terms of eligibility to service provision. This is determined by residence.

■ Could it be argued that if the local authority does not provide specific services then the assessment for those services need not be carried out?

The term 'any person for whom they may provide or arrange for the provision of community services' (section 47(11)) covers all those services under the Acts specified in section 46(3) which defines what is meant by community care services. The fact that the local authority does not supply all the services the client may require cannot be a justification for not carrying out the assessment. After all it could be argued that until the assessment has been carried out it cannot be certain which services the client will or will not require.

The duty to assess is owed to those who are ordinarily resident within the local authority area. Guidance on the possibility of making arrangements with other local authorities for the provision of services stresses the need to take into account the desirability of providing services in the locality.

Carrying out the assessment

Stages in the process

The summary of practice guidance included in both the *Manager's Guide*[9] and the *Practitioner's Guide*[10] sets out the stages which should be followed in implementing the care management and assessment process. These stages are shown in Figure 18.5.

Figure 18.5   Care management and assessment process.

stage 1: Information to carers and prospective clients on needs for which the agencies accept responsibilities and the range of services currently available.

stage 2: The level of the assessment required is decided.

stage 3: A practitioner is allocated to assess the needs of the individual and of any carers.

stage 4: The resources available from statutory, voluntary, private or community sources that best meet the individual's requirements are considered. The role of the practitioner is to assist the user in making choices from these resources and to put together an individual care plan.

stage 5: The implementation of the plan, i.e. securing the necessary financial or other identified resources.

stage 6: Monitoring of implementation of the care plan.

stage 7: Review of the care plan with the user, carers and service providers; firstly, to ensure that services remain relevant to needs and, secondly, to evaluate services as part of the continuing quest for improvement.

Levels of assessment

The *Practitioner's Guide* suggests that stage one requires an initial identification of the need and the determination of the level of assessment required. For example it sets out six possible levels of assessment:

- *level one* simple assessment
- *level two* limited assessment
- *level three* multiple assessment
- *level four* specialist assessment either simple or complex
- *level five* complex assessment
- *level six* comprehensive assessment

An example of an outcome from a level one assessment is a bus pass or disabled car badge. An example of an outcome from a level six assessment could be family therapy, substitute care or intensive domiciliary support.

Differing perceptions of need

The assessment of need is described in the *Practitioner's Guide* as being undertaken to 'understand an individual's needs, to relate them to agency policies and priorities, and to agree the objectives for any intervention'.

The practitioner is required by the guidance 'to define, as precisely as possible, the cause of any difficulty'. It recognises that need is unlikely to be perceived and defined in the same way by users, their carers, and any other care agencies involved. It suggests that:

'the practitioner must, therefore, aim for a degree of consensus but, so long as they are competent, the users' views should carry the most weight. Where it is impossible to reconcile different perceptions, these differences should be acknowledged and recorded...'

Who carries out the assessment?

There is an emphasis on a multi-disciplinary approach to the task of assessment with local authorities bringing in relevant professionals where necessary. The White Paper, *Caring for People: Community Care in the next decade and beyond* suggests:

'**3.25** All agencies and professions involved with the individual and his or her problems should be brought into the assessment procedure when necessary. These may include social workers, GPs, community nurses, hospital staff such as consultants in geriatric medicine, psychiatry, rehabilitation and other hospital specialties, nurses, physiotherapists, occupational therapists, speech therapists, continence advisers, community psychiatric nurses, staff involved with vision and hearing impairment, housing officers, the Employment Department's Settlement Officers and its Employment Rehabilitation Service, home helps, home care assistants and voluntary workers.

3.26 Assessments should take account of the wishes of the individual and his or her carer, and of the carer's ability to continue to provide care, and where possible should include their active participation. Effort should be made to offer flexible services which enable individuals and carers to make choices.'

Where the client is in hospital then the lead agency for carrying out the assessment will be the health services; where the client is in the community or in residential accommodation then the lead agency for carrying out the assessment will be the local authority.

What if the client refuses to co-operate in the assessment?

It would seem that there is a duty under section 47(1)(a) of the 1990 Act for the assessment to be made even if the client refuses. Clearly, however, this may lead to a less than satisfactory assessment and any later objection by the client to the assessment should take account of this lack of co-operation. Where the client is incapable of assisting in the assessment, e.g. as a result of mental disability, the co-operation of relatives, carers or other representatives should be sought. The Law Commission's recommendations on decision making on behalf of the mentally incapacitated adult should, when implemented, fill this vacuum. A consultation paper *Who Decides* was issued in December 1997. (see Chapters 22 and 24).

The physiotherapist and the assessment

In hospital
The physiotherapist is more likely to be involved in a health care led assessment, especially when the patient is being assessed prior to discharge from hospital. It is essential that the physiotherapist is able to take a full part in this multi-disciplinary process. She should also ensure that she records her assessment and the outcome.

Situation: Report ignored

> Prior to the discharge of a stroke victim, a physiotherapist carries out an assessment on the patient, together with an analysis of the carer's ability to cope with the patient at home. She recommends further in-patient care for the patient. To her surprise the Consultant ignores her report and states that the patient should be discharged that day.

This is becoming an increasingly common problem as the pressure on beds, especially during the winter months, leads to early discharges. All the physiotherapist can do in this situation is:

● ensure that her report has been seen by all relevant parties and in particular the Consultant;
● take all reasonable steps to provide support for the patient and carer in the community through liaison with social services, occupational therapy and other relevant departments;
● make arrangements to visit the patient if appropriate; and
● ensure that her records reflect the action which she has taken.

In the community
From April 1990 General Practitioners have had, as part of their terms of service, the duty to carry out an annual assessment of every patient on their list who is aged 75 years or more. This work is increasingly delegated to practice nurses but there is no reason why physiotherapists should not take a greater responsibility in the assessment of these groups.

Review of continuing care decisions

Each health authority in conjunction with local authorities and other agencies is required to establish a procedure for reviewing decisions in relation to the provision of continuing care. Guidance was published in 1995[11]. It sets out a recommended review procedure to be established in the context of high quality discharge policies based on proper assessment and the provision of all relevant information and sensitivity to the needs and concerns of patients and their families. The working of the review procedures has been monitored as part of the overall evaluation of the community care provisions (see below).

Community Care (Direct Payments) Act 1996

On 1 April 1997 the Community Care (Direct Payments) Act came into force which enables social services departments to make payments in cash instead of kind to certain groups in receipt of community care. This enables a person to purchase their own care. However the local authority retains its discretion and cannot be compelled to offer cash rather than services. The level of payment must be sufficient to enable the recipient to buy the services the payments are intended to cover.

Situation: Protecting the public purse

A physiotherapist helps parent/carers to apply to the Social Fund for a chair for their adult son, in order to aid maintenance of a good posture. The Social Fund agree and a cheque is sent to the parents. When the physiotherapist makes inquiries about the chair she discovers that, as it was Christmas time, the money has been used for other purposes. What action should she take? Does she have a duty to inform the Social Services?

The simple answer to the last question is 'No'. It is not her responsibility to ensure that Social Fund moneys are used for the purpose they have been allocated. She has no duty to inform the DSS. However, since the client is still without the chair, she could encourage the family to try and save up for it since, without it, the client's condition will deteriorate.

Assessment of carers

The Carers (Recognition and Services) Act 1995 which came into force on 1 April 1996 places a duty on local authorities to provide for the assessment of the ability of carers to provide care and for connected purposes. The basic provisions are shown in Figure 18.6.

Figure 18.6 **Carers (Recognition and Services) Act 1995 – section 1(1).**

[I]n any case where—

(a) a local authority carries out an assessment under section 47(1)(a) of the [1990] Act of the needs of a person ('the relevant person') for community care services, and

(b) an individual ('the carer') provides or intends to provide a substantial amount of care on a regular basis for the relevant person,

the carer may request the local authority, before they make their decision as to whether the needs of the relevant person call for the provision of any services, to carry out an assessment of his ability to provide and to continue to provide care for the relevant person; and if he makes such a request, the local authority shall carry out such an assessment and shall take into account the results of that assessment in making that decision.

The duty to assess the carer on request also applies where the local authority makes an assessment of the needs of a disabled child for the purposes of Part III of the Children Act 1989 or section 2 of the Chronically Sick and Disabled

Persons Act 1970 and a carer provides or intends to provide a substantial amount of care on a regular basis for the disabled child or person.

Excluded from those carers entitled to be assessed are those providing care by virtue of a contract of employment or other contract with any person, or as a volunteer for a voluntary organisation.

It is too early to evaluate the effect of this statutory duty to assess the carer. Inevitably the value of such a provision will to a considerable extent depend upon the resources provided to assist the carer. There are many concerns raised about the support which should be provided for carers, the lack of respite beds and the fact that where such respite provision is made by local authorities it is on a means tested basis. Yet it is clear that unless respite is made available many carers will not be able to continue for so long caring for a person at home.

Stress management for carers is discussed by Susan Gregory[12] who describes the setting up and running of a stress management group designed for people who are caring for an elderly confused person at home. She shows the value that the participants placed upon the sessions but

> 'from the facilitator's point of view it was difficult to know where to set the boundaries for a session. The sessions need to find a point somewhere between a "chat" and a defined psychotherapeutic structure for them to be effective.'

The group also provided valuable insight into the nature of caring at home, what causes most stress, and what needs are unfulfilled.

The Princess Royal has established an Association for Carers (see Address List).

Chapter 10 is relevant to legal issues relating to the carer's liability in negligence.

Community care plans

Section 46 of the 1990 Act requires each local authority to prepare and publish a plan for the provision of community care in their area. The section also requires the local authority to keep the plan, and any further plans prepared by them under this section, under review and empowers the Secretary of State to direct the intervals at which the local authority must prepare and publish modifications to the current plan or a new plan.

Consultation

There are statutory duties under section 46(2) for the local authority to consult the following organisations:

- any health authority whose district overlaps the area of the local authority
- every local housing authority in the area (where relevant) which is not the local authority itself
- voluntary organisations representing the interests of users or potential users of community care services within the area or the interests of private carers within that area

- voluntary housing agencies and other bodies providing housing or community care services in their area
- such other persons as the Secretary of State may direct.

A direction has been made that there should be consultation with the independent sector (see below).

Definitions of each of these terms are given and 'private carer' is defined as a person who is not employed to provide care in question by any body in the exercise of its function under any enactment.

Directions on Consultation were issued by the Secretary of State for Health on 25 January 1993 and for the Welsh Office on 22 February 1993. The Directions are intended to ensure that there is full and proper consultation between local authorities and independent sector providers on community care plans by requiring local authorities to consult with organisations which have declared themselves as representing independent sector providers. The second direction requires that local authorities state in their plans the arrangements for consulting all those parties with a statutory right to be consulted.

Initial policy guidance on the preparation of community care plans was given in *Caring for People: Community Care in the next decade and beyond; Policy Guidance*[13]. This advised local authorities on:

- the statutory requirements to consult in the planning process;
- the statutory requirements for publishing plans;
- the arrangements for monitoring plans; and
- the scope and content of Social Services Department plans.

The physiotherapist and the community care plans

These community care plans are central to the effective development of community care in partnership with all relevant statutory, voluntary and independent organisations. If carefully revised and monitored they can highlight any deficiency or surplus in the provision and ensure that the assessed needs of clients are being met. It is therefore essential that the physiotherapist should have a significant role in the preparation and revision of these plans and ensure that weaknesses which she is aware of in the provision of community care services are brought to the attention of those responsible for finalising the plans.

Monitoring of community care provision

The Audit Office and the Department of Health itself are continually monitoring the effects and implementation of the community care programme. Thus in 1995 a report was published on the national exercises carried out in 1994 on the community care monitoring[14]. The overall view was that there was evidence of a need for considerable progress to be made in a number of areas in order to deliver the full benefits of the new community care arrangements for users and carers. This is in accord with the findings of MENCAP which reported negatively in 1995 on the practice of care management and assessment for people with learning disabilities[15].

Long term care and NHS/social services responsibilities

The ideal of the 'seamless service'

In the Parliamentary debates on the community care provisions of the 1990 Act much emphasis was placed upon the need to secure a seamless provision of services from one organisation to another. Considerable difficulties however arose in the implementation of a seamless service and in ensuring close co-operation and collaboration between the various providers.

One difficulty was that of defining where the NHS statutory duty to provide ends and the statutory duty of the local authority begins. Whilst local arrangements could resolve many disputes, the fact that the NHS care must be provided free at the point of delivery (unless there is specific statutory provision, as with prescription charges) but that most social services can be means tested means that the distinction is extremely important from the client or patient's point of view.

There have been several cases brought before the Health Service Commissioner about the failures of health authorities to make provision for the continuing care needs of their patients. The Department of Health and Welsh Office issued advice setting the principles on which continuing care should be provided by the different statutory authorities. Each local authority was asked to prepare, in conjunction with the health authority and voluntary groups, local eligibility policies for continuing care.

Uneven provision

Situation: The right to live at home?

> Ben is paraplegic, being cared for in hospital, but wants to return home. His wife would be happy for him to be nursed at home. The health authority has said that the costs of caring for him at home would be four times the cost of his remaining in hospital and have refused. Residential accommodation has been offered to him. Ben learns that in a neighbouring health authority area, a patient with a similar condition has been allowed home. What is the law?

Unfortunately, although we have an NHS, there is a lack of uniformity of provision across the country and resources dictate the services which are available to local residents. In theory, Ben could seek judicial review of the refusal of the HA to provide the facilities for his home care. However on the basis of previous judicial decisions[16] (see Chapter 6), he is unlikely to succeed unless he can show that the health authority has failed to follow DoH guidance in providing the home facilities[17].

Future developments

Major changes are anticipated in the working together of health and social services. In an announcement on 16 September 1998[18], the health ministers stated that health and social services authorities were to be allowed to pool resources to provide integrated services. A Consultation document *Partnership in Action* was published with the intention that, following legislation, by April 2000 authorities would be able to delegate one as a lead commissioner to take overall responsibility.

Many commentators are agreed that as long as there is a distinction between the authorities in terms of payment, it is essential to have national criteria on the responsibilities of each, so that an individual in one part of the country does not obtain free a service which a person in another part of the country has to pay for.

Residential and nursing home provision

Physiotherapy input into the residential care sector can be very important. Accommodation is governed by the Registered Homes Act 1984 and further details can be found in other specialist books[19]. Jennifer Duthie and Rosemary Chesson[20] describe the results of research carried out on physiotherapy in private nursing homes in the Grampian Region of Scotland and showed that, although a high percentage of residents were found to have neurological and musculoskeletal conditions, in some homes there had been no physiotherapy in the six months prior to the investigation. This compared unfavourably to the physiotherapy input into the long-stay hospital wards in Aberdeen General Hospitals where physiotherapy was regularly available as part of a multi-disciplinary approach to care.

The authors emphasise the importance of planning a regular service.

'Intensive physiotherapy might then be a realistic option, especially for residents returning to a home after a hospital admission.'

A regular service would also facilitate early intervention. This regular service could be provided on an outreach basis from a specialised hospital base or a community care team could be developed with time set aside for visiting private nursing homes that would not be compromised by competing demands.

Significant recommendations to improve standards are put forward in the White Paper on modernising social services[21].

Inspection

Local Authorities have long had responsibility under the Registered Homes Act 1984 for inspecting residential care homes. These duties in respect of inspection were extended under the NHS and Community Care Act 1990. Health Authorities are responsible for registration and inspection of nursing homes and mental nursing homes under the 1984 Act.

Inspection units

Inspection Units Directions issued in 1990 required every local authority to establish an inspection unit. This inspection unit has an obligation to inspect:

- residential accommodation provided by the local authority under sections 21 and 26 of Part III of the National Assistance Act 1948 and under Schedule 8 of the National Health Service Act 1977; and

- residential accommodation within the area of the local authority which is required to be registered under Part I of the Registered Homes Act 1984 (residential homes), and any records kept pursuant to that Act.

In addition every local authority is required to establish an advisory committee to advise on the operation of the inspection unit. Membership of the advisory committee is determined by the local authority.

Since 1991 the directions have been extended to apply to community homes and registered children's homes within the meaning of the Children Act 1989.

Guidance

The policy guidance on community care required local authorities to carry out such inspections in a consistent and even-handed manner in respect of services in local authority, private and voluntary sectors. Guidance covered structure, accountability, staffing, collaboration with Health Authorities, and working practices. The Directions do not preclude the possibility of the use of agency arrangements but the making of agency arrangements will not release any local authority from its responsibility to comply with the Directions.

The Social Service Inspectorate of the Department of Health was given the task of monitoring the progress of inspection units, and further steps are now being taken in line with the Citizen's Charter to ensure independence, openness and lay involvement of the inspectorate.

Inspection advisory panels

These were originally recommended but left to the local authority to determine. The requirement now is that the number of places given to lay people is at least equal to the number of places given to service providers, including the officers mainly or wholly concerned with the provision of services. It is not intended that these advisory panels should have executive powers and the *Guidance*[22] states that where these advisory committees have been set up as sub-committees under section 4 of the Local Authority Social Services Act 1970 or section 102 of the Local Government Act 1972 they should be reconstituted on less formal lines. They should choose their own chairmen and the appointment should be for a fixed term, and made from among the provider, lay or consumer members of the group. The panel should meet at least twice a year.

Inspection reports

These should be clear, objective and accurate; they should avoid jargon and wherever possible contain a succinct summary of findings and recommendations. The inspection advisory panel should be given the opportunity to comment on the unit's annual report, before that report is presented to the Social Services Committee.

Follow up of inspection reports

Local authorities should have in place policy guidelines which explain how recommendations made in inspection reports on directly provided care homes will be acted upon. The policy statement should set out:

- who is responsible for following up the reports to ensure that any required action is taken on the recommendations;
- the time limits for follow-up action; and
- how the adequacy of the response to the reports is to be monitored.

Chief Executive's annual report

This must contain an assessment covering the work of the inspection unit and of the social services department's response to inspection reports on the services which it manages[23].

The future of inspection

A Consultation document was issued in 1995[24] which discusses different models for the organisational structure of regulation and inspection, including self-regulation by provider groups. The Labour Government has announced proposals to set up independent inspection of social services and of residential homes[25]. A White Paper has been published with proposals for a new Social Council of Care to regulate all workers in residential care and nursing homes. A Code of Practice will be published to cover all home helps and domiciliary workers. Independent regional inspectorates will be appointed to monitor both private and local authority homes.

Legal concerns of the community physiotherapist

No witnesses

One concern of physiotherapists working in the community, is that, if they visit homes on their own and they are falsely accused of theft or assault or another offence, then they are unlikely to have any witnesses to support them. In this situation it must be remembered (see Chapter 2) that in any prosecution it must be proved beyond all reasonable doubt that the accused is guilty. This will be difficult if there is no evidence against the physiotherapist other than the word of the client against that of the physiotherapist. If the physiotherapist is aware from the client's attitude that false accusations could be brought against her, then she should discuss with her manager being accompanied by another person or a colleague taking over that case.

Mileage and expenses

What if the employer accuses the physiotherapist of a fraudulent claim? The physiotherapist should be able to prove from her records and her diary, the length and time of each journey she has made to establish her innocence of the charge. She should keep a copy of each claim form she submits to the finance department for mileage and other expenses. If in practice for herself she will need to keep such records for tax purposes.

Health and safety

The physiotherapist who visits in the community will be entering onto premises which are not under the control or occupation of her employer. If therefore she suffers harm because of the condition of the premises, she would not be able to obtain compensation from her employer. She would be dependent upon the occupier having the funds or insurance cover (see Chapter 11).

It is therefore advisable for physiotherapists who visit in the community to have private accident insurance or check with their professional association that they are covered for such accidents. The CSP Industrial Relations Department has issued briefing papers on *Health and Safety*[26] and *Violence at work*[27].

Concern over elder abuse

There is growing awareness now of the extent of abuse of the elderly in the community. Unfortunately at present, there is no legislation comparable to the Children Act 1989 under which an elderly person or other mentally incompetent adult could be taken to a place of safety. The National Assistance Act 1948 enables a person to be taken to a place of safety on public health grounds (see Chapter 24) but this would probably not cover the possibility of more subtle abuse. The Law Commission[28] in 1995 recommended that there should be a statutory structure to make decisions for mentally incompetent adults and to care for them, but their proposals have not yet been given statutory force. The physiotherapist who suspected that a patient was being abused, would wish to seek the advice of social services and also of the health visitor to ensure that all reasonable action was taken to protect the elderly person.

Conclusions

It is probably still too soon to determine the effect of the community care programme and post 1990 developments on the role and identity of the physiotherapist. Nevertheless government policy is itself changing and as early as February 1996 the Secretary of State for Health Stephen Dorrell[29] referred to the need to use a term such as 'spectrum of care' rather than community care in discussing the provision of services for mentally ill persons who would originally have been cared for in institutions.

The Labour Government elected in 1997 have stated that the policy of care in the community has failed and at the time of writing (September 1998) are intending to publish new plans for health and social services. It must be pointed out, however, that talk of failure in community care relates, if at all, to those suffering from mental illness where too hasty a discharge from in-patient care or inability to admit early enough has caused considerable concern, suffering and, on some occasions, death. Community care, in its wider meaning of all non in-patient care, covers a much wider group than the mentally ill and for these people there are considerable benefits in having support to continue to live in the community.

 ## Questions and exercises _____

1 What impact has the NHS and Community Care Act 1990 had upon your practice? Are there any disadvantages which you can remedy?

2 An NHS physiotherapist carried out an assessment for a ventilated patient

being discharged to his home and prescribes certain equipment. She also considers that certain adaptations are necessary in the home. She then discovers that her recommendation has been changed by a disability officer employed by social services who is not a registered occupational therapist or registered physiotherapist. What action, if any, should she take?

3 Community care plans must be revised annually. What part should the physiotherapist play in the preparation of the plan and its revision?

4 What do you consider are the advantages to physiotherapy practice in the establishment of primary care trusts?

References

1 DoH (1997) *The New NHS: Modern Dependable.* HMSO, London.
2 *Wilshire* v. *Essex Health Authority* (CA) [1986] 3 All ER 801.
3 Seymour, J.C. & Kerr, K.M. (1996) Community Based Physiotherapy in the Trent Region: A Survey. *Physiotherapy* **82**, 9, 514–20.
4 Land, C. (1996) A Survey of How Community Physiotherapists Use their Time. *Physiotherapy* **82**, 4, 222–6.
5 Cross, J. (1996) *Letter to the editor: Audit for Community Physiotherapy. Physiotherapy* **82**, 7, 439.
6 Pope, P. (1997) Management of the physical condition in people with chronic and severe neurological disabilities living in the community. *Physiotherapy* **83**, 3, 116–22.
7 DoH (1989) *Caring for People: Community Care in the next decade and beyond.* Command Paper, 849. HMSO, London.
8 DoH (1990) *Caring for People: Community Care in the next decade and beyond; Policy and guidance.* HMSO, London.
9 DoH (1991) *Care Management and Assessment: Managers' Guide.* HMSO, London.
10 DoH (1990) *Care Management and Assessment: Practitioner's Guide.* HMSO, London.
11 HSG(95)39; LAC(95)17.
12 Gregory, S. (1991) Stress Management for Carers. *British Journal of Occupational Therapy* **54**, 11, 427–9.
13 DoH (1990) *Caring for People: Community Care in the next decade and beyond; Policy Guidance.* (pp 13–20) HMSO, London.
14 EL(95)39 and CI(95)7.
15 MENCAP (1995) *Britain's other Lottery: A report on the practice of Care Management and Assessment for people with learning disabilities.* MENCAP, London.
16 *R* v. *Secretary of State for Social Services, ex parte Hincks and others.* reported in *Solicitors Journal* 29 June 1979, 436.
17 *R* v. *North Derbyshire Health Authority, ex parte Fisher* [1997] 8 Med LR 327.
18 Mark Henderson, 'One-stop shop for care' *The Times* 17 September 1998.
19 Dimond, B. (1996) *The Legal Aspects of Care in the Community.* Macmillan, Basingstoke.
20 Duthie, J. & Chesson, R. (1996) Physiotherapy in Private Nursing Homes *Physiotherapy* **82**, 10, 566–72.
21 DoH (1998) *Modernising Social Services.* Cmnd 4169 1998, DoH, London.
22 DoH (1990) *Caring for People: Community Care in the next decade and beyond; Policy Guidance.* HMSO, London.
23 Annex A LAC(94)16, *Inspection Unit Directions 1994.*

24 DoH and Welsh Office (1995) *Moving Forward: A Consultation Document on the Regulation and Inspection of Social Services* DoH, London.

25 Jill Sherman 'Dobson will set standards for residential homes' *The Times*, 26 September 1998.

26 CSP Industrial Relations Department, Briefing Paper No. 7 (in: Stewards Handbook Part II) *Health and Safety*. CSP, London.

27 CSP Industrial Relations Department, Briefing Paper No. 2 (in: Safety Representatives Briefing Papers) *Violence At Work*. CSP, London.

28 Law Commission (1995) No. 231 *Mentally Incapacitated Adults* HMSO, London.

29 Dominic Kennedy 'Dorrell drops the term "care in the community".' *The Times*, 21 February 1996.

Chapter 19
The Physiotherapist as a Private Practitioner

An increasing number of physiotherapists are deciding to work as self-employed independent contractors and there is every likelihood that this number will grow as NHS Trusts, practitioners, other health service bodies, social services authorities and groups such as charitable organisations and private health care providers have the capacity to contract with self-employed individuals for services.

This chapter covers the following topics:

- Variety of contracting partners and CSP guidance
- Legal issues for the self-employed
- Running a business
- Accountability and the private practitioner
- Essential contract law
- The practitioner and health and safety
- Professional issues
- Private practice and the NHS
- Areas of concern
- Conclusion

Variety of contracting partners and CSP guidance

Figure 19.1 shows some of the different contracting partners for the physiotherapist who works as an independent contractor.

Figure 19.1 **Contracts and the private practitioner.**

- with private patients
- with NHS Trusts
- with health authorities
- with fund holding GPs
- with private hospitals
- with residential and nursing homes
- with agencies
- with local authorities
- with charities
- with solicitors

The Professional affairs Department of the CSP has issued guidance for private practitioners[1] which is considered where appropriate below. The Organisation of Chartered Physiotherapists in Private Practice (OCPPP) also actively supports the work of those in private practice by providing a forum for concerns to be explored and to develop standards of practice.

Legal issues for the self-employed

There are significant legal implications in becoming a self-employed practitioner and the CSP guidance warns practitioners very clearly about the implications of leaving the NHS or the independent sector and going it alone[2]. The most obvious one is that as self-employed professionals they do not have an employer who will be vicariously liable for their actions and therefore pay out compensation arising from their negligence. Instead as self-employed, independent practitioners who offer a contract for services with others, they are personally responsible for their own negligence and also vicariously liable for any harm resulting from the negligence or other wrongful acts of their employees (if any) which are committed in the course of employment. Some of the differences are shown in Figure 19.2.

Figure 19.2   **Legal issues and the private practitioner.**

Contract for Services **not** *Contract of Employment*

- No vicarious liability (except in respect of their own employees)
- No employee rights (except for those they employ)
- No indemnity *by* another (liability *for* others)
- Personal liability for health and safety of self and others
- Liability for breach of contract

If the private practitioner is an employer she will have the responsibility of complying with the statutory duties placed upon an employer and in accepting vicarious liability for the negligence of her employees.

The relationship between the independent contractor and the contracting party is not a contract of employment but a contract for services. All the benefits which the employment legislation gives to employees (see Chapter 17) such as sick pay, time off work for specific purposes, protection against unfair dismissal and redundancy and guaranteed payments are not there for the self-employed. Serious consideration should therefore be given to taking out insurance to provide all or some of the benefits that they would receive had they employee status. In addition they cannot look to an employer for protection in relation to health and safety and should take out their own personal accident cover.

Since private practitioners have to pay personally any compensation arising out of their negligence, it is crucial that they are insured in respect of public liability and that the cover is adequate for what might be a very high claim (see Chapter 10 for typical quantum figures)

As employers themselves they must ensure that they recognise the employment rights of their employees, have relevant insurance cover and also provide all reasonable care to protect their employees' health and safety.

Running a business

Practical business issues

CSP guidance assists any practitioner who is contemplating starting in private practice[3]. It sets out what should be the initial considerations and provides advice in determining the location, finding a position in the market, setting up trading arrangements, advertising and other considerations such as tax and insurance.

It is essential to plan the business. In the first of a series of management articles in *In Touch* Lesley McCann describes how a business plan can be put together, including carrying out a SWOT (Strengths, Weaknesses, Opportunities and Threats) analysis and preparing a budget[4]. The CSP has given guidance to its members who are intending to become independent practitioners on business planning[5]. As well as covering issues such as deciding on the location of premises, and the marketing of the service and choice of business name, it also gives advice on developing a business plan and writing it up. Reference should also be made to the CSP guidance on marketing[6] which covers such topics as services, clients, contracting, competition, environment, communication targets and the review.

David Grant[7], who is both a management consultant and business manager of his wife's physiotherapy practice, suggests using the SMART analysis for planning the objectives in the business plan:

- Specific
- Measurable
- Attainable
- Realistic
- Trackable

should be the characteristics of the chosen objectives.

Ethical/professional issues

The CSP has provided guidance on the *Standards of Business Conduct*[8] covering such issues as:

- conflict of interests,
- conflict of stance/position,
- changes in employment status,
- restrictive clauses,
- incentives,
- favouritism, and
- gifts and hospitality

which apply both in employed and self-employed practice, so that the physiotherapist is beyond reproach in her professional work. In American research quoted in Chapter 1 by Herman Triezenberg[9] identified present and future ethical issues arising in physical therapy practice and noted that many of the ethical issues relate to the financial relationship between therapist and patient. It is essential that any physiotherapist embarking on private practice clarifies from the start such issues as payment and services available from the NHS without payment, and is scrupulous to avoid any temptation to exploit her professional relationship for financial reward other than the receipt of appropriate fees.

Situation: Increasing private practice

Della, a registered physiotherapist with a private practice, received a referral from the mother of a child with severe neurological problems following a road accident. Della knew that the parents were extremely wealthy and she planned a course of treatment of several sessions a week. She was aware that there was little research evidence to suggest that her treatments would be effective.

Della should discuss with the parents frankly the lack of any evidence that her proposed treatment would be clinically effective. They may be prepared to commence it on an experimental basis but provision should be made for the progress to be evaluated at reasonable intervals and the interventions reassessed.

Financial rewards should not lead to physiotherapists recommending treatments which cannot be professionally justified. The CSP gives guidance on recommended salaries and fees in private practice[10].

Tax issues

It is also essential that at the very beginning of commencing business, the physiotherapist should have an accountant to guide her in setting up a practice and the tax laws which apply. Timothy Deykin[11] describes a battle which he has had with the inland revenue, where instead of the accounts being taxed on a cash and receipt basis they are taxed on an income and expenditure basis, and the problems of being taxed for medico-legal work on income which has not yet, and may never, be received.

Partnership issues

It is essential that the practitioner takes legal advice before deciding upon the type of arrangement she should have if working with another person or persons. For example, it may seem preferable to set up a partnership so that the profits and overheads can be shared. However each partner would be responsible for the debts of the partnership even if she has not personally incurred them. Advice is provided by the CSP on trading status, copyright and patents[12], but it emphasises that a practitioner should always take legal advice in determining the legal form that the business should take.

Summary

It is essential that all the legal responsibilities of becoming an independent practitioner are taken on board. Those intending to start on business on their own should seek professional help on the areas shown in Figure 19.3.

Figure 19.3 **The private practitioner and business law.**

- Income tax/VAT
- National Insurance:
  - self
  - others
- Insurance and indemnity:
  - Personal accident cover
  - Public liability insurance
- Health and Safety regulations

- Contracts for supplies/services
- Training and development
- Employment law (for own employees)
- Data Protection
- Pensions and sickness:
  - for self
  - for employees

Formation of business
- Type of business:
  - Sole trader
  - Partnership
  - Limited company
  - Co-operative
- Name
- Protection:
  - patents
  - registered designs

- Premises:
  - Planning permission
  - Building regulations
  - The lease
- Trading laws:
  - Sale of goods and services
  - Trade Descriptions Act
  - Unfair Contract Terms Act
- Taxation and starting up:
  - Capital allowances
  - Deciding on tax year

Accountability and the private practitioner

Figure 19.4 illustrates the arenas of accountability for the private practitioners. For the most part they are similar to those of the professional who works as an employee. However instead of being accountable to an employer the private practitioner has a contract of services with a purchaser (see Figure 19.1). If there is a breach of contract then the referral is not to the industrial tribunal but to the civil courts.

Figure 19.4 **Accountability and the private practitioner.**

To the public:	criminal law including Trade Descriptions legislation
To the patient:	civil law of negligence and contract law; and Sales of Goods and Services legislation
To the purchaser:	civil law; contract for services
To the profession:	disciplinary board of the CSP and the Physiotherapy Board of the CPSM

Essential contract law

The private practitioner must have a good understanding of the law of contract. Some of the essential features of contract law are shown in Figure 19.5 and are also discussed in Chapter 17.

Figure 19.5   **Elements of contract law.**

Formulation:	invitation to treat offer and acceptance	**Breach:**	remedies for breach right of election
Contents:	fundamental terms implied terms express terms	**Termination:**	by performance by breach by agreement by notice by frustration
Performance			

Formation of contract

There may often be a lengthy period of negotiation before a contract is formed. There may for example be an opening 'invitation to treat' by the one party which is on different terms to those eventually arrived at. The contract is eventually reached where one party can be said to have made an offer (either in response to the invitation to treat or as a 'counter offer') and the other party accepts that offer. If an offer is made and the other party responds by offering alternative conditions, this is a counter offer which, if accepted by the other party constitutes the agreement and therefore the contract. The contract may not be entirely in writing. It may be partly in writing and partly by word of mouth. If, following a dispute, one party argues that additional terms discussed during negotiations became part of the contract and are therefore binding, it is a question of interpretation of what was said and any other evidence to establish what are the agreed terms of the contract.

The three essential elements to make a contract binding are:

(1)   An agreement
(2)   Consideration
(3)   An intention to create legal relations.

Consideration need not necessarily be payment of money in return for the performance of the agreement by the other side. It could be a benefit in kind or it could be an agreement releasing the other from something which they had a duty to do.

It need not necessarily equate with what the other is prepared to do. For example a physiotherapist who has a private practice may agree that, because a client is extremely short of funds but runs an aromatherapy clinic, she will forgo any payment on the understanding that she will be given two sessions of aromatherapy. On that basis the agreement is made and she provides the physiotherapy. If the aromatherapist client then goes back on that agreement she is in breach of contract. The physiotherapist has the right to seek damages for breach of contract in the civil courts. In practice she may prefer not to attract the publicity which such an action would bring.

It is important that agreement upon fees payable should be reached before treatment commences and that this agreement is put into writing.

In commercial contracts the intention to create legal relations would normally be presumed. In domestic matters, there is a presumption that there is no such intention. Where a practitioner is carrying out private work it is essential for her to make it absolutely clear that it is the intention to create a binding agreement in order to be able to enforce the contract through the courts.

Where possible the private practitioner should ensure that all the terms of the contract are put in writing to protect herself in the event of a dispute. The CSP has provided guidance on an associate agreement for self-employed staff[13] which could also be used as the basis for private practice. It sets out clearly the essential terms on which agreement must be reached before a contract can be considered to exist.

Breach of contract

If it is claimed that one party is in fundamental breach of the contract then the innocent party has the right of election. She can either elect to see the contract as at an end and seek damages, i.e. compensation for the breach of contract, or she can elect to treat the contract as continuing but seek compensation for the loss to her (financial or otherwise) of it being less than she had bargained for. It is important that the innocent party makes it clear how she chooses since, if she delays and carries on regarding the contract as subsisting, it could be said that by her conduct she has treated the contract as continuing and has therefore lost the right of election.

Termination of contract

By performance/agreement/notice
It is advisable to consider at the beginning of the contract how it should end.

- Is it for a specific number of treatments?
- Is it for a certain length of time?
- Is it for a specified number of weeks after hospital discharge?
- Can it be ended on notice by one party to the other?
- How long should that notice be?

In the absence of notice provisions in an employment contract the courts will imply a reasonable notice provision into the contract and there are statutory minimum periods. However these statutory minimum periods do not exist for contracts for services and it would be more difficult to determine what is reasonable notice.

Frustration
Frustration of contract arises when an event takes place which is right outside the contemplation of the parties when the contract was made.

Situation: A cancelled match

A physiotherapist had a contract to provide assistance at a football match. Unfortunately the match was cancelled because of very heavy snow falls. The physiotherapist claimed that she was still available to provide services and was therefore entitled to a minimum payment. The club argued that the snow frustrated the contract and therefore brought it to an end.

In this situation it would be surprising if the contractual agreement did not cover the possibility of matches being cancelled or postponed because of weather conditions and, if there are provisions covering this, then the doctrine of frustration would not apply. If however the contract is silent on such a possibility then the law of frustration would apply and the contract, because of the existence of an event which makes the performance of the contract very different than that contemplated, would come to an end by operation of law. If the physiotherapist had actually spent some time or money, e.g. had travelled to the venue for the match, then she would be able to obtain reimbursement for the work she had already undertaken. As a result of the Law Reform (Frustrated Contracts) Act 1943 generally all sums paid before the contract was frustrated are repayable and any money due to be paid but not paid before frustration ceases to be payable. However, the court will look to the justice of the situation and work done will be paid for. This Act does not apply where the contract itself makes provision for any frustrating event and it would therefore be possible for the private practitioner to include in the agreement provision defining what rights would exist were a frustrating event to occur.

What if the client refuses to pay?

Payment is the passing of consideration from the one party to the contract in return for the provision of some service. Time of payment is not normally a fundamental term unless the contract clearly makes it so. It is therefore advisable for the professional to include in the contract a term in relation to when the fee should be paid – in advance, in instalments at each session, after each session, monthly, etc. When she is negotiating with a health service body or NHS Trust there might not be much choice for her, but it is essential that she should agree this, so it is clear when there has been a breach of contract and she is entitled to commence action for recovery.

Situation: Failure to pay promptly

A physiotherapist contracted with a NHS trust for physiotherapy services to be provided for four sessions a week on the basis that payment would be made every month in arrears on completion and submission of a return certified by the unit manager. The physiotherapist duly performed the services and submitted the return but several months later was still without payment. Should she cease to work?

Failure to pay could be regarded as breach of a fundamental clause of the contract and, looking back at the section on breach of contract, it will be recalled that the innocent party therefore has the right of election, i.e. to decide whether to continue to recognise the contract as continuing or see it ended by the breach of contract. The physiotherapist could therefore see the contract as at an end and sue for the outstanding payment and damages for the breach of contract. Alternatively, if there is every likelihood that she would eventually be paid, she might well prefer to elect to see the contract as continuing and continue to perform her sessions meanwhile chasing them for the outstanding payments. Should she eventually be forced into taking legal action she could, depending upon the amount outstanding, take the case to the small claims court, to the County Court or (in theory if the sums were large enough) to the High Court. With the contract in writing and evidence of the sessions she has carried out she should obtain her payments with no valid defence being available against her.

However, if she were suing an individual rather than an organisation, the practicalities of getting the money from someone who may have no assets and no job is another matter.

Case: physiotherapy debts

In a case[14] concerning judicial separation there were many debts which the husband had not paid. These included a debt of £2050 to the physiotherapist. The husband explained that he had not paid in accordance with the undertakings because he had not got the money.

It is essential that the physiotherapist does not allow debts owed by a private individual to build up, since the dangers of non-payment increase and, as seen from the above case, could become tied up in matrimonial settlements.

A physiotherapist who provides services for a private hospital will probably do so on the basis that she has a personal contract with the patient. It is important therefore that she keeps an account of the debt and ensures early payment.

Contract law and the tort of negligence contrasted

It may be bewildering to non-lawyers that there are two overlapping duties – the duty owed to a client under the law of negligence and the duty owed to a client under the law of contract. However this is the legal situation and an aggrieved client who had suffered harm as a result of the activities of the private practitioner could sue both for breach of contract and also for breach of the duty to care at common law.

The duties are not identical, since the former derives from the contract which has been agreed between client and practitioner, including the implied terms, and the latter is set by law. It has been stated by the Court of Appeal that, where a duty of care in tort arose between the parties to a contract, wider obligations could be imposed by the duty of care in tort than those arising under the contract[15].

The practitioner and health and safety

Responsibility for others

Whilst there exists no employer who is responsible for the self-employed practitioner, she may be an employer herself and therefore have responsibilities to her employees. The duty to take reasonable care of the health and safety of the employee exists whether the employee is full or part time. She also has a duty under the health and safety legislation to take care of the safety of others who may be affected by her work and if she operates from premises which clients attend she could be liable as 'occupier' if harm befalls them as a result of a forseeable hazard (see Chapter 11).

Regulation requirements

The Management of Health and Safety at Work Regulations refer specifically to the self-employed as shown in Figure 19.6.

Figure 19.6   **Regulation 3(2) and (3) – the self-employed.**

(2) Every self-employed person shall make a suitable and sufficient assessment of—
(a)   the risks to his own health and safety to which he is exposed whilst he is at work; and
(b)   the risks to the health and safety of persons not in his employment arising out of or in connection with the conduct by him of his undertaking,
for the purpose of identifying the measures he needs to take to comply with the requirements and prohibitions imposed upon him by or under the relevant statutory provisions.

(3) Any assessment such as is referred to in paragraph (1) [employers] or (2) shall be reviewed by the employer or the self-employed person who made it if–
(a)   there is reason to suspect that it is no longer valid; or
(b)   there has been a significant change in the matters to which it relates;
and where as a result of any such review changes to an assessment are required, the employer or self-employed person concerned shall make them.

Threatened violence and self-defence

Situation: Violence in private practice

> A private practitioner, who has her own premises which clients attend, was carrying out a session when a client became extremely violent and threatening. The professional was working on her own and there was no-one who could come to her aid.

In such a situation she is entitled to use reasonable force in self-defence. What is reasonable depends upon the circumstances:

- the danger she is in and the amount of violence which she faces;
- the nature of the training she has received;
- her own size and that of her assailant; and
- the type of weapons to hand.

Where grievous bodily harm is feared, more force might be justified. Her actions should however always be defensive not aggressive.

Professional issues

Client-led practice

Situation: Unjustified demands

> A physiotherapist works as a self-employed practitioner and has a case load of clients for whom she provides services. One client is extremely demanding and is very anxious to obtain a chair lift from the social services. The physiotherapist forms the view that a lift is neither appropriate nor practicable and in fact given the client's particular circumstances could be dangerous. The physiotherapist is told by the client that unless she is prepared to support her claim their contract for services will be ended. What should the physiotherapist do?

The answer should be clear: she must abide by her professional standards and not be demand-led by the client into recommending equipment which is entirely unsuitable. The difference between the employee status and the self-employed status however is apparent. If NHS employees refuse to agree with patients on professional grounds, their employment should not be endangered. If it is the employer who is putting pressure on them to act unprofessionally then, provided they have the continuous service requirement, they could claim constructive dismissal in the industrial tribunal (see Chapter 17). However the self-employed professionals have no such protection. If they keep to their professional standards then they might lose that client and suffer economically. However there is no alternative if they wish to remain as registered professionals.

NHS refusal to purchase services

Not everyone is content with health care developments outside the National Health Service. There may for example be some practitioners who refuse to contract with private practitioners. What action can the private practitioners take? Even under the NHS following the White Paper[16], primary health care groups will have the freedom to buy services from those providers that they consider would be best for their patients. They cannot be forced to go outside the NHS nor can they be forced to stay within it. If a GP practice refuses to use the services of the private sector there is no action which can be taken other than to hope that in terms of quality and price the private service will eventually succeed in providing services to those within the NHS.

Compensation claims – expert witness and witness of fact

An increasing part of the practitioner's work is the provision of expert reports for those who have been involved in litigation and are seeking compensation. The practitioner might be asked by the plaintiff's solicitor or the defendant's solicitor for an expert report on the situation and the prognosis in order to assess the amount of compensation (known as quantum). This and the need to give the true picture even if it does not 'help' the client's case is considered on Chapter 13 on giving evidence in court.

Complaints and unprofessional conduct by others

Because the private practitioner often works on her own, she is more vulnerable in pointing out low standards of care provided by other professionals. She lacks a management hierarchy and does not belong to a large organisation (other than her own professional association) to be able to take action effectively and without herself becoming a scapegoat or losing out financially.

Situation: Unacceptable standards in residential care

A physiotherapist provides private services at a residential care home. She is horrified to discover that the residents have a very low standard of care. Some seem to be in pain and there is evidence of low standards of cleanliness both of the residents and the premises. She tries to point this out discreetly to the manager, but unfortunately the manager reacts badly at the implied criticism, and says the funds do not exist for more carers and cleaners to be appointed.

There are several options open to the physiotherapist but all are likely to end her association with the home.

- She could report the situation to the owners or senior management.
- She could complain to the Registration Authority under the Registered Homes Act 1984 which would have to investigate her complaint. This would be the local authority.
- She could report the situation to the contract department of the local authority which purchases places in the home for clients.
- In extremely serious cases where it would appear that criminal activities are taking place, she could report the situation to the police.
- She could report the situation to the Social Services Inspectorate of the Department of Health.

Unfortunately, none of these courses of action are likely to ensure that her work with the home will continue.

■ What if the unsound or unsafe practice she witnesses is the conduct of another professional?

Situation: Unacceptable practice by colleagues

A physiotherapist visits an elderly person who lives alone and is always profusely grateful for the help and attention she receives. She notices that on the dresser the client keeps a few notes of money. She questions her about the advisability of keeping money in the house and on the dresser. The client explains that she always gives the ambulance driver £5 after each visit to the day hospital. The physiotherapist fears that the ambulance man might be exploiting the old lady. What action, if any, should she take?

One course would be to explain to the client that the service provided by the ambulance is free and no payment need be made. If the client says that the ambulance men expect it, what does the physiotherapist do then? One possibility is for her to take up the complaint to the director of the ambulance service. This would be preferable to writing an anonymous letter or complaining indirectly. However she may find that she becomes ostracised as a result.

It is essential, however, that she takes appropriate action and does not ignore the dangers to the client. She has a duty of care to the client and if harm were eventually to befall the client and it were ascertained that the professional had been aware of the situation but had taken no action, she could face professional misconduct proceedings (see section on whistle blowing in Chapter 17).

Private practice and the NHS

Purchasing and providing in the internal market

Since the internal market was established following the NHS and Community Care Act 1990 private practice and NHS care have become more and more linked. Thus NHS health service bodies increasingly purchase services from the private sector, including individual private practitioners. Thus a GP might purchase physiotherapy services from an independent physiotherapist. This trend is likely to continue after the implementation of the 1998 White Paper even though the internal market as such is to be abolished. The CSP has given advice on the use of such services and suggested a model agreement[17].

Shared facilities

Private practitioners such as independent midwives and physiotherapists in private practice might make use of NHS facilities. The CSP has provided guidance on the use of NHS facilities for private practice[18] emphasising that members should avoid a conflict of interest. NHS facilities may be used by private practitioners outside of NHS hours, e.g. for sports injuries, but the basis on which they are so used must be made absolutely clear and a proper contract should be drawn up setting out the responsibilities of both parties. Fees charged should reflect the value of the services provided.

Shared clients

Difficulties can arise for both physiotherapists within the NHS and in private practice where their clients are receiving help from both sectors. The CSP has given advice on this issue[19], emphasising the importance of the therapists communicating with each other and not being derogatory of the other to the patient. If it becomes apparent that the two practitioners are using different and possibly conflicting methods of treatment, then it is essential that this is discussed with the patient and the patient invited to choose. The same problem can arise when an NHS patient or patient being treated by an independent physiotherapist seeks treatment from a person practising in an alternative or complementary therapy, e.g. osteopathy or reflexology. Issues in connection with complementary medicine are considered in Chapter 27.

Accreditation of private practice

The accreditation process endeavours to identify standards of practice for physiotherapists and also provides a form of reassurance for members of the public.

The Organisation of Chartered Physiotherapists in Private Practice (OCPPP) has established an Accreditation Manual which was revised in 1996 following a review of the accreditation process. The OCPPP has set up an Accreditation Management Panel which offers advice and help to those participating in the scheme[20]. Numerous questions relating to the justification of accreditation on a steam roller basis of members of OCPP are answered in *In Touch*, the Autumn Issue for 1994[21].

Part time private practice

Some physiotherapists might try to develop a private practice as well as being employed part time. In such a situation they must ensure that they do not exploit their employed situation to increase their private practice by taking clients away from their employer. This would be regarded as a breach of the implied term of loyalty to their employer in their contract of employment (see Chapter 17). Similarly they should keep their private practice entirely separate from their employment and not attempt to see private clients in working hours without the express consent of their employer nor use any of the employer's facilities for their private work (e.g. telephones, equipment, secretarial services or stationery). In the case of *Watling* v. *Gloucestershire County Council*[22] (see Chapter 17 for the full facts), Mr Watling, an occupational therapist employed by the County Council, was fairly dismissed since he continued to see private clients during his working hours.

If the physiotherapist has the agreement of her employer to her undertaking private practice in her own area, there should be no difficulty in doing private work. However it is essential that she makes sure that patients are aware of their entitlements to have NHS treatment without paying. There are dangers in the physiotherapist or a colleague treating the same patient as part of NHS at the same time as the patient is receiving private treatment from the physiotherapist. However it depends upon the circumstances.

Situation: Private and NHS?

> The mother with a child with cystic fibrosis was concerned that, because she was working full time, the child was not receiving sufficient physiotherapy. She mentioned this to a physiotherapist at the hospital who said that she did private work and would come in her off duty hours to give physiotherapy to the child. The mother was not told that there was a community physiotherapy paediatric service.

In this situation the mother may well have grounds for complaint if she was not told that the child could be given physiotherapy in the community under the NHS. If, however, the kind of service the mother wanted would not have been available, then the offer of private help would be acceptable. The physiotherapist should ensure that her employer knows of the arrangements and that the mother has been offered full information of what is available within the NHS.

Areas of concern

Insurance

The Guidance of the CSP[23] recommends that insurance should be obtained for private practice from the CSP's insurance brokers, Frizzells. The scheme for surgery cover includes equipment, loss of business money and employer's and public liability insurances. There is optional cover for other liabilities and risks.

Lasers and licensing

The CSP has provided an information paper[24] on the use of lasers by a chartered physiotherapist in private practice. It describes the anomalous position whereby although the Registered Homes Act 1984 requires that the use of Class 3B laser product is specified as a specially controlled technique and can only be carried out in a registered Nursing Home, there are so many exemptions from the registration requirements that

> 'It is almost wholly random as to whether a chartered physiotherapist using a laser requires a licence. For instance, a chartered physiotherapist practising from rooms which form part of their own home, or who use the treatment room at a football club is exempt; whereas a member who practised from a chalet in their garden would probably have to have a licence.'

Individual practitioners have to decide if it is necessary for them to have a licence and to seek further advice from the Chief Executive of the CSP.

Documentation

It should be obvious from the many conflicts which can arise in private practice that the documentation which the private practitioner keeps is extremely important – not only in establishing the care that is given to each patient and the terms on which it is to be given in the event of any referral or dispute, but also in relation to the management of a small business. She needs to ensure that she is able to respond to the many statutory requests for information about her practice from the Inland Revenue and Customs and Excise as well as answering any queries from statutory health and social services providers. (Record keeping is discussed in Chapter 12.)

Going abroad

Some physiotherapists may wish to consider working abroad. With a shortage of physiotherapists worldwide and freedom of work within the European Union the opportunities are considerable. Often they will be taking employment overseas but, where they consider offering services privately, then the topics covered in this chapter are essential, bearing in mind the fact that they will be working in a different legal context and therefore local advice will be necessary on the legal implications of offering services privately. The CSP has prepared guidance on going abroad[25]. It strongly advises its members to have at least two years good rotational experience before going overseas and gives advice on tax, insurance and pensions. Information is also provided by the CSP on facilitating exchanges[26]. Advice is also provided about the use of physiotherapists from outside the UK working within the UK[27].

Conclusion

There is likely to be an increase in the numbers of physiotherapists who are self-employed offering their services in the community and to hospital trusts. To move outside employed status is often a courageous step and the physiotherapist who is considering taking such step should seek professional advice and take note of the topics briefly discussed in this chapter. Reference should be made to general law books (see bibliography) and to the publications recommended by the Chartered Society of Physiotherapy[28].

 Questions and exercises

1 Identify the differences in law between the situation of the physiotherapist in private practice and the employed physiotherapist.
2 A colleague has suggested that there may be considerable advantages in the physiotherapists withdrawing from employed status within the NHS and setting up a group of private practitioners to sell their services to the Trusts and GP consortia. Draw up a list of benefits and weaknesses of this suggestion.
3 A physiotherapist in private practice has two sessions at a private nursing home. She is concerned at the low standards of patient care. What action could she take?

References

1 CSP Professional Affairs Department (various) PA No. 3 *Use of NHS Facilities for Private Practice* (January 1995); PA No. 5 *Seeking Treatment – Public and Private* (November 1994); PA No. 7 *Thinking of Private Practice?* (April 1998); PA No. 25 *Legalities of Laser Use in Private Practice* (January 1995); PA No. 26 *Standards of Business Conduct* (May 1995); PA No. 43 *Recommended Salaries and Fees in Private Practice* (September 1996); PA No. 44 *Self-employed status* (no date); PA No. 45 *Trading Status, Copyright and Patents* (no date); PA No. 46 *Associate Agreement (Self-employed staff)* (April 1998). CSP, London.
2 CSP Professional Affairs Department (no date) PA No. 44 *Self-employed status*. CSP, London.
3 CSP Professional Affairs Department (1998) No. PA 7 (April 1998) *Thinking of Private Practice?* CSP, London.
4 McCann, L. (1998) The Practice Management Series – Putting Together a Business Plan *In Touch* Winter Issue 1996/7, 82, 16–17.

5   CSP Professional Affairs Department (1996) No. 42 (September 1996) *Business Planning.* CSP, London.

6   CSP Professional Affairs Department (1998) No. PA 38 (March 1998) *An Introduction to Marketing.* CSP, London.

7   Grant, D. (1995) Thriving on Chaos? *In Touch* Summer 1995, 76, 22–4.

8   CSP Professional Affairs Department (1995) No. PA 26 (May 1995) *Standards of Business Conduct.* CSP, London.

9   Triezenberg, H.L. (1996) The identification of Ethical Issues in Physical Therapy Practice. *Physical Therapy* **76**, 10, 1097–1108.

10 CSP Professional Affairs Department (1996) No. PA 43 (September 1996) *Recommended Salaries and Fees in Private Practice.* CSP, London.

11 Deykin, T. (1994) Medical-legal work. *In Touch* Summer 1994, 72, 18–19.

12 CSP Professional Affairs Department (no date) No. PA 45 *Trading Status, Copyright and Patents.* CSP, London.

13 CSP Professional Affairs Department (1998) No. PA 46 (April 1998) *Associate Agreement (Self-employed staff).* CSP, London.

14 *W* v. *W (Judicial separation ancillary relief)* [1995] 2 FLR 259.

15 *Holt and Another* v. *Payne Skillington (a firm) and Another* (1995) *The Times* 22 December 1995.

16 DoH (1997) *The New NHS: Modern Dependable.* HMSO, London.

17 CSP Professional Affairs Department (1998) No. PA 46 (April 1998) *Associate Agreement (Self-employed staff).* CSP, London.

18 CSP Professional Affairs Department (1995) No. PA 3 (January 1995) *Use of NHS Facilities for Private Practice.* CSP, London.

19 CSP Professional Affairs Department (1994) No. PA 5 (November 1994) *Seeking Treatment – Public and Private.* CSP, London.

20 England, S. (1996) Accreditation – take a new look – we have it. *In Touch* Winter Issue 1996/7, 82, 26.

21 Editorial (1994) Accreditation: Your questions answered. *In Touch* Autumn Issue 1994, 73, 22–3.

22 *Watling* v. *Gloucestershire County Council* EAT/868/94 17 March 1995, 23 November 1994, Lexis transcript.

23 CSP Professional Affairs Department (1996) No. PA 32 *Chartered Physiotherapist and Insurance.* CSP, London.

24 CSP Professional Affairs Department (1995) No. PA 25 (January 1995) *Use of lasers by Chartered Physiotherapists in private practice.* CSP, London.

25 CSP Professional Affairs Department (1994) No. PA 12 (October 1994) *Going Abroad – Questions to ask.* CSP, London.

26 CSP Professional Affairs Department (1994) No. PA 11 (October 1994) *Facilitating Exchanges.* CSP, London.

27 CSP Professional Affairs Department (1997) No. PA 10 (November 1997) *Working in the United Kingdom.* CSP, London.

28 See end note 1 above.

Section E
Specialist Client Groups

Chapter 20

Care of Those with Physical Disabilities, Sports and Road Traffic Injuries and Neurological Disorders

This chapter considers legal issues which mainly arise in the course of caring for those with physical disabilities, with sports and orthopaedic injuries and suffering from neurological disorders, but there are, of course, many clients with multi-handicaps and who therefore come under other client groupings covered in Chapters 21 to 24. Reference should also be made to the general chapters in sections B and C which discuss legal issues arising across all client groups. Possible situations of negligence in relation to this group and in relation to equipment and adaptations are considered in Chapters 10 and 15 and complaints from this client group are discussed in Chapter 14. Legal issues arising in relation to children are considered in Chapter 23.

This chapter will look at the following issues:

- The Chronically Sick and Disabled Persons Act and related legislation
- Inter-agency and inter professional co-operation
- Limitations on resources and priority setting
- Legal issues arising from sports injuries
- Legal issues arising in musculoskeletal conditions
- Road traffic victims and legal issues
- Legal aspects of respiratory care
- Legal issues arising in patients with neurological conditions
- Pain management
- Smoking and the physically disabled
- Conclusions

Chronically Sick and Disabled Persons Act 1970 and related legislation

The general duties placed upon local authorities in respect of the needs of the disabled are set out in the Chronically Sick and Disabled Persons Act 1970. The principal duties are shown in Figure 20.1. It should be noted that the provisions apply to those suffering from mental disabilities as well as those with physical disabilities, but for convenience these are dealt with here and not repeated in Chapters 21 or 22.

Figure 20.1 **Duties under the Chronically Sick and Disabled Persons Act 1970 – section 1.**

(1) It shall be the duty of every local authority having functions under section 29 of the National Assistance Act 1948 to inform themselves of the number of persons to whom that section applies within their area and of the need for the making by the authority of arrangements under that section for such persons.

(2) Every such local authority—
(a) shall cause to be published from time to time at such times and in such manner as they consider appropriate general information as to the services provided under arrangements made by the authority under the said section 29 which are for the time being available in their area; and
(b) shall ensure that any such person as aforesaid who needs any of those services is informed of any other *service provided by the authority (whether under any such arrangements or not)* which in the opinion of the authority is relevant to his needs *and of any service provided by any other authority or organisation which in the opinion of the authority is so relevant and of which particulars are in the authority's possession.*

[words in italics introduced by the 1986 Act (see below)]

Section 2 of the 1970 Act lists the provisions that the local authority has a duty to make in the following circumstances:

- The local authority has the functions under section 29 of the National Assistance Act (NAA) 1948.
- It is satisfied that the section applies to an individual.
- The person is ordinarily resident in their area.
- It is necessary, in order to meet the needs of that person,
- To make arrangements for all or any of the matters set out in Figure 20.2.

(The duties referred to in section 29 of the NAA 1948 are that the local authority may make arrangements for promoting the welfare of persons over 18 who are blind, deaf, dumb, or who suffer from mental disorder, and other persons who are substantially and permanently handicapped by illness, injury or congenital deformity or such other disabilities.)

Figure 20.2 **Arrangements which the local authority has a duty to make – section 2.**

(a) the provision of practical assistance for that person in his home;
(b) the provision for that person of, or assistance to that person in obtaining, wireless, television, library or similar recreational facilities;
(c) the provision for that person of lectures, games, outings or other recreational facilities outside his home or assistance to that person in taking advantage of educational facilities available to him;

Continued

Figure 20.2 Continued.

(d) the provision for that person of facilities for, or assistance in, travelling to and from his home for the purpose of participating in any services provided under arrangements made by the authority … or in any services provided otherwise than as aforesaid which are similar to services which could be provided under such arrangements;

(e) the provision of assistance for that person in arranging for the carrying out of any works of adaptation in his home of the provision of any additional facilities designed to secure his greater safety, comfort or convenience;

(f) facilitating the taking of holidays by that person, whether at holiday homes or otherwise and whether provided under arrangements made by the authority or otherwise;

(g) the provision of meals for that person in his home or elsewhere;

(h) the provision for that person of, or assistance to that person in obtaining, a telephone and any special equipment necessary to enable him to use a telephone.

The right to enforce provision under section 2 was considered by the High Court, Court of Appeal and House of Lords in a case[1] where disabled persons applied for judicial review of the decision by Gloucester County Council to cut social services for the disabled (see the section on resources and priority setting below).

It is inevitable, given the range of services required and the limited resources of local and health authorities that services for individual patient groups will vary.

Social security provisions for the disabled

It is impossible to cover in detail the benefits which are available to those suffering from mental and physical disabilities and reference must be made to the publications of the Royal Association for Disability and Rehabilitation (RADAR) and others which are updated on an annual basis. An excellent guide to the rights and benefits which are available is provided by the Disability Rights Handbook. This provides far more detail that can be given in this chapter.

The main benefits include:

- Social Fund:
  - Loans which are repayable
    - budget loans
    - crisis loans
    - funeral payments
  - loans which are not repayable
    - maternity payments
    - cold weather payments
- Independent Living Fund
- Disability Living Allowance:
  - care component
  - mobility component

- Attendance allowance
- Invalid care allowance
- Income support.

The physiotherapist should be careful to ensure that she knows the limitations of her knowledge in this very complex area which is constantly changing. She could be liable for giving negligent advice if clients relied on her advice to their financial loss. It is preferable for her to ensure that she knows how to guide the client to the best sources of advice available.

Accommodation

Local authorities have a duty to provide accommodation for those suffering from physical and mental disabilities under the provisions of section 21 (as amended) of the National Assistance Act 1948 and other legislation.
  Directions issued under the amended section 21 cover:

- Residential accommodation for persons aged 18 or over who by reason of age, illness, disability or any other circumstances are in need of care and attention not otherwise available to them.
- Temporary accommodation for persons who are in urgent need where the need for that accommodation could not reasonably have been foreseen.
- Accommodation
  ○ for persons who are or have been suffering from mental disorder, or
  ○ (to prevent mental disorder) for persons who are ordinarily resident in the area or have no settled residence.
- accommodation in order to
  ○ prevent illness
  ○ care for those suffering from illness; and
  ○ provide after care of those so suffering.
- Arrangements specifically for persons who are alcoholic or drug-dependent.
- Residential accommodation for expectant and nursing mothers (of any age) who are in need of care and attention which is not otherwise available to them.

Services for residents
Further arrangements (in relation to persons provided with accommodation) cover all or any of the following purposes:

- The welfare of all such persons
- Supervising the hygiene of the accommodation so provided;
- Enabling such persons to obtain:
  ○ medical attention
  ○ nursing attention
  ○ services provided by the National Health Service

The local authority is also required to review the accommodation and the arrangements. However it is not required to provide any accommodation which it is the duty of the NHS to provide.

Local authorities may also, in such cases as the authority considers appropriate, provide for the conveyance of persons to and from the accommodation which is provided.

Developments after the 1990 Act

The result of changes introduced by the 1990 Act was that, whilst the basic duties of the local authority to provide accommodation to specific categories of people have been slightly modified, the range of organisations with whom they can contract has increased.

In addition the purchasing of the accommodation for persons since 1 April 1993 is the responsibility of the local social services authorities, who can recover fees from residents on a means tested basis, rather than the Department of Social Security.

Reference should also be made to Chapter 18 on community care.

Factors in the placement decision

Psychological needs as well as physical ones have to be taken into account.

Case: *R. v. Avon County Council, ex parte M.*[2]

> The applicant was 22 and suffered from Down's Syndrome. In 1989 the local authority began an assessment of the applicant's needs. In 1991 he was offered a place at Milton Heights where he spent three weeks. He and his family were set on his going there, but the local authority proposed various alternatives which were not acceptable. In January 1992 a review panel recommended that he should be placed at Milton Heights. The social services committee rejected the recommendation. After the threat of judicial review proceedings and further delay for a joint assessment of the applicant's needs the review panel in January 1993 found that the applicant had formed an entrenched wish to go to Milton Heights and recommended that he should be placed there. The social services committee declined to accept this recommendation and decided to place the applicant elsewhere. As a result the applicant revived his application for judicial review to challenge the local authority's decision.

The High Court held (quashing the local authority's decision)

(1) Residential accommodation should be appropriate to the needs of the individual applicant which properly included his psychological needs. In the present case the applicant's entrenched wish to go to Milton Heights was not mere personal preference, but part of his psychological needs.

(2) The social services committee could not overrule the recommendation of the review panel without a substantial reason. The review panel had properly arrived at its decision on the evidence before it and the strength, coherence and apparent persuasiveness of that decision had to be addressed head on if it were to be set aside and not followed. Anybody required, at law, to give reasons for reconsidering and changing such a decision must have and show a good reason for doing so. The local social services committee had failed to do so and its decision must be quashed.

Disabled facilities grants

Under section 114 of the Local Government and Housing Act 1989 the local housing authority had a duty to approve applications for grants for facilities for the disabled. These are known as disabled facilities grants (DFGs). The Housing, Grants, Construction and Regeneration Act 1996 replaced many of the mandatory grants under previous legislation by discretionary grants, except for DFGs which remain mandatory. Section 23(1) of the 1996 Act now details the provision of DFGs for the purposes shown in Figure 20.3.

Figure 20.3 **The Housing, Grants, Construction and Regeneration Act 1996 – section 23.**

(1) The purposes for which an application for a disabled facilities grant must be approved ... are the following—

(a) facilitating access by the disabled occupant to and from the dwelling or the building in which the dwelling or, as the case may be, flat is situated;

(b) making the dwelling or building safe for the disabled occupant and other persons residing with him;

(c) facilitating access by the disabled occupant to a room used or usable as the principal family room;

(d) facilitating access by the disabled occupant to, or providing for the disabled occupant, a room used or usable for sleeping;

(e) facilitating access by the disabled occupant to, or providing for the disabled occupant, a room in which there is a lavatory, or facilitating the use by the disabled occupant of such a facility;

(f) facilitating access by the disabled occupant to, or providing for the disabled occupant, a room in which there is a bath or shower (or both), or facilitating the use by the disabled occupant of such a facility;

(g) facilitating access by the disabled occupant to, or providing for the disabled occupant, a room in which there is a washhand basin, or facilitating the use by the disabled person of such a facility;

(h) facilitating the preparation and cooking of food by the disabled occupant;

(i) improving any heating system in the dwelling to meet the needs of the disabled occupant or, if there is no existing heating system in the dwelling or any such system is unsuitable for use by the disabled occupant, providing a heating system suitable to meet his needs;

(j) facilitating the use by the disabled occupant of a source of power, light or heat by altering the position of one of more means of access to or control of that source or by providing additional means of control;

(k) facilitating access and movement by the disabled occupant around the dwelling in order to enable him to care for a person who is normally resident in the dwelling and is in need of such care;

(l) such other purposes as may be specified by order of the Secretary of State.

A comment by the judge in the case brought against Birmingham (see below) was

'In enacting the 1996 Act Parliament chose to downgrade statutory duties to discretions in relation to the approval of other types of grant, save for the disabled facilities grants for section 23(1) purposes. In making the decision to treat section 23(1) disabled facilities grants differently, it recognised the importance of obliging local housing authorities to approve grants to disabled occupants whose applications fulfilled the purposes enumerated in section 23(1).'

There is also provision for a disabled facilities grant to be available for making the dwelling or building suitable for the accommodation, welfare or employment of the disabled occupant in any other respect (section 23(2)).

Disabled occupant is defined as 'the disabled person for whose benefit it is proposed to carry out any of the relevant works' (section 20).

Disabled person is a person, over 18 years, registered under section 29(1) of the National Assistance Act 1948, or is a person for whose welfare arrangements have been made under section 29 or, in the opinion of the social services authority, might be made under it (section 100(2) of the 1996 Act).

The social services authority, means the council which is the local authority for the purposes of the Local Authority Social Services Act 1970 for the area in which the dwelling is situated (section 100(4) of the 1996 Act).

A grant is not automatic. By section 24(3), (4) and (5) the local authority in making a decision can consider whether:

- the relevant works are necessary and appropriate to meet the needs of the disabled occupant;
- it is reasonable and practicable to carry out the relevant works, having regard to the age and condition of the dwelling or building;
- the dwelling is fit for human habitation;
- (in the case of an application that requires works to the common parts of a shared building) that building meets the requirements of section 604(2) of the Housing Act 1985
- (in respect of works to the common parts of a building containing one or more flats) the applicant has a power or is under a duty to carry out the relevant works.

These statutory provisions can give rise to many difficulties for physiotherapists. Although the local housing authority should ensure that the social services authority is consulted over the decision to give a grant this is not always implemented. It may happen that applications go straight to the housing authority which places them upon a waiting list without first obtaining the advice and assessment of a registered physiotherapist or occupational therapist.

It is inevitable that priorities have to be established to meet the demand for DFGs and physiotherapists may be encouraged to make an assessment in the light of the available resources rather than in the light of the needs of the disabled person.

Nevertheless it was held by the High Court in the case of *R.* v. *Birmingham City Council*[3] that financial resources are not relevant when a local authority is deciding whether to provide someone with a disabled facilities grant under section 23(1) of the Housing, Grants, Construction and Regeneration Act 1996. The judge allowed an application for judicial review of a decision of Birmingham City Council which took account of financial resources when deciding whether to offer the applicant a disabled facilities grant. However entitlement to receive a disabled facilities grant is means tested, and this fact may dampen demand.

It should also be remembered that, in addition to its powers under section 23(1), the local housing authority also has the power to make grants in respect of improvements and repairs depending upon the age of the property, its condition and the nature of the applicant's interest in the property.

It is possible that where parents are separated a dispute could arise between them over which house should be adapted to meet the disability needs of a child. This situation is considered in Chapter 23 on children.

Education and training and employment facilities

Duties are placed upon local authorities under the National Assistance Act 1948, the Chronically Sick and Disabled Persons Act 1970 and the Disabled Persons (Employment) Acts 1944 and 1958 (as amended by subsequent legislation) to provide education and training and employment facilities for those with physical and mental disabilities.

Sheltered employment facilities for the seriously physically or mentally disabled have therefore been established by local authorities. The local authority's duty extends to those disabled people who are resident within its catchment area.

Physiotherapists may have a role in the management and planning of such facilities and in bringing to the attention of the social services authority deficiencies and shortcomings in the arrangements and facilities, as well as being involved in the assessment of clients for the use of such facilities.

Inter-agency and inter professional co-operation

Joint Consultative Committees

Local authorities have a statutory duty to co-operate with other statutory authorities and the voluntary sector in the provision of services. Under the NHS and Community Care Act 1990 they also have the responsibility of preparing and each year revising, in conjunction with health authorities and voluntary agencies, a community care plan setting out the provision for those receiving community care services (see Chapter 18). The Joint Consultative Committee (JCC) is the body which is set up between health authorities and the relevant local authorities, together with other organisations in the area, to consider the joint planning of health and social services.

In practical terms the co-operation between health staff and local authority staff is vital to the interests of the client and can cause the physiotherapist considerable problems. The work of Geoffrey Barnes and Fiona Lee in the co-ordinating and planning services for stroke patients in hospital and the community[4] is an interesting example of cross-agency co-operation.

Integrated care pathways

The physiotherapist will also be part of a multi-disciplinary team and must be aware of the contributions of others to patient care. Pam Poole and Sue Johnson[5] applied the principle of integrated care pathways (ICPs) to the work in a typical orthopaedic unit. ICPs are both a management and clinical audit tool. They can be used to setting out in a pathway all the activities of the various disciplines involved in the care of a patient with a particular condition within an expected time frame. Managerially the aim is to ensure that the care and treatments given are delivered at the right time, by the right professional, in the right way. As a means of clinical audit the use of ICPs highlights variance from the typical pathway. The authors showed that when this model was applied to an orthopaedic unit the length of stay was reduced without compromising the quality of care as measured by pain and mobility. Other benefits were:

- Smoother progress through the hospital for the patient
- Greater communication and team work between the different disciplines
- Much improved co-ordination of care
- An educational tool for the induction of new staff and students
- Audit data constantly available
- Monitoring standards.

It is of course essential that therapists should ensure that they record clearly any deviation in their treatments from the norm. The authors note that

'The ICP document within orthopaedics does not as yet replace the physiotherapy notes, and physiotherapists currently sign the ICP document as well as writing out their own notes. This is necessary because these pathways do not yet provide the physiotherapists with a means of recording their own notes in full while adhering to the legal requirements.' (See Chapter 12 on record keeping.)

Use of volunteer agencies and other non-statutory bodies

Local authorities are increasingly using non-direct labour for the provision of services and entering into contracts with other organisations, usually of a non-profit making kind, for them to provide the services which the local authority has a statutory duty to ensure exist. Such arrangements can create complex issues relating to responsibility and accountability. It is advisable for the physiotherapist who may have to deal with complaints about the services provided by these non-statutory organisations to have sight of the agreements drawn up with the local authority in order to be certain of the terms on which their services are given and to be aware of which duties are enforceable.

The use of such organisations and agencies does not, however, remove the primary responsibility from the local authority to ensure that the services are available.

Limitations on resources and priority setting

In 1995 certain disabled people in Gloucester challenged, by judicial review, the decision by Gloucestershire County Council to reduce or withdraw certain welfare assistance provided to them under section 2 of the Chronically Sick and Disabled Persons Act 1970.

The court had to decide the issue of resources and statutory duties.

Case: *R. v. Gloucester County Council, ex parte Mahfood and others*[6]

Disabled persons complained when services had been curtailed following withdrawal of a government grant upon which the County Council's plans had been based and the Council gave greater priority to the more seriously disabled. The Council had not reassessed in the light of the cutbacks but had simply sent out a standard letter withdrawing services.

The High Court at first instance refused to grant a declaration that in carrying out the reassessment the local authority was not entitled to take into account the resources available to it. A local authority was right to take account of resources both when assessing needs and when deciding whether it was necessary to make arrangements to meet those needs.

One applicant, Mr Barry, appealed to the Court of Appeal.

The Court of Appeal[7] allowed the appeal, granting a declaration that in assessing or reassessing whether it was necessary to make arrangements in order to meet the needs of a disabled person, a local authority was **not** entitled to take into account the resources available to it. The local authority appealed to the House of Lords.

The House of Lords[8] held that, for the purposes of section 2 of the 1970 Act, the needs of a chronically sick or disabled person were to be assessed in the context of, and by reference to, the provision of certain types of assistance for promoting the welfare of disabled persons using eligibility criteria (decided upon by the local authority) as to whether the disability of that particular person dictated a need for assistance, and if so at what level. Those criteria were to be set by taking into account:

- current acceptable standards of living,
- the nature and extent of the disability, and
- the relative cost balanced against the relative benefit and the relative need for that benefit.

In deciding how much weight was to be attached to the cost of providing the benefit, the authority had to make an evaluation about the impact which the cost would have on its resources, which in turn would depend on the authority's financial position. It followed that a chronically sick and disabled person's need for services could not sensibly be assessed without having some regard to the cost of providing such services, since his need for a particular type or level of service could not be decided in a vacuum from which all considerations of cost were expelled.

The House of Lords therefore allowed the appeal.

At the same time the court heard an application by Mr McMillan[9] for judicial review of the decision of Islington Borough Council not to provide him with home help cover, when his carers were ill or away. This application failed on the grounds that the Council had conducted a proper balancing exercise taking into account resources and the comparative needs of the disabled in its area. The court held that the Council was not in breach of the duty which it owed to the applicant.

Reference should also be made to Chapter 18 on community care[10].

Legal issues arising from sports injuries

The Association of Chartered Physiotherapists in Sports Medicine

The ACPSM was founded in 1971 to provide quality sports physiotherapy, rehabilitation and counselling to athletes and recreational participants before, during and after injury[11]. Its objectives are shown in Figure 20.4.

Figure 20.4 **Objectives of the ACPSM.**

- To improve the techniques and facilities for the prevention and treatment of sports injuries.
- To inform all interested individuals and bodies of the existence and availability of Chartered and State Registered Physiotherapists.
- To provide a specialised service to meet the demands of sports people.
- To encourage education, and to develop and publish research in the field of sports physiotherapy in the UK.

Sports injuries were surveyed by David Ball of Middlesex University[12] and he found that rugby was the most dangerous with the risk of injury occurring 440 times out of 100 000 participating in comparison with swimming with two injuries per 100 000 participating. On the other hand fatalities were more likely to occur in swimming with 191 fatalities between 1988 and 1992 in comparison with two in rugby.

Numerous legal issues arise in this field of physiotherapy practice including:

- The liability of those who volunteer help and take on the duty of care (this is considered in Chapter 10).
- The liability of the unregistered physiotherapist who provides help at sports event (see below on initiatives to ensure that only chartered physiotherapists provide services on the football field).
- The physiotherapist in private practice specialising in sports injuries (the problems relating to private practice are considered in Chapter 19).
- Keeping within one's competence (this is discussed in Chapter 4 on the scope of professional practice).
- Giving advice as to whether the patient should continue on the field (liability arising from negligent advice is considered in Chapter 10 but a situation relating to a sports injury is discussed below).
- Administration of pain killers on the field (see below).
- Acting as an expert witness in a case brought by an international sports person against another player on the field (the role of the expert witness is considered in Chapter 13).

Negligent advice on the sports field

A physiotherapist specialising in sports physical therapy could be liable in three different circumstances:

- providing treatment designed to enable continued play with an injury before it is fully healed;
- informing athletes of the potential health risks on continued athletic activity in their physical condition; and
- evaluating and advising athletes on their ability to resume athletic activity[13].

Situation: Tension stress fracture

Alan, a registered physiotherapist, assists a local football team. He is not paid a fee for his work, but is allowed free entrance for all matches including away games. He is called onto the pitch following an injury to one of the players, Billy. He gives Billy a speedy examination. Billy is clearly in a lot of pain in the groin region and Alan sprays an analgesic over the affected area and when asked by Billy if he should come off, he says that Billy could carry on playing. Subsequently, Billy is diagnosed as having a tension stress fracture and his continuing to play has exacerbated his injury. Billy who is likely to be off work for many months is claiming compensation from Alan for the extra work time he has lost because of Alan's negligent advice. Is he likely to succeed?

In the above situation, whether the footballer's case will succeed will depend upon whether he can prove that he was given advice which no reasonable physiotherapist would have offered. In addition he will have to prove that he relied on the advice he received and would have come off the field if that advice had been given instead. It is possible that, with the adrenalin of the match, he was anxious to continue and would have ignored advice to come off if the physiotherapist had so advised him.

Liability of the unregistered physiotherapist

What would be the legal situation if, in the above situation, the physiotherapist assisting at the game was not registered? At present there is no legal requirement that those providing physiotherapy support services in sports should be registered. The danger is that the injured person would be dependent upon the person calling himself a physiotherapist having the insurance cover to pay compensation. There is also doubt about the standard of care: it is hoped that, were such a case to come to court, the judge would not apply a lower standard of care, because the physiotherapist was not registered. The Football Association has ruled that all new therapists employed by Premiership clubs should be registered and from 2000/01 they will also need to have completed the FA's postgraduate certificate in Football Sport Medicine[14]. Alan Hodson, Head of Medicine at the FA, emphasised that clubs should also allow sports therapists, athletic trainers, masseurs and sports scientists to have their place in the multi-disciplinary sports medicine team.

The club's liability

What of the local team? Does it have a duty to confirm that it is insured for Billy's injuries and that it only employs a registered physiotherapist?

Much would depend upon Billy's status – whether he is an amateur or an employee of the club. The club itself would not necessarily be defined as a legal entity and capable of being sued (it depends upon how it has been formed and its constitution), but individuals who had specific responsibilities may be liable. The fact that players are amateurs rather than professionals would not automatically change any principles in relation to insurance cover. However much will depend upon what the players are told. If they are told to obtain their own insurance cover then they could not look to the club for that protection.

The fact that they have not used a chartered physiotherapist may be significant if club members consider that they are entitled to have a reasonable standard of professional care. The courts have not, to the author's knowledge, considered a case where the different professional standard between a chartered physiotherapist and a non-chartered physiotherapist was in issue. The importance of maintaining competence is clear from an article by Roger Hackney who describes the sports hernia[15] and identifies the different possible causes of groin pain.

Children

Clearly no player should be compelled to return to a game and care should be taken with children. In a school situation Corinne Williams[16], 16 years old, obtained damages of £1500 when she was forced to join in a PE class despite having an injured ankle. The girl's mother, an orthopaedic nurse, had written to the school notifying them that the girl had a sprained ankle but, believing the letter to be forged by the girl, the school teacher forced her to take part. (See also Chapter 23.)

Sports preparation

A physiotherapist may be involved in the preparation for sports activities as well as dealing with the aftermath. Liz Mendell describes how a physiotherapist can assist a person prepare for skiing[17]. (See Chapters 10 and 26 on liability for negligent advice and instruction.)

Dance specialists

There are other areas of specialism which could involve physiotherapists. For example Dance UK has established a national list of health professionals who are used to working with dancers and so will understand their needs and problems. Any physiotherapist wishing to be on the register has to complete a form of application and provide a recommendation from a dancer or dance company.

Representing the multi-disciplinary team

The physiotherapist should be aware of any limits on her own competence in rehabilitation and recognise the contribution that other professionals could make.

Britt Tajet-Foxell and Lynn Booth[18] emphasise the value of giving equal importance to the psychological factors as well as the physical factors in rehabilitation of the athlete. Other factors such as environmental, historical, educational and social variables must also be taken into account. It becomes important therefore to recognise the need for a multi-disciplinary approach to the management of injuries. Often, however, a physiotherapist may be the only contact with the injured athlete and it is important that she recognises when referral to other professionals is appropriate.

Further reading

Medicine Sport and the Law edited by Simon D.W. Payne[19] provides more detailed information relating to specific conditions such as patients with organ transplants and the transplant games, rowing, golf, water sports and most other sports including Firearms Act and mental health. See also *Sports Medicine: Ethics and Law* by E. Grayson and C. Bond[20].

Legal issues arising in musculoskeletal conditions

This is one of the most difficult areas of physiotherapy practice including back pain, rheumatology and other conditions. Of frequent concern are such issues as:

- Deception by patient
- Limits of competence
- The use of other specialists in this field, e.g. osteopaths, chiropractors, neurologists and neurosurgeons
- Giving advice
- Prognosis decisions and advice
- Sickness and disability laws
- Management of chronic pain and legal aspects which arise
- The scope of professional practice, e.g. TENS (transcutaneous electrical nerve stimulation) being applyed by the physiotherapist
- Acupuncture and electro-acupuncture (see Chapter 27 on complementary therapies).

The Manipulation Association of Chartered Physiotherapists

This Association was formed in 1967 to provide a specialist approach in the treatment of musculoskeletal disorder and is a member of the International Federation of Manipulative Therapy (IFOMT)[21].

The aims of the Association are shown in Figure 20.5.

Figure 20.5   **Aims of the Manipulation Association of Chartered Physiotherapists.**

- To promote the concept of a broad based approach to the overall management of musculoskeletal disorders.
- To develop highly skilled clinicians who are able to draw upon a vast bank of knowledge, and analyse, evaluate and treat often extremely complex problems of neuromusculoskeletal origin.
- To provide an opportunity for those actively engaged in the practice of manipulative therapy to exchange knowledge and improve their professional skills.

Membership of the Association is gained via either a postgraduate diploma or MSc in manual therapy, or a membership examination. A minimum of two weeks clinical supervision under someone with an MACP education is strongly recommended. The Association has adopted a continuing education policy for members. It also encourages research into manipulative therapy and to this end has appointed a research officer and allocated funds to assist individual members with their projects.

In 1992 the Manipulation Association of Chartered Physiotherapists together with related organisations formed an umbrella organisation known as the British Association of Chartered Physiotherapists in Manipulation (BACPIM). It aims to maintain connections with all the manipulative groups, to promote manipulative skills amongst its members and to make the public, the government and medical practitioners aware that there are several thousand highly trained Chartered Physiotherapists capable and willing to treat patients with neuromusculoskeletal problems by manipulation and associated therapies[22].

Advice the physiotherapist specialising in this field might give would include:

- advice on posture
- advice on dynamic lifting
- instruction on ergonomics
- muscle strengthening exercises e.g. abdominal exercises
- flexibility exercises
- advice on overall fitness[23].

Communication problems

'The patient's knowledge of anatomy may be poor, and he is likely to use colloquial expressions. When pain is felt "in the hip" it usually means the buttock or greater trochanteric region. Patients rarely volunteer "the buttock". When pain is felt 'in the shoulder' it often means the supraspinous region of the scapula.'[24]

The way in which a patient might refer to symptoms may be extremely important in ensuring good communication between professional and patient. Liability can arise for negligence on the part of the professional in the duty to inform and communicate (see Chapters 7 and 10).

Hutson gives a list of headings in history taking for back pain. They include:

- longevity of symptoms
- onset of symptoms
- intensity of symptoms
- change in symptoms
- site of pain
- accompanying symptoms
- terminology
- relationship to activity
- general health enquiry
- past health
- effect on lifestyle

Lower limb amputation and risk management

J. Kulkarni and others describe[25] a study of patients attending the Manchester Disablement Service Centre. 58% of patients with unilateral amputations and 27%

of patients with bilateral amputations reported at least one fall in the last 12 months. Of the unilateral patients, 12% of these falls related to prosthesis alone. The authors recommend a multi-disciplinary intervention for all such patients and education for both patients and professionals.

Only a quarter of patients recall being instructed in how to get up from a fall and the authors have prepared a small booklet with diagrammatical illustrations showing patients how to do this with the physiotherapist providing supporting demonstration and instruction. Risk management is considered in Chapter 24 on the care of the elderly and in Chapter 11 on health and safety law.

Road traffic victim and the legal issues

The following situation is an example of a case (taken from Lynch and Grisogono[26]) giving rise to multiple legal issues. The text in italics emphasises the legal problems which arise and where they are considered in this book.

Situation: Dawn an RTA victim

Dawn was a 26 year old victim of a road traffic accident in which her friend, who was driving a sports car in which she was a passenger, died. She was resuscitated at the accident site and placed on life support. She needed a transfer to a nearby hospital so that she could be given a CAT scan. *Dawn's parents had to give their written permission for the transfer, which added to their anxieties about the situation (Chapter 7 on the law of consent). This chapter shows that relatives do not have the power to give or withhold consent on behalf of a mentally incapacitated adult. The professionals should have acted in the best interests of the patient and not sought the consent of the relatives.*

The parents were initially told that she would not be likely to survive. CAT scan showed no brain damage. When she came round from the coma, she was found to be suffering from a left hemiplegia. The parents never understood at what stage she suffered brain damage. They found this confusing, and, to a certain extent, it became a cause of resentment. *Reference should be made to the law relating to giving information to relatives, the duty of care and liability for negligent information (see Chapters 7 and 10).*

She suffered from bouts of severe depression and at one stage was referred to a clinical psychologist for counselling. *The standard of care to which the patient is entitled requires the involvement of other health professionals and a physiotherapist would be failing in her duty of care if she failed to bring in the appropriate person at the correct time.*

The psychologist worked on the basis that Dawn would always be dependent and referred her to a neurosurgeon who promised that he could operate to cure the spasticity which kept causing her muscles to tense up involuntarily. The parents only discovered that the operation would leave her paralysed and wheel bound for the rest of her life when they questioned the neurosurgeon about the operation. *There is a duty to inform according to the reasonable standard of care; the duty includes not simply information about serious risks but also inevitable consequences of any operation (see Chapters 7 and 10).*

Most of her treatment was done privately, because she could not obtain adequate long term treatment through the National Health Service.' *The right to have care is considered in Chapter 6 and responsibilities for the provision of rehabilitation and continuing care is considered in Chapter 18.*

She had to make a claim against the insurers because her friend had not had full cover for his sports car. *See Chapter 16 for mention of the Motor Insurer's Bureau which covers liability where driver is not insured or in a hit and run case, but only provides compensation for personal injuries and death not property.*

The case dragged on and the insurers made an offer of settlement. *It is important to consider the effect of court proceedings on patients; the role of the physiotherapist who may have to give evidence in court about the patient's condition is considered in Chapter 13. The dangers that patients are unwilling to do exercises, because any improvements might reduce the amount of compensation, are considered in Chapter 7 and in this chapter. Legal significance of a settlement is considered in Chapters 2 and 10).*

Dawn was advised that she might obtain more money if she went to court, but she felt that this would be too hard for her emotionally, even though she had no memory of the accident or indeed of the friend who had died. She accepted the offer. *See Chapter 13 on giving evidence in court.*

She was able to buy a specially adapted car. *See Chapter 16 about transport and disabled drivers, Road Traffic Act rules and insurance issues. The physiotherapist may be involved in providing confirmation that a disabled person is fit to drive.*

She took up sports, javelin, shot and discus, but her coach misunderstood the nature of her spasticity and believed that controlling spasticity was a matter of trying harder. As a result of his persuasion to run into a throw, she fell over and suffered a broken ankle. *See Chapter 10 for liability of people who do not understand the condition give advice and instructions which cause harm. See also Chapter 26 for liability of the instructor. The possibility that a patient might assume the risks of harm (volenti non fit injuria) is discussed in Chapter 10.*

She married. *In order to be able to give consent to marriage she must be mentally capable, otherwise the marriage would be void. There are social security provisions for a married person with disabilities.*

Non-compliance in RTA cases

Physiotherapists often come across situations where patients are awaiting compensation following road accidents to be settled and there is a reluctance on the patient's part to make rapid progress which would reduce the amount of compensation they receive.

Situation: Non-compliance following a road traffic accident

Jim had severe leg injuries following an accident on his motor bike for which he was not to blame. He was hesitant to take part in mobility exercises since he was anxious to obtain maximum compensation for his injuries. What is the legal situation of the physiotherapist?

The physiotherapist should do all she can to encourage Jim to make as full a recovery as possible as quickly as possible. She should advise Jim

- that the law requires an injured person to mitigate their loss, i.e.
- to do as much as is reasonable to reduce the effects of the harm which has been suffered;

- that the courts will take into account the pain and suffering that the patient has borne during the recovery process; and
- that ultimately money is a poor substitute for the loss of amenities.

The courts could find that there has been contributory negligence by Jim in failing to follow a recommended treatment and exercise plan thus reducing the compensation. (This is discussed in Chapter 10.) Ultimately, however, the physiotherapist cannot force Jim to undertake the exercises if persuasion and reasoning fail (see Chapter 7 on the law of consent).

Problems for medical staff

The care of young adults following road traffic injuries can present special problems for the physiotherapist as the following situation shows.

Situation: Joking around

> Tom, a lad of 19 years, had severely fractured his leg in a road accident and hated being confined in hospital for traction. He was full of high spirits and encouraged other patients to play jokes on the nursing and therapy staff. What action can be taken?

Legally an occupier of premises is entitled to ask any person whose presence has become intolerable to leave the premises. Even a patient can be asked to leave if their conduct is unacceptable, unless the cause is mental disorder. There will therefore be certain limits beyond which Tom's behaviour need not be accepted and he could be warned of this possibility. Even though it is clinically inadvisable for him to leave hospital, if his conduct becomes dangerous to others then in an extreme situation it may be necessary to discharge him.

Legal aspects of respiratory care

The Association of Chartered Physiotherapists in Respiratory Care have prepared clinical guidelines on physiotherapy management of the spontaneously breathing, acutely breathless, adult patient[27]. Topics covered include: assisted ventilation, entonox, humidification, bronchodilation, NFR (which in this context means neurophysiological facilitation of respiration – and not 'Not for Resuscitation') and TENS. If it were alleged that a physiotherapist providing respiratory care was negligent reference could be made to these guidelines in determining the reasonable standard of care which should have been followed, on the understanding that the guidelines were kept up to date and reflected the reasonable standard of care at the time.

Situation: a tetraplegic

> Mavis, a tetraplegic, is extremely abusive to staff, especially the physiotherapy staff and this has led to several physiotherapists applying for posts in other hospitals. What action can be taken?

Unlike the 'Situation: Joking around' described above, it would be impossible to tell Mavis that if she continued such abuse she would have to leave hospital.

However, it is possible that her agggression arises from underlying factors of depression and the non acceptance of her condition. It may be that a psychologist or other counsellors could provide assistance. It is essential that senior management provide support to staff, ensuring that the care of Mavis is shared around the department, since employers can be liable for mental illness arising from stress at work (see Chapter 11).

Legal issues arising in patients with neurological conditions

This covers a vast group of patients including those who have had strokes, cerebral palsy, Parkinson's Disease and many forms of brain damage. Each of these fields give rise to many different legal issues. Thus in Parkinson's Disease[28] the legal issues which arise include:

- consent from a patient who may not be able to communicate but is able to understand the clinical situation (see in Chapter 7);
- the rights of the patient to receive appropriate care, including the right to receive drugs or surgery as appropriate (see in Chapter 6);
- the standards of care to be provided (see Chapter 10).

Treatment of undressed patients

One well known method for treating patients with muscle weakness and neurological disorders is the Bobath method of treatment. Its philosophy is for a hands on approach to patient treatment. Many legal concerns can arise for the Bobath physiotherapist.

Situation: Accused of assault

The mother of a child with severe cerebral palsy made a complaint about the actions of a physiotherapist when she discovered that the physiotherapist took off her son's clothes in order to carry out the treatment. She had assumed that the exercises would be carried out with the boy fully clothed.

There has been a clear failure of communication in this situation between physiotherapist and mother. Had the mother been properly informed about the nature of the treatment, she could have refused on behalf of her son, or she could have made sure that she was present during the treatment and saw that no assault was taking place. The physiotherapist must be highly sensitive to any discomfort felt by a patient during such treatments and examinations which involve intimate procedures and clarify the patients' or parents' consent or cease to provide that personal treatment (see Chapter 7).

Clinical effectiveness

Situation: Slow progress

A Bobath physiotherapist considers that she has made considerable progress with realigning muscles in a patient and she is supported by the mother. However she has now learnt that resources for the work she is doing are to be discontinued on the grounds that there is no identifiable clinical progress.

Many treatments in physiotherapy show only gradual progress and there is a danger that, with the emphasis on clinical effectiveness, minute stages of progress in patient comfort and care may be ignored and resources refused because identifiable results are not apparent. Moreover often treatments may prevent further damage or distortion rather than leading to a complete cure. Record keeping is essential so that the physiotherapist can point to a clear record of benefit to such patients, as expressed by the patients themselves or by the relatives.

Litigation fears

Situation: Fears of litigation

A physiotherapist trained in the Bobath method was so concerned at the possibility of litigation for assault or for negligence that she decided to give up practice.

It would be unfortunate if the increase in litigation and complaints led to practitioners withdrawing their services or turning to other careers. It is impossible to prevent a person deciding to sue (although in extreme cases, an order of the court can be sought to ban a vexatious litigant from pursuing a worthless claim). However the physiotherapist should be able to defeat any such claim by pointing to her records, and to the fact that she has followed a reasonable standard of care and has obtained the consent of the patient (or parent) to any touching of the person.

Pain management

Physiotherapists are involved in all aspects of pain management with all client groups, so this topic has been placed in this chapter for convenience. This is a field where major developments are taking place and the management of pain relief is becoming less of an ad hoc process of trial and error and more systematically managed. Hospices have developed considerable expertise in pain control amongst the terminally ill. Physiotherapists will be expected to be aware of developments in understanding which treatments are clinically effective. The Bolam test (see Chapter 10) requires that the individual physiotherapist will be providing the reasonable standard of care in the circumstances of the case. Thus it is essential that treatments which are no longer seen to be effective are only provided where there are clear clinical indications for them. Thus treatments such as infra red treatments and shortwave diathermy may still have their place, but are in very restricted use. Similarly wax treatments may have only limited application. The physiotherapist has to keep up to date with research developments.

Back pain[29]

Bill and Geoff Tancred[30] consider the role of exercise in the prevention and treatment of low back pain. They conclude that, providing certain considerations are applied, findings overwhelmingly advocate the use of exercises in the treatment of such afflictions. Personalised exercise programmes for the restoration and maintenance of adequate lumbar function are required. These would include flexibility, stamina, strength, skill, speed and specificity. The legal implications of this paper are that contributory negligence in a patient failing to follow a treatment plan and carry out the programme of exercises could be an important factor in determining the amount of compensation payable in a case of litigation. (This issue of patient non-compliance because compensation has not been settled is considered above.)

Smoking and the physically disabled

Situation: Assisted smoking

> A patient who is tetraplegic insists on being assisted in smoking. Does the physiotherapist have to help? What if she disagrees with smoking?

Often the physiotherapist might find that her personal views conflict with those of her patients/clients. She does not have any right to impose her beliefs on others (although the law does recognise a statutory right for medical personnel to object to involvement in the termination of pregnancy or fertilisation and embryology). On the other hand there is no statutory right for the patient to smoke and some NHS trusts have introduced a no smoking policy. However it would seem to be reasonable for a tetraplegic patient to be permitted to smoke provided that any dangers to safety were resolved.

Situation: Smoking dangers in the community

> A severely disabled person at home wishes to smoke but because of his condition drops the cigarette and causes fires. He has been burnt on several occasions, but still continues to smoke. Fire alarms and smoke detectors have been fitted to his premises and they keep going off. Even if social services try to prevent him having access to matches, he obtains them from neighbours. What is the law? Can he be allowed to remain a menace to public safety?

Unlike the preceding situation where the patient is in hospital, here the person is in the community, presumably living on his own. There are provisions to take a person to a place of safety under the National Assistance Act 1948 and the Mental Health Act 1983 if the statutory conditions are present (see Chapters 21 and 24). However it is likely that these conditions would not be present in these circumstances and it may be necessary to prepare a care package which takes account of the dangers from his smoking and the need for persons to be in attendance. Neighbours could be warned of the dangers of giving him matches and then leaving him on his own.

Situation: Enveloped in smoke

> A physiotherapist visits a patient with MS. Both he and his wife smoke and the room reeks of tobacco. The physiotherapist is concerned about her own health as a passive smoker in this environment. Does she have any rights?

The physiotherapist cannot be compelled to enter a situation which damages her health. It would be uncertain how damaging spending half an hour in this environment three times a week is likely to be. Certainly it would be reasonable for the physiotherapist to ask the couple not to smoke whilst she is visiting. However it is unlikely that the circumstances here are sufficient to justify any refusal to attend.

Conclusions

It is not possible in a work of this kind to consider every possible type of physical disability and physical injury or condition which physiotherapists might treat and consider the legal implications of each. Emphasis has to be placed on the general principles. However it is apparent that considerable criticisms can be made about the facilities which are available for those suffering from physical disabilities. However, as the Disability Discrimination Act 1995 (see Chapter 17) is implemented the situation will improve. Regulations such as the *Building Regulations (Amendment) Regulations 1998*, SI No. 2561 (which further amend existing regulations in relation to access and facilities for disabled persons and detail new requirements in relation to sanitary conveniences in dwellings) will make considerable improvements in the quality of life of those physically disabled.

The National Audit Office reported on health services for physically disabled people aged 16 to 64[31] in 1992 and concluded that more action needed to be taken to provide more rehabilitation services generally and in particular the treatment of incontinence and prevention of pressure sores. Specific recommendations were made for health authorities to ensure that rehabilitation services were provided to meet identified need including services for brain damaged people. Gaps in the provision of respite care should be identified and action taken to fill them. In addition there should be improvements in the timeliness, quality, and availability of information on services available for physically disabled people. Physiotherapists have a key role to play in identifying the gaps and ensuring that the appropriate services are provided and monitored.

 Questions and exercises _____

1   A client suffering from multiple sclerosis who lives on her own complains to you that her home help visits have been reduced to three a week. What advice do you give her and what action do you take?
2   Your assessment of the physical needs of a person suffering from arthritis and your treatment plan for physiotherapy is rejected by the general practitioner who considers that only six sessions rather than the 12 you have recommended should be provided. What is the legal situation? (See also Chapters 6 and 10.)

3 Draw up a protocol which identifies the role and function of the physio-therapy assistant in the care of those suffering from physical disabilities.

4 You have been asked by your local rugby club to provide a service on the field. What considerations would you take into account before accepting the offer?

5 You are involved in the care of a patient suffering from back pain, but are not convinced that her symptoms are real. You see her shopping in a supermarket with no apparent discomfort. What action, if any, would you take?

6 Following a serious stroke the parents of a 25 year old boy are asked to give consent to brain surgery. They refuse to give consent. What is the legal situation?

References

1   *R* v. *Gloucester County Council, ex parte Mahfood (et al)*. The Times Law Report, 21 June 1995.

2   *R* v. *Avon County Council, ex parte M* [1994] 2 FLR 1006.

3   *R* v. *Birmingham City Council, ex parte Mohammed* The Times Law Report, 14 July 1998.

4   Barnes, G. & Lee, F. (1995) The Coordinating and Planning Services for Stroke Patients in Hospital and the Community. *British Journal of Occupational Therapy* **58**, 4, 158–60.

5   Poole, P. & Johnson, S. (1996) Integrated Care Pathways: An Orthopaedic experience. *Physiotherapy* **82**, 1, 28–30.

6   *R* v. *Gloucester County Council, ex parte Mahfood, et al. R* v. *Islington London Borough Council, ex parte McMillan* (QBD) The Times Law Report, June 21 1995.

7   *R* v. *Gloucester County Council and another, ex parte Barry* [1996] 4 All ER 421.

8   *R* v. *Gloucestershire County Council* [1997] 2 All ER 1.

9   *R* v. *Gloucestershire County Council* [1997] 2 All ER 1.

10   For further information on statutory duties and community care see Dimond, B.C. (1997) *The Legal Aspects of Care in the Community*. Macmillan, Basingstoke.

11   Evans, P. (1995) Association of Chartered Physiotherapists in Sports Medicine. *In Touch* Winter 1995, 74, 29.

12   Ian Murray 'Sports Injuries show rugby is the riskiest'. *The Times* 14 September 1998.

13   Mitten, M.J. & Mitten, R.J. (1995) Legal considerations in treating the injured athlete. *Journal of Orthopaedic and Sports Physical Therapy* 21 January (1), 38–43.

14   News Item (1998) *Frontline* **4**, 13, 1 July, 17.

15   Hackney, R. The Sports Hernia. *In Touch* Winter Issue 1995/6, 78, 2–3.

16   Virginia Fletcher 'Damages for injured girl made to do PE'. *The Times*, 6 August 1998.

17   Mendell, E. (1995) Preparing your patient for skiing. *In Touch* Winter Issue 1995/6, 78, 10–11.

18   Tajet-Foxell, B. & Booth, L. (1996) An 'Equal Expertise' Approach to Rehabilitation of Athletes. *Physiotherapy* **82**, 4, 264–6.

19   Payne, S.D.W. (ed.) (1990) *Medicine Sport and the Law*. Blackwell Scientific Publications, Oxford.

20   Grayson, E. & Bond, C. (1996) *Sports Medicine: Ethics and Law*. Butterworth-Heinemann, Oxford.

21   Exelby, L. (1994) The Manipulation Association of Chartered Physiotherapists. *In Touch* Autumn 1994, 73, 17.

22 Saunders, S. (1994) British Association of Chartered Physiotherapists in Manipulation. *In Touch* Summer 1994, 72, 10.

23 Taken from Hutson, M.A. (1993) *Back Pain Recognition and Management.* (page 51) Butterworth-Heinemann, Oxford.

24 Hutson, M.A. (1993) *Back Pain Recognition and Management.* (page 39) Butterworth-Heinemann, Oxford.

25 Kulkarni, J. *et al.* (1996) Falls in Patients with Lower Limb Amputations: Prevalence and Contributing factors. *Physiotherapy* **82**, 2, 130–5.

26 Lynch, M. & Grisogono (1991) *Strokes and Head Injuries.* John Murray, London.

27 The Association of Chartered Physiotherapists in Respiratory Care (1996) *Clinical guidelines: physiotherapy management of the spontaneously breathing, acutely breathless, adult patient.* ACPRC, Solihull.

28 Sagar, H. (1991) *Parkinson's Disease.* Macdonald Optima, London.

29 Hutson, M.A. (1993) *Back Pain Recognition and Management.* Butterworth-Heinemann, Oxford.

30 Tancred, W. & Tancred, G. (1996) Implementation of Exercise programmes for Prevention and Treatment of Low Back Pain. *Physiotherapy* **82**, 3, 168–173.

31 National Audit Office (1992) *Report on Health Services for Physically Disabled People aged 16 to 64.* HMSO, London, *see also* NAHAT Briefing Summary, September 1992.

Chapter 21
Care of the Mentally Ill

This chapter aims to give the physiotherapist an understanding of the law in relation to the care of those suffering from a mental illness (both the detained and the informal patient). Legal issues arising from the care of those with neurological conditions are considered in Chapter 20. Reference should also be made to text books on physiotherapy and mental health[1]. Useful sources of law relating to the care of the mentally ill are given in the bibliography.

The following topics are covered in this chapter:

- Physiotherapists practising in the field of mental health
- The Mental Health Act 1983
- Care in the community
- Informal patients
- General issues involving physiotherapists
- The future

Physiotherapists practising in the field of mental health

Physiotherapy has been seen in the past as essentially dealing with the physical and therefore its role in mental illness has been doubted. Thus in 1992, in reporting the results of research into the recruitment of physiotherapists into psychiatry, Helen Ainsworth[2] stated that psychiatry had not been part of physiotherapy training and even then was covered patchily, that senior physiotherapists therefore had little or no experience in the field and were reluctant to take on the unknown.

The situation is changing however. Inevitably the main contribution of physiotherapists in the field of mental health has been a traditional one with the emphasis on physical problems, but physiotherapists realise that they can make a significant contribution in the treatment of psychiatric and psychological problems. The physiotherapist working in the field of mental health needs to be multi-skilled with a knowledge of mental illness as well as physical problems. For example Pat Massey[3] explored the role of autogenesis (passive concentration on the relaxed body which promotes changes in attention, consciousness, thought and emotion) in treating anxiety states.

Some physiotherapists who specialise in the care of the mentally ill will be working in secure psychiatric units where most patients will be detained under the Mental Health Act 1983. Other physiotherapists specialising in mental health care may be involved in community care and/or with long-stay chronic mentally disordered patients who are not detained under the Act and others who suffer from depression, anxiety states and behavioural problems.

The ACPMHC

An Association of Chartered Physiotherapists in Mental Health Care (formerly the Association of Chartered Physiotherapists in Psychiatry formed in 1982) facilitates the exchange of information and the development of the understanding of physiotherapists practising in this field. Its aims are shown in Figure 21.1.

Figure 21.1   Aims of the Association of Chartered Physiotherapists in Mental Health Care

- To provide a representative body of physiotherapists in psychiatry.
- To establish standards of good practice through education and research.
- To facilitate the exchange of ideas and information.
- To improve multi-disciplinary communication and understanding.
- Formation of Regional Groups.
- To encourage communication and interaction with physiotherapists in other spheres.
- To encourage the involvement of community physiotherapists with psychiatric patients.

The ACPMH has prepared guidelines for good practice for physiotherapists working in this area. This covers the role of the physiotherapist in mental health care, standard setting and quality, key points of competence, quality measures, developing a physiotherapy service in mental health and examples of physiotherapy input[4].

Examples of input include:

- Assessment of difficulties of mobility and function associated with physical, mental or psycho-social problems.
- Assessment of problems of mobility and function related to chronic mental illness and associated with drug induced symptoms of abnormal muscle tone, posture and gait.
- Setting realistic goals with client and/or carers.
- Planning and implementing treatment programmes for clients including those who are unable or unwilling to communicate or co-operate.
- Individual or group exercise programmes to:
  - promote physical and mental health
  - improve functional ability, confidence and self-esteem
  - maintain fitness and maximise physical independence
  - give purposeful use of energy
  - release aggression

○ promote relaxation
○ prevent/delay deterioration of physical ability.

Projects undertaken by members are published by the Association. For example Ann Chapman has looked at physiotherapy intervention in the treatment of anorexia nervosa[5] and Elizabeth Coleman has studied a holistic physiotherapy approach to treatment in chronic low back pain and anxiety/depression[6].

Further information is available through the CSP (see list of addresses).

The Mental Health Act 1983

The philosophy of the Mental Health Act 1983 is that admission to a psychiatric hospital should be avoided if there is alternative treatment and care available outside and compulsory admission should not be used if the patient will agree to be admitted as an informal patient or if alternative services outside the hospital are possible. Since only about 5 to 10% of psychiatric patients are detained under the statutory provisions, the physiotherapist working with the mentally disordered is more likely to be caring for informal rather than detained patients unless she works in a regional secure unit or special hospital. However they should all have an understanding of the basic provisions of the Act.

Definition of mental disorder

Nobody can be compulsorily detained under the Mental Health Act 1983 unless they are suffering from mental disorder as defined in the Act. The definition is set out in Figure 21.2.

Figure 21.2   Mental Health Act 1983 – section 1.

'Mental disorder' means mental illness, arrested or incomplete development of mind, psychopathic disorder and any other disorder or disability of mind ...

[All these terms, except mental illness, are further defined]

The Act makes it clear that a person cannot be dealt with under the Act as suffering from mental disorder 'by reason only of promiscuity or other immoral conduct, sexual deviancy or dependence on alcohol or drugs'. This means that if a patient is abusing drugs he cannot be detained under the Mental Health Act 1983 unless he is shown to be suffering from mental disorder apart from the drug abuse.

Compulsory admission

There are three main sections for the compulsory admission of the mentally disordered person (other than through the courts). These are shown in Figure 21.3.

Figure 21.3 **Compulsory admission for mental disorder.**

Section 4   emergency admission for assessment for up to 72 hours.

Section 2   admission for assessment for up to 28 days.

Section 3   admission for treatment for up to 6 months – this section can be renewed, initially for six months, and thereafter for twelve months at a time.

Admission for assessment – sections 4 and 2

The requirements for the medical recommendation for admission under sections 2 and 4 are shown in Figure 21.4.

Figure 21.4 **Medical requirements for section 2 or 4 admission.**

(a)   [The patient] is suffering from mental disorder of a nature or degree which warrants the detention of the patient in a hospital for assessment (or for assessment followed by medical treatment) for at least a limited period; and

(b)   he ought to be so detained in the interests of his own health or safety or with a view to the protection of other persons.

The applicant is usually an approved social worker (ASW) though, as with the other two sections, it could be the 'nearest relative' (a term defined by the Act – see below). ASWs are 'approved' because they have had to undergo a special training in mental health.

Section 4 is an emergency admission section and enables a person to be detained for up to 72 hours on the basis of one medical recommendation. In applying for a section 4 emergency admission the ASW has to explain why a second medical recommendation for admission could not be obtained. The application is made to the managers (see below) of the appropriate hospital and the application gives authority to the ambulance men or police to transfer the patient to the hospital. When a second doctor can be contacted the admission under section 2 with the longer period for assessment can be made.

Section 2 is an application for assessment and under this the person can be detained for up to 28 days. There must be two medical recommendations, one of them from a doctor who is recognised as having the required expertise in psychiatric medicine, i.e. he is approved under section 12 of the Act – colloquially called 'a section 12 approved' doctor. One of the two doctors should have had previous acquaintance with the patient and, if this is not possible, the ASW must explain the reasons why on the application form. The medical requirements shown in Figure 21.4 must be present.

Admissions for treatment – section 3

This is an admission for treatment (sometimes following an initial assessment under section 2) and can last up to six months, and it can be renewed. Two medical recommendations are required but, unlike section 2, a specific form of mental disorder must be stated (see Figure 21.5). The other requirements shown in Figure 21.5 must also be present. Again one of the medical recommendations must be by a section 12 approved doctor and preferably at least one of the doctors should have had previous acquaintance with the patient. The nearest relative should be consulted over the application by the ASW and has the right to object to the application being made.

Figure 21.5   **Medical requirements for section 3 admission.**

(a)   [The patient] is suffering from mental illness, severe mental impairment, psychopathic disorder or mental impairment and his mental disorder is of a nature or degree which makes it appropriate for him to receive medical treatment in a hospital; and

(b)   in the case of psychopathic disorder or mental impairment, such treatment is likely to alleviate or prevent a deterioration of his condition; and

(c)   it is necessary for the health or safety of the patient or for the protection of other persons that he should receive such treatment and it cannot be provided unless he is detained under this section.

Definition and powers of the nearest relative

The nearest relative has a significant role to play in the statutory provisions for compulsory admission of the mentally disordered. The relative who is 'nearest' is defined by statute. (section 26 of the Mental Health Act 1983). The order of priority in determining the nearest relative is shown in Figure 21.6.

Figure 21.6   **Definition and order of priority of nearest relative.**

(a)	husband or wife	(e)	grandparent
(b)	son or daughter	(f)	grandchild
(c)	father or mother	(g)	uncle or aunt
(d)	brother or sister	(h)	nephew or niece

A cohabitee would count as the nearest relative where the couple had been living together for a period of not less than six months. A person other than a relative could be classified as a relative if he or she had been ordinarily living with the patient for at least five years. A relative who ordinarily lives with or cares for the patient would take precedence over the others.

The functions and powers of the nearest relative include the following:

● Application for admission of the patient: under section 2 for assessment, or section 3 for treatment, or section 4 emergency admission for assessment – in practice the ASW usually makes the application.
● Application for the patient to be placed under guardianship (section 7).
● Must be consulted by the ASW and can object to an application by an ASW for admission for treatment or for a guardianship order.

- Must be notified of application for admission for assessment and in an emergency (sections 2 and 4).
- Has the power to discharge the patient from compulsory admission under section 2 or 3 but must give 72 hours notice to the Managers of such an intention.

Treatment for mental disorder

Compulsory treatment for mental disorder can be given under the Act to the patient detained under either section 2 or section 3 but not to the patient who is detained under section 4. This is so even though section 2 is described as admission for assessment. Figure 21.7 shows the treatments which can be given and the conditions required.

Figure 21.7   **Treatment for mental disorder.**

Section 57   Surgery destroying brain tissue, hormonal implants to control sexual urge. The patient must consent and the understanding of the patient to consent should be certified by three persons appointed by the Mental Health Act Commission, one of whom must be a registered medical practitioner. The latter must certify that the treatment should be given.

Section 58   Medication after three months and electro convulsive therapy (ECT). The patient must either consent or a second opinion must be obtained from an independent doctor appointed by the Mental Health Act Commission.

Section 63   Any treatment not covered by section 57 and 58 which is given for mental disorder under the direction of the responsible medical officer.

Section 62   The provisions of the above sections to be dispensed with in an emergency situation.

The second opinion appointed doctor

It should be noted that if medication is required after three months and the patient is either unable or unwilling to give consent, a second opinion appointed doctor (SOAD) must be called in to decide if the treatment should be given. The SOAD has a duty:

- to examine the patient;
- to determine whether the patient is incapable of giving consent or is refusing consent;
- to talk to the responsible medical officer about the proposed treatment; and
- to decide whether the treatment should be given against the patient's will.

Before the SOAD decides he or she must consult with two persons – one a nurse who is professionally concerned with the treatment of the patient and the other who is neither doctor nor nurse who is also professionally concerned with the patient.

Involvement of the physiotherapist

The second person whom the SOAD is obliged to consult before agreeing to treatment under section 58 could be a physiotherapist if she is professionally concerned with the treatment of the patient. The SOAD merely has to record on the statutory form (form 39) the names of the nurse and the other professional whom he has consulted. Their advice does not have to be recorded. If the physiotherapist were to be the second professional to be consulted it would be advisable for her to ensure that she records in her patient records the content of her advice to the SOAD.

A physiotherapist may also be consulted in a treatment decision involving brain surgery for mental disorder or hormonal implants to reduce sexual drive in the male. Before she consents to be formally consulted she must have a good knowledge of the patient and the earlier treatments and be able to give her views on the use of section 57 treatments.

Definition of treatment

Treatment is defined in the Act: 'Medical treatment' includes 'nursing, and also includes care, habilitation and rehabilitation under medical supervision' (section 145(1)).

It has been held[7] that preliminary care given to enable the treatment for mental disorder to be given was within the definition and so covered by section 63. Thus a detained patient who was anorexic could be given tube-feeding, even though that was not the treatment that justified admission under section 3.

This definition would, of course, cover most of the therapy provided by physiotherapists, which in theory could therefore be given compulsorily under section 63. However there are very few treatments offered by physiotherapists which in practice can be given compulsorily against the will of the patient. For the most part treatments rely for their success upon the active involvement and participation of the patient.

There are considerable difficulties in persuading acutely ill or chronically sick patients to accept attendance at therapy sessions. However the patient's involvement can be obtained through a quasi contract in the form of an agreement whereby the treatment plan includes attendance at various sessions and rewards are then forthcoming. Turning up at the treatment venue does not necessarily imply consent by the patient to the treatment and the physiotherapist should be aware of the legal status of the patient and any rights to give treatment under a section. In Chapter 7 the nature and form of consent to treatment is considered in detail.

Individual treatment plans

The physiotherapist may be involved in the multi-disciplinary preparation of a patient's treatment plan. Where this involves medication or electro convulsive therapy, and the detained patient has originally agreed to the plan but then changes his mind, treatment can be continued under section 62 if discontinuance of the treatment would in the view of the responsible medical officer cause serious suffering to the patient (section 62(2)). Arrangements should be made for the SOAD to attend as soon as possible.

Treatment and common law powers

If life saving treatment is required for the patient who is admitted under section 4 then it could be given under the powers which exist at common law under the *Re F* ruling (for further discussion on this see Chapters 7, 22 and 24).

The informal in-patient and the Mental Health Act 1983

Many patients enter psychiatric hospital voluntarily and section 131(1) of the Mental Health Act 1983 emphasises that there is nothing in the Act to prevent patients being admitted without any formality or remaining in hospital after being discharged from their detention. In a recent decision, however, the Court of Appeal[8] interpreted this section as requiring the consent of the patient. As a result guidance[9] was issued that patients not under section should be assessed to determine their competence to consent to admission. If they were judged mentally incapacitated, then they should be examined with a view to admission under the Mental Health Act. As a result many patients had to be compulsorily detained under the Mental Health Act provisions. The House of Lords[10] upheld the Department of Health's appeal against the Court of Appeal decision and confirmed that mentally incapable adults can be admitted to and cared for in hospital under the common law powers to act out of necessity recognised by the House of Lords in *Re F*. (see page 355).

If the patient is already in hospital as an informal patient and wishes to take his own discharge and it would be dangerous to his health or his safety or to the safety of other people for him to do so, he could be detained.

Holding power of the nurse – section 5(4)

This enables an appropriately qualified nurse to prevent an informal patient who is being treated for mental disorder from leaving the hospital. The detention can continue for up to six hours but it will end as soon as the patient's own doctor (or the doctor's nominee) arrives to see the patient. The doctor may then, following an examination of the patient, decide to detain the patient further.

Power of doctor to detain an in-patient section 5(2)

This enables the patient's doctor or the doctor's nominee to detain the patient for up to 72 hours to enable an application to be considered for admission under the Mental Health Act 1983. It may be that after the doctor has examined the patient it is decided that compulsory admission is not necessary. The effect of the section will then end and the patient will revert to informal status. Alternatively, following examination by the patient's own doctor, by another doctor and an ASW an application may be made under section 2 or section 3.

Limitations on these powers

It must be emphasised that the provisions set out in section 5(2) and section 5(4) apply only to in-patients – the doctor's power applying to any in-patient, the nurse's only to in-patients being treated for mental disorder. This means that if a physiotherapist is working in an out-patient day hospital, or other such facility, and an informal patient becomes dangerous to himself or others, the patient can only be detained under section 5(2) or 5(4) if the patient is an in-patient and, in the case of section 5(4), being treated already for mental disorder.

The physiotherapist must be very clear about which category the patient comes under. If an out-patient becomes very disturbed and it appears that statutory powers of detention need to be investigated, then an ASW would have to be summoned together with one registered medical practitioner for detention under section 4 (in an emergency) or two registered medical practitioners for detention under section 2 or 3 to be considered.

Renewal

Section 4, section 2, section 5(4) or section 5(2) are not renewable. A patient on section 2 who needs to be detained for longer can only be further detained on section 3. Section 3 can be renewed for a further six months and then for one year at a time. The procedure for the renewal is that the responsible medical officer in charge of the patient's care examines the patient, within the period of two months ending with the date the section is due to end and, if it appears to him that the specific condition of mental disorder is present and the other conditions required by section 20 (similar to those set out in Figure 21.5) are present, he must furnish to the Managers (a defined term – see below) a report to that effect and the patient's detention is then renewed. The Managers in their review can later decide that the patient should be discharged.

Appeals against detention

The patient can appeal to a Mental Health Review Tribunal (MHRT) for discharge or to the Managers of the hospital. There are set times for applying to the MHRT but not to the Managers. The nearest relative also has the right to apply to an MHRT if his or her attempt to discharge the patient under section 23 (the power to apply for a detailed patient's discharge) has been barred by the responsible medical officer under section 25 (the option to veto that application if certain specified circumstances seem to justify doing so). Either patient or nearest relative can apply to the MHRT if the specific form of mental disorder is reclassified under section 16.

Where a patient has not applied himself for an MHRT hearing during the first six months (and after that at least once every three years) the Managers of the hospital have a duty to refer the patient to the MHRT. (In the case of patients under 16 years, the time limit is every year.)

It may be that the physiotherapist is asked to provide a report and/or oral evidence at the hearing, whether MHRT or Managers' hearing, to give her views upon the discharge. Reference should be made to Chapter 12 on record keeping and to Chapter 13 on report writing and giving evidence in court for the professional principles to be followed.

Information

To the patient
One of the duties on the Managers introduced by the 1983 Act is to ensure that patients receive, both in writing and orally, information relating to the section under which they are detained, the right to apply to the Managers and the MHRT,

and the rules relating to consent to treatment. This duty is usually delegated by the Managers to the nursing staff or the medical records staff. Leaflets are available giving the information for each of the different sections and are available in a wide variety of languages.

A physiotherapist who is concerned that a detained patient does not appear to understand the provisions of the Act or the section he is under, should ask to see the leaflet so that she herself understands the implications of the section the patient is under and can explain it to him.

To the nearest relative

The information which is given to the patient must also be given in writing to the nearest relative. However the patient has a statutory right to object to this information being given to the nearest relative.

The Managers

In respect of a NHS trust these are the non-executive board members and only they, with their co-opted members, can carry out the function of hearing appeals to the Managers by the patient against detention or renewing the patient's detention following a report from the responsible medical officer. These functions of hearing appeals from patients or approving a renewal cannot be delegated to officers. Other functions in respect of the Mental Health Act can however be so delegated.

The Mental Health Act Commission

In 1983 a watchdog for detained patients was established known as the Mental Health Act Commission. It consists of about 90 different professionals and lay people whose jurisdiction is to visit detained patients and to take up any complaints from them where they are not satisfied by the response from the Managers, or any other complaint relating to the exercise of powers and duties under the Mental Health Act.

It also has statutory duties in relation to the withholding of mail in the special hospitals (i.e. Broadmoor, Rampton and Ashworth). The Managers at special hospitals can withhold any postal package sent by the detained person if they consider it likely that it will cause distress to the addressee or to any other person (except hospital staff and other specific public persons such as MPs) or if it is likely to cause danger. Equally, packages sent to a detained patient in a special hospital may be withheld if, in the opinion of the Managers, it is necessary do so in the interests of the safety of the patient or for the protection of other persons. These decisions are subject to review by the MHAC.

It also has a duty every other year to provide a report to the Secretary of State which he must place before each House of Parliament.

Role of the physiotherapist in assessment

Even though the physiotherapist is not amongst those professionals who have the responsibility of admitting the patient for treatment or assessment, she may have a role to play in taking part in the multi-disciplinary work of assessment of the patient's mental health and treatment. In addition she will have her own assessment procedures with regard to:

- health and fitness;
- mobility; and
- physical assessment of musculoskeletal injuries.

The Code of Practice

The Secretary of State has a duty to prepare a Code of Practice. A second edition was published in 1993 and physiotherapists who care for those suffering from mental disorder would find this (or the new edition when produced) a useful tool of reference. Some of its comments and recommendations apply also to the care of the informal patient.

Care in the community

Mental Health Act patients

Even physiotherapists working in the community may find that they are caring for patients who are under the provisions of the Mental Health Act 1983.

Section 17 leave

Some patients who have been detained under the Mental Health Act 1983 may be on section 17 leave. This is leave of absence granted by the responsible medical officer (RMO), i.e. the registered medical practitioner in charge of the treatment of the detained patient. Whilst there is no statutory requirement for the leave to be granted in writing, there are strong reasons in practice why this should be so[11]. The RMO decides the conditions on which the patient can have leave of absence – escorted or unescorted, overnight or any other terms. The RMO has the right to withdraw the leave of absence at any time but this revocation has to be put in writing. The patient must then return to the hospital. If he fails to do so, then he is unlawfully at large and could be returned under section 18 or under the Police and Criminal Evidence Act[12].

If a physiotherapist is attending a patient who is under section 17 leave and is concerned about a deteriorating mental condition, she should ensure that she takes the appropriate action for his return to hospital to be considered. The length of time a patient could be given leave of absence used to be a maximum of six months. This has now been amended by the 1995 Act (see below) and the present situation is that the patient may be given leave for up to 12 months.

An absconding patient who is liable to detention under the Act or refuses to return to hospital when leave of absence under section 17 expires or is revoked can be brought back to hospital under the provisions of section 18. This does not apply to an informal patient who can only be returned to the hospital if he satisfies the compulsory admission provisions of the Act and the correct procedures are carried out.

Section 117 after care

Certain detained patients have a specific right under the Mental Health Act 1983 to receive after care. The right is given by section 117 which is shown in Figure 21.8.

Figure 21.8 The Mental Health Act 1983 – section 117.

(1) This section applies to persons
- who are detained under section 3 [admission for treatment],
- or are admitted to a hospital in pursuance of a hospital order made under section 37 [a court order]
- or who transferred to a hospital [from prison]

and then cease to be detained and leave the hospital.

(2) It shall be the duty of the Health Authority and of the local social services authority to provide, in co-operation with relevant voluntary agencies, after-care services for any person to whom this section applies until such time as the Health Authority and the local social services authority are satisfied that the person concerned is no longer in need of such services. [They cannot be so satisfied if the patient is under after-care under supervision – section 117(2A) added by 1995 Act requiring a section 12 CMRO and supervisor to be provided at all times.]

(3) In this section 'the health authority' and 'the local social services authority' are the health authority and the local social services authority for the area in which the person concerned is resident or to which he is sent on discharge by the hospital in which he was detained.

[subsection (1) is broken down with bullet points for clarity]

This statutory right exists alongside the provisions of the NHS and Community Care Act 1990 which are discussed in Chapter 18. The statutory right is enforceable by the patient against the health authority and/or the local authority[13].

The physiotherapist and after care planning

Ideally care planning for post-discharge should be given before the admission of the patient, so that the treatment aims of the in-patient stay can be decided and the long-term care planned. The physiotherapist will have a role to play in this multi-disciplinary planning and care and should ensure that her involvement is weighty and meaningful. She should also make certain that her input and the outcome in terms of the team's decision is recorded. She has a further important role in ensuring the involvement of patients in after care planning and should discuss with them long-term plans for rehabilitation, employment and accommodation.

Mental Health (Patients in the Community) Act 1995

This Act was introduced to meet the concerns which arose from situations where long-term mentally disordered patients who had been discharged from detention in hospital deteriorated in the community to the extent that they became a serious danger to themselves or other people – Ben Silcock (who was seriously mauled in the lions' enclosure in London Zoo) and Christopher Clunis (who attacked and killed a total stranger at an underground station). The Act introduced an arrangement whereby after care under supervision (known as 'supervised discharge') could be provided.

The grounds for the application

An application can be made for a patient over 16 years who is under sections 3 or 37 or 47 and 48 of the 1983 Act with the aim of ensuring that he receives the after care services to be provided for him under section 117.

It must be shown that

- the patient is suffering from a specific form of mental disorder;
- there would be a substantial risk of serious harm to the health or safety of the patient or the safety of other persons, or of the patient being seriously exploited, if he were not to receive the after-care services to be provided for him under section 117; and
- his being subject to after care under supervision is likely to help secure the after care services to be so provided.

The application can only be made by the responsible medical officer and is addressed to the health authority which has the duty of providing the section 117 services.

Consultation

Before making the application the responsible medical officer must take into account the consultation with:

- the patient;
- one or more persons who have been professionally concerned with the patient's medical treatment in hospital;
- two or more persons who will be professionally concerned with the after care services to be provided under section 117; and
- any person who will play a substantial part in the care of the patient, but will not be professionally concerned with any of the after care services to be provided.

The responsible medical officer must ensure that steps have been taken to consult the nearest relative of the patient and take into account any views expressed by the person so consulted.

The health authority must consult with the local social services authority before accepting a supervision application.

Documentation

The supervision application must be accompanied by a written recommendation of a registered medical practitioner who will be professionally concerned with the patient's medical treatment after he leaves hospital and by the written recommendation of an ASW. There must also be:

- a statement in writing by the person who is to be the community medical officer in relation to the patient after he leaves hospital that he is to be in charge of the medical treatment provided for the patient;
- a statement in writing by the person who is to be the supervisor in relation to the patient after he leaves hospital that he is to supervise the patient;
- details of the after care services to be provided for the patient; and
- details of any requirements to be imposed on the patient under section 25D (a new section introduced into the 1983 Act by that of 1995).

Requirements – section 25D

The requirements which can be imposed upon the patient who is subject to aftercare under supervision include:

- that he reside at a specified place;
- that he attend at specified places and times for the purpose of medical treatment, occupation, education or training; and
- that access to the patient be given, at any time where the patient is residing, to specified persons.

These requirements can be enforced by an authorised person having the power to take or convey the patient to the place of residence or occupation.

Review and appeal

The after care services must be kept under review and can be modified by the responsible after care bodies. The after care supervision lasts for six months beginning with the day on which the supervision application was accepted. It can be renewed for a further six months and then for further periods of one year at a time. The community responsible medical officer may at any time direct that a patient subject to after care under supervision shall cease to be so subject. A patient subject to after care under supervision shall cease to be so subject if he is admitted to a hospital following an application for admission for treatment or is received into guardianship.

The patient can apply to a Mental Health Review Tribunal for the supervision to be ended:

- when the application is first accepted,
- if his diagnosis is changed, or
- whenever the supervision order is renewed.

Involvement of the physiotherapist

The physiotherapist may be involved in these provisions in two ways:

- She may be involved in the discussions which precede an application for the patient to be placed under after care under supervision and therefore contribute to the formulation of the decisions on the required after care services.
- She may be one of the persons specifically consulted (in respect of her professional involvement with the patient) before the responsible medical officer makes an application for after care under supervision.

She needs to be familiar with the implications of the statutory framework for the rights of the patient and her own legal duties and powers.

Multi-disciplinary team and key worker

In certain cases the physiotherapist may be the identified key worker for the care of the patient in the community. If she takes on this role she should ensure that she works within her professional competence. She must have an understanding of the role and competence of other health professionals and also those in other spheres in order to make appropriate referrals for further interventions. There should be clear operational policies on the terms of referral.

The physiotherapist working in the field of mental health may also find that she is relied upon by nurses who are not dual-trained, but only trained in mental health nursing and look to the physiotherapist for expert advice on the physical care of the patient. Again it is essential that the physiotherapist does not work outside her professional competence.

Informal patients

If a patient is not formally detained under the provisions discussed earlier in this chapter or prevented from leaving under section 5(2) or 5(4), then the patient can leave hospital at any time. Many patients however remain in hospital without their active consent simply because they do not have the capacity to make a decision for themselves. There are concerns about the large number of persons who are not detained, and who are outside the provisions of the Mental Health Act 1983 but remain in hospital as passive patients. In 1995 the Law Commission made recommendations[14] which, if implemented, would fill the vacuum which at present exists in relation to decision making on behalf of the mentally in competent adult. Pending such legislation the House of Lords[15] in a recent decision has confirmed that it is lawful for adult patients, who lack the mental capacity to agree to admission, to be admitted informally to psychiatric hospital by the powers which exist at common law, but the need for reform to provide protection for such patients was noted. (This case is further discussed above and in Chapter 22.)

Nevertheless the physiotherapist would have a duty to ensure that she takes action if she is aware that a mentally incompetent informal patient would benefit from the protection provided by the Mental Health Act 1983. There are several advantages to the patient if he is formally detained under the Act including:

- Visits from Mental Health Act Commissioners.
- Provision for the Mental Health Act Commission to investigate complaints made by him or on his behalf.
- Automatic regular review of his detention by the Mental Health Act Commission.
- The appointment of a SOAD before any treatment is given compulsorily or without his consent (after the first three months of medication).
- Being formally notified of these and other rights under the Mental Health Act.

She should also ensure that she is aware of the provisions of the *Code of Practice*[16] prepared and monitored by the Mental Health Act Commission on behalf of the Department of Health which has useful guidance for the care of informal patients. For example there may be informal patients who are cared for behind locked doors. This could constitute a false imprisonment of these patients unless an emergency situation exists. Chapter 18 of the *Code of Practice* gives advice on the care of difficult to manage patients and includes guidance on locked doors and informal patients.

The seclusion of patients must be closely monitored and there should be in existence a clear policy which sets out the maximum intervals within which a patient should be examined by a registered medical practitioner. Managers should review both the policy and its implementation and physiotherapists should ensure that they have copies of the policy and are involved in both its implementation and monitoring.

General issues involving physiotherapists

Danger to the physiotherapist from aggressive patients

The tragic death of the occupational therapist who worked at the Edith Morgan Unit is a sad reminder of the fact that working with the mentally disordered can be dangerous. Those physiotherapists working in acute and specialist units should be aware of the recommendations of the Blom-Cooper report[17]. The employers have a duty to ensure that reasonable care is taken of the health and safety of each employee and also of the general public and this is further discussed in Chapter 11. Physiotherapists should be involved in the risk assessment of any unit for the care of the mentally ill and take active steps to ensure that recommendations for improving health and safety and preventing accidents are implemented. A risk assessment should also be carried out of dangers resulting from home visits. Where the risk assessment indicates it, physiotherapists should also have training in control and restraint procedures and receive regular training in the management of aggression and potential violence.

It is essential that careful records should be kept of any incident, including near misses, since these are vital in carrying out a useful and productive risk assessment.

Danger to patient from equipment

The physiotherapist who works with the mentally ill should also be aware of the dangers of any equipment she is using, not only from the point of view of the patient accidentally or intentionally harming himself, but also from the dangers of the patient harming another person.

She needs to have full information regarding the patient's clinical condition and the risks of any harm which could arise. She must be prepared to carry out this risk assessment and management. Should harm befall a person in a department under her control, she may have to answer for that, both professionally and in relation to her employer and the civil courts. She therefore needs to know the differences which exist in law in relation to her powers and duties towards detained patients compared with informal patients.

Clinical risks may be different from health and safety risks and the physiotherapist must assess for both.

Death of a patient – suicide fears

In the event of an untoward death of an informal patient or the death of a detained patient, the coroner would be informed. In the case of a detained patient, the MHAC would also be informed. The physiotherapist may be required to give a statement on her knowledge of the patient and the events leading to the death (see Chapters 13 and 25).

Monitoring and evaluation

It is essential that the physiotherapist takes part in the monitoring process and assesses the quality and output of her work. Where possible she should try to obtain patient feedback on the services since this could lead directly to improvements.

Relationship with patients

Any improper relationship with a patient would be regarded as misconduct and could therefore be subject to disciplinary proceedings by the Disciplinary Board of the CPSM. This would cover not only sexual impropriety but also the exploitation of vulnerable and mentally incapable adults. There should be a clear procedure relating to the acceptance of gifts (see Chapter 4) so that no suspicions could arise.

Elderly mentally infirm patients

One of the biggest difficulties in caring for the mentally ill is that fact that many patients lack the competence to give consent, or suffer from intermittent mental capacity. Where there are doubts about the mental competence of a patient, it is advisable to obtain a determination of competence by a person not directly involved in the care of the patient. Reference should be made to Chapter 24 on the elderly and consent issues and to Chapter 25 on living wills.

The future

The impact of the Mental Health (Patients in the Community) Act 1995 is being closely monitored and the results are leading to fresh proposals for the care of the long-term mentally ill. Many organisations, such as the Mental Health Act Commission, have called for a radical review of the Mental Health Act 1983. This Act is primarily based on the institutional care of the compulsory detained patient and does not have the focus on community care. Major rethinking is required. In 1998 the Government announced the setting up of an Inquiry to consider the drafting of a new Mental Health Act and there are likely to be significant proposals for revision over the next few years, starting with the White Paper, *Modernising Mental Health Services: Safe, Sound and Supportive*, published in December 1998[18]. Physiotherapists should be aware of these developments and ensure that they play their full part in the important debates which will be taking place.

Questions and exercises

1   An out patient, who has a history of mental health problems, comes to the physiotherapy department and is clearly highly disturbed and may need to be detained. What is the legal situation?

2   A physiotherapist is asked by the second opinion appointed doctor (SOAD) for her views on the giving of electro convulsive therapy to an elderly patient who is extremely depressed and has been starving herself. What information should she obtain and what principles should she follow in providing her recommendation?

3   A detained patient asks a physiotherapist to accompany her to a Managers' hearing on her application for discharge. What action should the physiotherapist take?

4   The physiotherapist is a member of a community mental health team which is caring for a former detained patient who has been placed under after care under supervision. What are the implications of this for the work of the physiotherapist?

References

1   Everett, T., Dennis, M. & Ricketts, E. (eds) (1995) *Physiotherapy in Mental Health*. Butterworth-Heinemann, Oxford.

2   Ainsworth, H. (1992) Recruiting physiotherapists into psychiatry. *Journal of the Association of Chartered Physiotherapists in Psychiatry*. September 1992, IX, 31–4.

3   Massey, P. (1990) Autogenesis – the way forward. *Journal of the Association of Chartered Physiotherapists in Psychiatry*. September 1990, VII, 4–11.

4   ACPMH (1995) *Physiotherapy in Mental Health Care*. CSP, London.

5   Chapman, A. *Physiotherapy intervention in the treatment of anorexia nervosa*. ACPMH, CSP, London.

6   Coleman, E. *A holistic physiotherapy approach to treatment in chronic low back pain and anxiety/depression*. ACPMH, CSP, London.

7   *B* v. *Croydon Health Authority* [1994] The Times Law Report, 1 December 1994, [1995] 1 All ER 683.

8   *L* v. *Bournewood and Community and Mental Health NHS Trust* reported in *The Times* 3 December 1997; [1998] 2 WLR 764.

9   Mental Health Act Commission Guidance Note (issued March 1998) 1/98. *L* v. *Bournewood Community and Mental Health NHS Trust and the Mental Health Act*. MHAC, London.

10   *R* v. *Bournewood Community and Mental Health NHS Trust, ex parte L* (HL) *The Times* 30 June 1998, (also available on the internet).

11   Blom-Cooper, L., Hally, H. & Murphy, E. (1995) *The Falling Shadow – One patient's*

mental health care 1978–1993. Duckworth, London (Report of an Inquiry into the death of an Occupational therapist at Edith Morgan Unit, Torbay 1995).

12 *D'Souza* v. *DPP, sub nom. R* v. *D'Souza* (HL) [1992] 4 All ER 545.

13 *R* v. *Ealing District Health Authority, ex parte Fox* [1993] 3 All ER 170.

14 Law Commission (1995) Report No. 231 *Mental Incapacity*. HMSO, London.

15 *R* v. *Bournewood Community and Mental Health NHS Trust, ex parte L* reported in *The Times* 30 June 1988 (also available on the internet).

16 DoH (1993) *Code of Practice on the Mental Health Act.* 2nd edn. HMSO, London.

17 Blom-Cooper, L., Hally, H. & Murphy, E. (1995) *The Falling Shadow – One patient's mental health care 1978–1993*. Duckworth, London.

18 DoH (1998) *Modernising Mental Health Services: Safe, Sound and Supportive.* HMSO, London.

Chapter 22
Care of Those with Learning Disabilities

The topics to be covered in this chapter include:

- Philosophy behind the care of those with learning disabilities
- Physiotherapy and learning disabilities
- Living and working in the community
- Risk assessment and risk taking
- Horse riding for the disabled
- Decision making and incapacity
- Non-compliance or refusal by client or carer
- Sexual relations and related issues
- Property and exploitation
- Conclusion

It should be pointed out, that whilst for convenience the different client groups (those with physical disabilities, mental illness, learning disabilities, children and the elderly) are considered in separate chapters, many clients may come into more than one category and reference should be made to the other relevant chapters.

Some clients with learning disabilities, for example, also suffer from a mental illness, and these can present some of the most challenging behaviour for physiotherapists to deal with – a challenge which is made more difficult because of the health and social services organisations may classify the client groups differently so that the physiotherapist could be having to deal with different teams and even different NHS Trusts.

The physiotherapist should also be aware of the provisions of the Mental Health Act 1983 which may become relevant in the situation where compulsory powers are needed. The definition of mental disorder includes those who suffer from mental impairment with associated specified conditions (see Chapter 21 on mental illness). It should also be noted that the statutory duties which are placed on local and health authorities in respect of those with disabilities apply to both physical and learning disabilities. To avoid repetition, an account of these duties and the financial benefits which are available is included in Chapter 20 on physical disabilities.

Reference should also be made to Chapter 23 on children for a discussion on the assessment and statementing of children with special educational needs.

Chapter 11 covers the law relating to health and safety, including manual handling. *Learning Disabilities: A Handbook of Care*[1] covers the basic principles applying to all health and social professionals in the care of those with learning disabilities. Chapter 13[2] of this handbook in particular considers the ethical issues which arise and the principles which can be applied in the resolution of moral problems in decision making. Some of the situations which are discussed can also be related to the legal principles considered here.

The Association of Chartered Physiotherapists for People with Learning Disabilities (ACPPLD) (up to 1991 the Association of Chartered Physiotherapists in Mental Handicap) provides a forum for the interchange of information and research developments between members and also publishes a news letter/ journal. Following the death in 1991 of Ann Russell, founder member of the ACPMH which preceded the ACPPLD, a memorial trust was established and there are annual prizes for members who make a contribution to the advancement of the practice of physiotherapy in services for people with learning disabilities. The Association is exploring the establishment of a post-graduate course.

The role of the physiotherapist in learning disabilities was considered in an article by Rita Fraser for MENCAP and reprinted in the ACPPLD newsletter for October 1994[3]. She gives the example of a person being discharged from a long-stay hospital who wanted to be able to fasten the buttons on her coat. This was assigned to the physiotherapist who treated the patient holistically, a treatment which involved dieting and exercise. Physiotherapists can

- help with movement problems,
- help prevent deformity,
- encourage maintenance of good posture,
- promote good health, and
- support and advise carers.

Philosophy behind the care of those with learning disabilities

Autonomy

A basic principle which has been accepted by most 20th century Western Philosophers is that the autonomy of the adult person should be respected and enhanced. Autonomy or self-rule or self-determination is based on the principle of respect for the person. It does not follow that because a person has learning disabilities that he or she is unable to act autonomously. There may be some decisions which are within the person's competence and the aim of any carer – informal or professional – should be to maximise the person's ability to enjoy his or her autonomy. It therefore follows that the rights of the person with learning disabilities should be protected.

The rights shown in Figure 22.1 were identified by Knapp and Slade[4] in relation to the socio-sexual developmentally disabled person.

Figure 22.1   **Rights of the socio-sexual developmentally disabled person.**

- The right to equal educational opportunity.
- The right to education and habilitation which include the right to receive information about sex and contraception.
- The right to be free unless proven dangerous.
- The right to privacy, especially concerning one's intimate bodily functions, including the right to sexual expression.
- The right to equal access to medical services.
- The right to have relationships with one's peers, including the members of the opposite sex – this right includes the right to sexual expression.
- The right to equal opportunities for housing.
- The right to equal and fair treatment by public agencies and officials.

Normalisation

It follows from the principle that the autonomy of an individual should be respected that, as far as is possible, those with learning disabilities should be supported in enjoying as 'normal' a life as possible.

Figure 22.2 shows the rights which these same authors considered essential to implement the principle of normalisation.

Figure 22.2   **Rights to implement the normalisation principle.**

- The right to a normal rhythm to the day (regular mealtimes, work and leisure time).
- The right to experience the normal life cycle.
- The right to grow up, to leave parents and to move into the community.
- The right to live in and experience male/female relationships.
- The right to the same economic standards.
- The right to make choices.
- The right to fail – if developmentally disabled persons are offered as much autonomy as they are capable of, this necessarily will include the possibility of failing, just as everyone experiences this possibility.

Normalisation has as its aim to ensure the full potential of such clients and to attempt to prevent any restriction on their life and opportunities which is not an inevitable consequence of their condition. In this work the physiotherapist has an important role to play. It is clear that in the setting of priorities considerable sums should be available for staffing and equipment.

However, carers always have a duty to act in the best interests of their clients and these are not necessarily achieved by forcing a concept of 'normality' on clients who may be distressed by pressure to make decisions for themselves. Also it is often the case that learning disabilities are accompanied by physical problems and so a 'normal' lifestyle might not be that which is most comfortable for clients or, indeed, best for their physical health.

Situation: Being normal

The physiotherapist assessed a patient as requiring a shoe raise. However the staff in the community home considered that it was not normal to have a raise on one's shoes so, in the interests of the normalisation principle, these shoes were withdrawn. What is the legal situation?

This would appear to be an extremely odd implementation of the normalisation principle – comparable to denying spectacles to a person with extreme short-sightedness because people do not usually wear glasses. The physiotherapist has a responsibility to show the staff the importance to the physical health and safety of the patient that she should wear shoe raises, that long-term damage could occur if they were not worn and advise on how shoes could be obtained which took into account aesthetic or fashion considerations.

Maximum development of potential

The principles which govern the care of those with learning disabilities include not only that of normalisation but also the aim of ensuring the maximum development of the potential of each individual. This requires individual assessment and the preparation of an individual care plan covering all aspects of life – education, health, and social and economic development. The physio-therapist must play her part in this strategic planning for each individual as part of a multi-disciplinary team.

Physiotherapy and learning disabilities

Direct patient contact

Physiotherapy treatments often require more intimate contact with patients than those of other health professionals. Clients may be asked to remove their clothes. Often those with learning disabilities are unable to give a valid consent to such treatments and the removal of clothing.

Situation: Massage for constipation

A physiotherapist advises that massage might assist an extremely constipated client, who suffers from severe learning disabilities. She is concerned that her treatment could be misinterpreted both by the client and others.

Every effort should be made to explain to the patient what the physiotherapist is intending to do. There would be strong reasons to ensure that the physiotherapist is chaperoned, both for her own protection and for that of the client. Clearly if the client refused this treatment, then its value would have to be reassessed.

Equipment for those with physical learning disabilities

Chapter 15 considers legal issues arising from the use of equipment. In this chapter further situations relating to those with learning disabilities will be considered.

Situation: A bad case of housemaid's knee.

A 24 year old patient with severe cerebral palsy, no verbal communication, extremely poor sitting balance and very strong extensor thrusting on excitement was fitted with a Gill II seating system. However due to his fluctuating tone when excited or anxious his extensor thrusting was so strong he broke the hinge between the back and the base. This was repaired with reinforcing struts. A knee brace was used to limit his extensor thrust but the carers were unable to strap his feet to the foot plates. His athetoid movements resulted in his shins pistoning up and down against the knee brace resulting in a bad case of double housemaid's knee. He was treated with ultrasound and resting from the knee brace for 10 days.
[Taken from Maureen Grimmer][5]

The lesson learnt from the above case was that an athetoid patient should not be fitted into a Gill II seating system with knee brace unless one can strap the feet securely to the footplate. One would expect this lesson to be incorporated into the standard of care as measured by the Bolam test (see Chapter 10). One concern raised by this situation is whether the strapping of the feet would be classified as restraint. On the other hand, if the only safe way of transporting such a patient in a wheel chair was by using this strapping, then it would be seen as restraint, but justifiable in the best interests of the patient, like a seat belt in a car. If the patient refuses to agree to the strapping then it should be made clear that he could not go in the wheel chair. If the patient lacked the mental competence to appreciate this reasoning, then the temporary restraint might be justified on the basis that the physiotherapist was acting in the best interests of the patient according to the principle of *Re F*[6].

Situation: Tied to the toilet

In order to preserve the privacy and dignity of the client, a physiotherapist used a belt to tie the client to the toilet. This was so that she would not fall off and could be left alone. Is this lawful?

This would appear to be a degrading practice even if the intention was laudable. It would seem preferable to stay with the client, providing personal support, than to use such a dangerous method of restraint.

Situation: Splints to prevent harm to the face

Rachel, a woman of 32 with severe disabilities, scratches her face and eyes and arm splints are used to protect her.

There would appear to be justification in the short term to prevent Rachel from harming herself, but long-term methods of behavioural therapy and other treatments should be used to obtain a fundamental change in the patient's behaviour. Records should be kept of the use of the splints and regular monitoring should take place to ensure that alternative ways of preventing her harming herself, e.g. by staff being in attendance on her, are used as often as possible.

Manual handling

Care for those with learning disabilities may often involve manual handling. Chapter 11 looks at this subject in more detail and also considers the physiotherapist's liability in instructing staff and providing guidance on manual handling in residential homes. Negligent instructions could give rise to liability if in reliance upon those instructions and a person was harmed or caused harm to others.

Situation: Lifting a patient with cerebral palsy

> Social services staff sought guidance from a physiotherapist in lifting a client who has cerebral palsy. He is well able to walk, but insists upon sitting down on the pavement and even in the road. What legal aspects arise?

Unless the behaviour of this client can be changed, it may be that a risk assessment would result in a recommendation that he should only be permitted outside the grounds of his home if he is in a wheel chair. He could possibly be taken to a safe area such as a park and assisted in walking. Much depends upon the practicality of staff lifting him off the road and to his feet. If he were of any significant weight this may not be safe practice unless there were at least three staff able to carry out the manoeuvre.

Any physiotherapist who is involved in instructing others in manual handling or in giving guidance on specific situations, should ensure that she keeps records of this instruction or guidance, including the details of those present and what was said.

Restraint

Any restriction on the liberty of a person is a false imprisonment unless there is a lawful justification. Such justification could include a lawful arrest by a police constable or citizen exercising the right to arrest under the Police and Criminal Evidence Act 1984. Acting temporarily in the best interests of an adult who lacked mental capacity could also be lawful: thus to hold back a person with learning disabilities from running across the road would be defensible under the doctrine of necessity, recognised at common law.

Situation: Restraint

> John Turner has severe learning disabilities and is always trying to leave the home. Staff tie him to the chair to keep him from wandering off. What is the law?

To tie a person into a chair would be an unlawful act, a false imprisonment, and also a breach of the Human Rights Act 1998 as degrading treatment under Article 3. In exceptional circumstances restraint may be justified as a temporary measure, but:

- it must be in the best interests of the mentally incapacitated adult,
- it must be of short duration, and

- it must be the minimum necessary to protect the health and safety of the person.

Records should be kept and any restraint should be regularly monitored.

In certain situations restraint may be required by law such as the wearing of seat belts.

GP contacts

A physiotherapist working with people with learning disabilities is part of a multidisciplinary team providing care. An important member of this team, though unfortunately not always playing a full part, is the general practitioner. The following situation may be familiar to many.

Situation: No response

A patient with learning disabilities is referred to a physiotherapist by social services. She informs the GP of her involvement, and her planned treatment and asks if there is any reason why the patient should not receive the proposed treatment or participate in a certain activity. She receives no reply and wonders if she can assume that the absence of a reply implies that there is agreement to the treatment plan.

Silence does not imply agreement. In this situation to ensure that no harm occurs to the patient the physiotherapist needs to have access to the patient's medical records. The referral form should also include on it any information relating to the patient's condition of which the physiotherapist should be aware but this cannot be relied on.

In this situation of getting no reply to a request for information the physiotherapist would have to act as a reasonable physiotherapist would do in the circumstances (i.e. in accordance with the Bolam test), which might well be not to commence treatment but consult with her managers for them to take the issue further. If the patient's condition would seriously deteriorate if the treatment did not start immediately, the physiotherapist would have to weigh the risk of delay against the risk of proceeding without possibly relevant information.

Gender issues

A female physiotherapist caring for an adult client with learning disabilities can be confronted with practical difficulties arising from different genders.

Situation: Swimming pool problems

A female physiotherapist uses a standard public swimming pool with a male client who needs help to undress. What should she do?

There are various choices in this situation:

- she could go with him into the male changing room, which would probably embarrass her more than the men in the room;

- she could take the patient into the female changing room which would disturb any other females changing there;
- she could ask the manager if there are any available rooms where she could take the client to change him (the possibility is extremely unlikely).

The answer would appear to be that only a male physiotherapist takes this particular client to the swimming pool or the female physiotherapist ensures that, if she goes, she is accompanied by a male care assistant.

Situation: Undressing in an adult training centre

A physiotherapist attends an adult training centre and considers that treatment is best provided for a patient with learning disabilities if she is undressed. What is the law?

If the treatment is clearly indicated according to the Bolam test (see Chapter 10) and any reasonable physiotherapist would require the patient to be undressed, then this would be justified. However it is essential that the patient's dignity and privacy are respected and a chaperon is recommended.

Situation: Suspected abuse

A physiotherapist visits a patient who lives with her parents and brother and suspects that she may be the victim of sexual abuse. What action should she take?

She has a duty of care to the client and this would include taking appropriate action if she suspected physical or mental abuse. There is no clear mechanism for the protection of the mentally incapacitated adult as there is under the Children Act 1989, although some local authorities now have procedures for dealing with the abuse of the elderly. The physiotherapist should discuss her concerns with the multi-disciplinary team and ensure that social services are brought in (if not already represented on the team). In some circumstances, it may become a police matter and lead to prosecution.

Outcome measures

Ilias Papathanasiou and S. Jane Lyon-Maris[7] discuss outcome measures and case weightings in physiotherapy services for those with learning disabilities. They developed a case weighting system:

- to evaluate the cost of the service,
- to predict the need for physiotherapy,
- to balance and prioritise the caseload between physiotherapists, and finally
- to use as an outcome measure.

They investigated service level and client level and concluded that this problem solving specific therapy approach can be used widely with people who have learning disabilities.

The appropriate adult

It is a requirement that where a person with learning disabilities is involved in any police investigations or court proceedings an appropriate adult should be appointed to protect their interests.

Situation: An appropriate adult

A physiotherapist was asked to attend the police station with a client with severe learning disabilities whom she had known for many years. He was suspected of committing the offence of indecency. What action should she take?

Such a request could be very unnerving for the physiotherapist. It may well be that in the actual situation here described she would need to ensure that a solicitor attended to represent the client legally. She could however, as a person known to the client, ensure that the client was not harassed or bullied and ensure that practical arrangements were made for his care. She should keep records of her involvement.

Living and working in the community

Community homes for those with learning disabilities

The effect of the community care initiative has meant that fewer clients with learning disabilities are cared for in institutions administered under health service organisations and more are cared for either within the family setting or in community homes especially built or adapted for the needs of those with learning disabilities. Some of this accommodation has been provided by Housing Associations which may work in conjunction with care organisations which undertake the day to day management of the home. These organisations often provide a code of practice covering the rights which the client/tenant/resident should enjoy and setting quality standards.

Many clients with learning disabilities are therefore under the care of professionals employed by the social services departments rather than NHS trusts.

At present only a small proportion of those with learning disabilities have been found accommodation in community homes. The physiotherapist, within the context of the multi-disciplinary team, should have a role to play in these community homes, not only in the selection of clients for each home but also in providing support and guidance on the health and mobility of those clients.

Sheltered workshops

Clients, whether living in their family homes or in community homes should have the facility of attending sheltered workshops and other forms of industrial therapy. However provision is patchy across the country. Physiotherapists can work with the multi-disciplinary team and provide expert advice on the most appropriate activities, taking into account any physical handicaps of the client group.

Record keeping

Health professionals visiting on an occasional basis need to be aware of changes in the client's condition.

Situation: 'I was not informed'

Each time a physiotherapist visited a client in a residential home, she said to the staff, please notify me of any changes to the patient's condition and provided an information sheet for any changes to be recorded. On her next visit, she noted that nothing had been recorded and commenced her treatment with the client, who screamed loudly when she touched his shoulder. She was then told that he had had a bad fall two days before.

The physiotherapist clearly understood the importance of knowing the client's recent history and tried to meet this by providing the information sheet and asking the question. Unfortunately the staff asked might not have been on duty at the time and might themselves have had no cause to consult the records where the fall should have been noted. The physiotherapist's own information sheet left at the home for noting such changes, while a laudable attempt to get relevant information, might have confused the issue. It would amount to a second and separate place where the incident should be noted – always difficult when staff are working under pressure (see Chapter 12 on the problems of more than one set of records).

The above situation is an example of the importance of record keeping. At each visit to the Home the physiotherapist should see the patient records and should therefore have read of this incident. She should herself be noting her own treatments and care in these records so that other professionals are aware of her interventions. If records are not being kept, then, through the multi-disciplinary team, she should be urging higher standards of patient care and record keeping.

Conflict with carers

Refusal to grant accommodation

The rights of relatives to refuse to take back an adult client who has been in respite care also need to be considered. In the case of an adult person suffering from mental impairment, if the relatives refuse to take the person back home this is their right and they cannot be compelled to look after him or her. Health and social services professionals would have to look for other accommodation for the client.

Reference should be made to the discussion in Chapter 18 on the guidelines for the division between health services and social services responsibilities on continuing care.

Protection of the autonomy of the client

It may happen that an extremely diligent parent/carer is unwilling to allow a son or daughter with learning disabilities to leave home and enter sheltered accommodation. In an extreme case a mother had been placed under an injunction not to visit her son who had been moved to alternative accommodation. The Court of Appeal ruled that the injunction should be lifted as it was not appropriate to threaten her with imprisonment but the case illustrates the difficulties of 'letting go'.

The role of the physiotherapist

If physiotherapists are aware of a conflict between the rights (as shown in Figure 22.2) of the person with learning disabilities and the wishes of the carer, they should (within the context of the multi-disciplinary team) ensure that action is taken to protect the client and endeavour to secure a harmonious outcome, bearing in mind the rights of the client. Again this is another area, where if the recommendations of the Law Commission (see below) were to be implemented, the client who lacks the mental capacity to make his own decisions would be protected.

Risk assessment and risk taking

The philosophy of normalisation requires that health and social services professionals working with those with learning disabilities should be acquainted with and implement a risk assessment strategy in relation to each individual client. It would be possible to prevent any harm arising by keeping the client indoors under close supervision and denying him or her opportunities to go shopping, to go to work and to undertake every day activities. However the quality of life would be severely reduced if the opportunities were not taken for holidays, trips and other activities.

The law requires that reasonable precautions are taken to prevent reasonably foreseeable risks of harm. Thus a risk assessment in respect of each individual client would be required to identify the risks of possible harm to the client or other people arising and to determine what action would be reasonable to prevent such risks occurring.

It is essential that records are kept of this risk assessment so that should the client's condition deteriorate or improve, it is possible to identify the significance of these changes to the proposed participation in the activities and so that other health care workers can identify through the treatment plan what a client should or should not be encouraged to do. Records are also of extreme importance if harm arises to the client or another person and the professional is required to justify her action before the civil courts, criminal courts, disciplinary proceedings, or professional conduct proceedings. If it can be established that the actions of the professional were reasonable in relation to reasonably foreseeable risks, then civil liability should not exist.

In Chapter 11 the use of a risk assessment strategy is considered in the context of health and safety and this strategy could also be used in relation to individual care planning.

Risk assessment and client compliance

Situation: Cycle helmet – a necessity

> The physiotherapist has carried out a risk assessment of cycling and recommended that cycle helmets should be worn. One particular client refuses to wear a cycle helmet.

What is the legal situation? Can he be allowed to cycle without a helmet at his own risk or should he be refused the chance of cycling?

If the client's learning disabilities make it impossible for him to appreciate the risks of cycling without a helmet, he cannot, in law, voluntarily accept the risk of being harmed. The defence of *volenti non fit injuria* (see Chapter 10) would therefore not apply. Those caring for this person must ensure that all reasonable care is taken during any activities. Reasonable care would include wearing a helmet. Failure to wear a helmet would therefore preclude cycling. It may be that skilful teaching, showing the client other persons wearing helmets, letting him choose the colour and other ways of involvement may lead to his co-operation in accepting that cycling requires that helmets have to be worn.

Situation: Water sports

A physiotherapist arranges with a local yacht club that the club facilities can be used by clients with learning disabilities. She is concerned about the safety of one client who often fails to obey instructions. Would it be too risky to permit this client to take part in activities?

At the heart of the answer to this situation should be a risk assessment. The physiotherapist has a duty to take reasonable care of the safety of the client. She can reasonably foresee that this client might refuse to obey extremely important instructions and jeopardise his own safety and that of others. She needs therefore to balance the risks with the benefits and also consider how any risks could be reduced. If on balance the risks of harm cannot be avoided or reduced, then it would be reasonable to refuse to permit the client to take part. Much of course depends upon the mental capacity of the client and it could be that behavioural therapy methods could lead to compliance by the client, so that the risks were reduced.

Risk management and rebound therapy

Rebound therapy has been found useful in work with clients with learning disabilities. A clear risk assessment should be carried out before the therapy commences. Draft Rebound Therapy Guidelines were published in July 1996 by the ACPPLD. They suggest that the client is screened for many problems including cardiac or circulatory problems, respiratory problems, vertigo, epilepsy, spinal cord and neck problems, etc.

Situation: Rebound therapy and pregnancy

A physiotherapist assessed a client for rebound therapy following the guidance issued by the ACPPLD. She failed to ascertain whether the client was pregnant. During the therapy, the client complained of severe stomach cramps and subsequently miscarried. The client's parents are now threatening to sue the physiotherapist for negligence.

It was ascertained that the physiotherapist had asked the client if she had had any recent medical attention, but did not ask her specifically if she was pregnant. Her failure to ask this specific question would be judged against the reasonable practice of a competent physiotherapist practising in the field of rebound therapy, whether or not a specific question on pregnancy was on the guidelines set by the ACPPLD.

If a client is incapable of understanding the question or the importance of it, enquiries should be made of the parents or carers as to the client's situation and whether pregnancy is a possibility.

Horse riding for the disabled

Horse riding can be a useful activity in the care and treatment for both the physically and mentally handicapped, but for convenience the topic is included in this chapter on learning disabilities. There are three classifications recognised by the Association of Chartered Physiotherapists in Therapeutic Riding:

- Therapeutic riding – where the client is taught to ride by an instructor and the physiotherapist assesses the rider.
- Hippotherapy – treatment using the movement of the horse.
- Recreational riding.

Jan Eastburn reviews the work of four years of hippotherapy with learning disabilities[8] and the value of setting tasks to be achieved and presenting certificates of achievement.

Such activities inevitably involve some element of risk and, particularly in working with those with learning disabilities, there is a duty on the health professionals to be vigilant on behalf of clients who might lack the capacity to appreciate and accept risks for themselves. The defence of *volenti non fit injuria*, or the voluntary assumption of risk on the part of the plaintiff, would not be available (see Chapter 10). The benefits are to be weighed against the risks in accordance with the Bolam test and changing circumstances kept under review.

Situation: Biting the horse[9]

Cathy, recently discharged from a long-stay hospital joined a Riding for the Disabled Group. People were nervous about how she would cope. She stroked the horse and was placed upon it and then suddenly leant forward and bit the horse.

In this situation it was explained that this was Cathy's way of indicating that she liked someone. However if as a result the horse had bolted with Cathy upon it would those responsible have been liable? There is no doubt that they would have a duty of care for Cathy. However liability would depend upon the extent to which they could have foreseen the specific risk of Cathy biting the horse and the horse therefore bolting. Once, of course, the event has occurred, the risk is foreseeable and should be taken into account. Thus in Cathy's case the author noted that Cathy was banned from riding, but proved to be a great water baby.

Situation: Assessing for competition categories in riding for the disabled

A physiotherapist, who assisted in riding for the disabled, was asked to provide an assessment profile of a disabled person for the correct category for a competition.

Subsequently the disabled person challenged the physiotherapist for a negligent assessment, disagreeing with the category within which she had been placed. Would the disabled person win any case?

The fact that the physiotherapist has volunteered her services does not imply that she has no duty of care to the client. Once she voluntarily accepts that task then she would be obliged to use all reasonable care, relevant to the circumstance, in fulfilling the duty of care. It would have to be shown that no reasonable physiotherapist would have assessed in the way in which she did. If the volunteer has carried out her duties reasonably according to the Bolam test (see Chapter 10) she should not be liable. Moreover the disabled person would also have to show that harm has been suffered as the result of the negligent assessment. Harm could include financial loss, and this may mean proving that had the disabled person been in a different category then prizes could have been won. This might be difficult to establish.

However this scenario shows the advisability of the physiotherapist keeping clear, comprehensive records even in situations where she is volunteering help.

Situation: Recommending an activity

A physiotherapist suggested that a particular client would benefit from horse riding. When the appointment came, the horse riding exacerbated a pre-existing shoulder injury. Whose responsibility is it to ensure that the client is fit to undertake the activity?

A physiotherapist would not be following the Bolam test in providing a reasonable standard of care for a client, if she recommended a particular activity without ensuring that the client was fit to undertake it. However once her assessment has been made, any subsequent changes in the client's condition should be assessed by the carer, or the individual supervising the activity, to ensure that the client is still safe in undertaking it.

Decision making and incapacity

Many clients with learning disabilities may still have the capacity to make decisions on their own account. Clearly the client's capacity must be related to the nature of the decision to be made. The client may be able to choose what clothes to wear or to buy but may not have the capacity to decide whether or not to undergo an operation to be sterilised. The basic principle of law is that a mentally competent adult has the right to give or refuse consent and cannot be compelled to have treatment even if it is life saving (see Chapter 7). At present, however, for adults of 18 and over who lack the capacity to make their own decisions, there exists a vacuum in law. No person has the legal power to make decisions in their name.

The *Re F* principle

In one case carers wanted a woman with learning disabilities to be sterilised in her best interests. Since no person had the legal right to give consent the issue was brought to court. The House of Lords[10] recognised the vacuum in law but stated that a professional had the duty to act in the best interests of any adult person who lacked the necessary mental capacity and should follow the Bolam test (see glossary) in providing a reasonable standard of care. The House of Lords recommended that a decision relating to an operation for sterilisation or similar treatment should be brought to the court and a Practice Direction (see glossary) has been issued and has since been updated.

The Law Commission proposals

The Law Commission, following an extended period of consultation on the issue of decision making and mental incapacity, prepared draft legislation[11] in 1995 which, if implemented, would ensure that a statutory framework would be established for decisions to be made in accordance with their seriousness. Court approval would be required for decisions relating to sterilisations, abortions, etc. However at the other end of the hierarchy, decisions could be made by a carer who would have a statutory power to make them on the client's behalf.

Recent developments

The Lord Chancellor issued a consultation document in December 1997[12] *Who Decides*. Following this consultation it is anticipated that a Bill will be introduced into Parliament to enact the Law Commission's recommendations. In the meantime, carers and health professionals in giving treatment and care to those who do not have the capacity to give a valid consent are protected by the powers recognised at common law in the case of *Re F.*, provided that they act in the best interests of the client and follow the reasonable standard of care (see Chapter 7 and the law relating to acting out of necessity).

A recent House of Lords decision[13] has confirmed that the power of acting out of necessity in the best interests of a person who lacks mental capacity can also apply to the admission of such patients to psychiatric care. The House of Lords overruled a Court of Appeal decision which had held that any adult who lacked the mental capacity to give consent to voluntary admission to psychiatric care had to be examined with a view to detention under the provisions of the Mental Health Act 1983 (see Chapter 21).

Non-compliance or refusal by client or carer

The client

The care of those with learning disabilities should be aimed at ensuring the maximum autonomy and decision making by the clients (see above). However difficulties can arise if the client refuses to undertake exercises which are necessary as part of a treatment plan designed by a physiotherapist. There is no statutory power to compel clients to co-operate in treatment unless the patient is formally detained under the Mental Health Act 1983 (see Chapter 21) and the treatment is seen as part of the treatment for mental disorder. There would, however, be power at common law to act out of necessity to provide treatment without their consent provided it is in their best interests (see above). However this is usually not practicable with physiotherapy treatments and it is clearly preferable to secure the client's cooperation. It may be possible as part of a treatment plan to build in incentives for the client to be involved and thus encourage participation.

Situation: Compulsory treatment?

> A client, with severe learning disabilities, has a fractured femur and was attended by a physiotherapist after surgery. The client refused to come out of bed to commence mobilisation. Can he be compelled to do so?

If the client were mentally competent the answer would be 'No' (see Chapter 7). However here the client lacks the mental capacity to make an appropriate decision. The House of Lords decision in *Re F*[14] would enable the physiotherapist to act in the best interests of the client following the reasonable standard of care. In these circumstances some limited coercion would therefore be permitted. However it is essential that all non-forceful means of compulsion should first be employed to persuade the client to co-operate in attempting to walk. A risk assessment would be necessary to ensure that the risks of harm were avoided or reduced and to identify the number of staff needed to walk the patient safely.

Non compliance by carer

Situation: Non-cooperation by carer

> The physiotherapist, following an assessment on a patient with learning disabilities, makes several recommendations as to what she thinks is best for the client, including daily passive movements to be carried out by the carer. She fears however that the care workers who look after the client may not carry out these exercises. What is the legal situation?

In this situation a distinction has to be made between the carer as an employee and the carer as a relative/friend in a non-employment situation.

Carer as an employee

If the physiotherapist has recommended a treatment plan which is to be implemented by the care worker, this should be discussed with the multi-disciplinary team as part of the treatment plan for that patient, taking into account the resources available. The home manager would then have the responsibility of ensuring that staff implemented the agreed care plan. Care assistants should be supervised to ensure that treatment plans were carried out. Failures by the care assistant should be followed by disciplinary measures, initially counselling and subsequently oral or written warnings.

Carer as a relative/friend

Where the carer is a relative or volunteer, then there is no contract which is enforceable against them to ensure that a treatment plan was implemented.

Clearly explanations would be given of the importance of following any recommendations by the physiotherapist (see Chapter 7). If they fail to comply and this lack of compliance affects the health and safety of the patient, then action could be taken with social services co-operation to remove the adult patient to other accommodation where the necessary care and treatment could be provided. Clearly this would only take place in an extreme situation. If the patient is a child, then the Children Act 1989 provides the mechanism for such action (see Chapter 23). Until the recommendations of the Law Commission[15] on a framework for decision making on behalf of the mentally incompetent adult are implemented, there is no easy procedure to be followed.

Situation: Deliberate obstruction by a relative

> David was 35 years old with severe learning disabilities and epileptic fits. He lived in a community home but was regularly visited by his mother, who insisted on playing a major decision-making role in all aspects of his life. She stated that he was not safe to walk and objected when staff helped him to walk unaided. She also refused to let him attend at the day centre for assessments and treatment by the physiotherapist. It was suggested that David should wear a helmet because of the frequency of his epileptic fits, but his mother objected to that. What is the legal position?

David is over 18 years. He appears to lack the mental capacity to make decisions for himself. Carers and professionals looking after him have a duty under the *Re F* principle to make decisions on his behalf and act in his best interests. It is clear that the mother is not, according to professional opinion, acting in his best interests. In theory it would be possible to obtain a declaration of the court about his best interests and the action which health professionals should take. Unfortunately in the absence of the statutory framework recommended by the Law Commission[16], there is no clear procedure by which there can be an absolute determination of the care of a mentally handicapped adult. The difficulty in this case is that David is probably gaining considerable benefit for the continuing relationship with his mother and any attempt to overrule her, albeit in David's best interests, might lead to difficulties between them. This is essentially a balancing act: would David benefit more by action being taken to enforce the mother to accept the treatment recommended by the physiotherapists for David, with a possible loss of contact or at least strained relations between them; or would David benefit more from the continued contact with his mother, unchanged without the treatment? Clearly all should be done to persuade the mother of the value to David of having the assessments, treatment and helmet. (See above for a case where the court intervened to prevent a mother from visiting her son.)

Sexual relations and related issues

Implicit in the concept of normalisation is the view that those suffering from learning disabilities should be able to participate in sexual activity according to their mental understanding.

Protection by the criminal code

The law protects those who do not have the capacity to give consent to sexual intercourse. It is an offence for a man to have unlawful sexual intercourse with a woman who is a defective (Sexual Offences Act 1956, section 7). However it is a defence if a man is able to prove that he did not know and had no reason to suspect that the woman was defective. In the case of *R* v. *Hudson*[17] the Court of Criminal Appeal allowed the appeal of the defendant against conviction on the grounds that a subjective test should have been applied to determine whether he had reason to suspect this.

Section 128 of the Mental Health Act 1959 (which was not repealed by the 1983 Act) makes it an offence for a man on the staff of or employed by a hospital or mental nursing home to have extra-marital sexual intercourse with a woman who is receiving treatment for mental disorder in that hospital or home either as an out-patient or an in-patient. It is also an offence for a man to have extra-marital sexual intercourse with a woman who is subject to his guardianship or is otherwise in his custody or care. (There is a defence if the man did not know and had no reason to suspect that the woman was a mentally disordered patient.)

The Criminal Law Revision Committee investigated sexual offences including those involving mentally disordered persons[18] in 1984 and recommended that the law should cease to make it illegal for a severely mentally handicapped man to have sexual intercourse with a severely mentally handicapped woman.

Protecting the vulnerable

The practical problem for carers is on the one hand protecting a person with learning disabilities from abuse and exploitation and on the other hand ensuring that where the capabilities exist the client should enjoy the rights set out in Figure 22.1.

Physiotherapists, working within the multi-disciplinary team, should be aware of the importance of protecting vulnerable people who may not have the capacity to consent and who may be exploited in sexual relationships. It is also important to ensure that they are protected against the risk of AIDS/HIV or other infections. Preventing pregnancy is only one aspect of safe sex[19].

The right to procreate

The rights set out in Figures 22.1 and 22.2 relate only to the client, no other person's rights are affected. However the right to procreate involves the rights of the future child. There is considerable debate as to whether a person with severe learning disabilities has a right to procreate[20].

Sterilisation

As the result of the case of *Re D* in 1976[21] (where a mother sought a declaration that her daughter, a sufferer of Sotos Syndrome, could be sterilised) it became a requirement that those seeking non-therapeutic sterilisations (i.e. one which was not required for the physical ill-health of the patient) should first obtain a declaration of the court. In this case, the judge refused to permit the sterilisation of a girl of 11 years, since it was not established that the child would not have the ability to make a decision for herself at a later date. On the other hand, in Jeanette's case[22] the House of Lords gave its approval to the sterilisation of a girl of 17 years who suffered from learning disabilities and in the case of *Re F*[23] (see above) the House of Lords declared that it would be lawful to sterilise a mentally incompetent adult woman if it were in her best interests and the doctors acted according to the Bolam test.

If there is a request from a relative that the client be sterilised then the professional should raise this issue with the multi-disciplinary team and ensure that, if necessary, an application is made to the court in accordance with the Practice Note[24]. The decision to sterilise an individual is one of the most significant which can be taken and it is essential that any health professional who is involved in the court proceedings and the evidence which is required should follow the principles considered in Chapter 13.

Abortion

A person with learning disabilities who has the capacity to give a valid consent could sign the form for an abortion to be carried out provided that the requirements of the Abortion Act 1967 (as amended by the Human Fertilisation and Embryology Act 1990) are met, unless an emergency situation exists. Where the person with learning disabilities lacks competence, then at common law the doctors have the power to act in the best interests of the patient under the principle of necessity set out by the House of Lords in the case of *Re F* (see above). However in contentious circumstances a declaration of the court should be sought before the abortion is undertaken.

Property and exploitation

The duty of care owed by the health professional to care for a client would also include a duty of care in relation to any property of the client. Where the client has the capacity to look after his or her own property, then the health professional does not become responsible for that property unless it has been specifically entrusted to her care or unless the client has become incapacitated and cannot care for the property him or herself.

Situation: Care of property

> A physiotherapist visits a community home for five persons with learning disabilities. Her client has wealthy parents who have provided him with expensive electrical goods. She sees him in his room and suggests that they go outside to carry out some exercises. When they return, a compact disc player, stereo system and cassette player have been stolen. Does the physiotherapist have any liability for these missing goods?

Normally such goods would be the responsibility of the resident but where the mental competence of the resident was such that he could not be expected to take care of the property the home would be expected to arrange safe custody. The physiotherapist, before leaving the room, should have checked if it were normal practice for the room to be locked and who had custody of the key. If, on the other hand, the resident had the mental capacity to secure his own room and had been provided with a key but failed to do so, then neither the physiotherapist nor the home manager would be liable.

Special precautions have to be taken in the care of those with learning disabilities who may be vulnerable to exploitation and who may not have the capacity to care for their own property. Any moneys belonging to the client and handled by staff must be strictly accounted for and records kept. Facilities should be provided for cash or other valuables to be safely stored and care should also be taken to prevent one client misappropriating property belonging to another. The Court of Protection and the Public Trustee Office provide for the security of property of those who, by reason of mental disorder, are unable to care for it themselves. Because these offices are not suitable for administering small amounts of property recommendations have been made by the Law Commission for new procedures for decision making in relation to property matters as well as treatment and other decisions[25]. Their recommendations have not yet been implemented. (See Chapter 10 for further discussion on liability for property.)

For a discussion of the Community Care (Direct Payments) Act 1996 see Chapter 18.

Conclusion

It is apparent that this topic could form a book in its own right and it has only been possible to touch the surface of the many legal issues which arise for the physiotherapist who cares for those with learning disabilities. Reference should be made to the other general chapters covering areas such as professional accountability, health and safety and the different rights of the client, and to the more specialist works included in the bibliography.

 Questions and exercises

1   It is suggested that one of your clients with learning disabilities should go for a week's holiday by the sea-side. In carrying out a risk assessment for this client, what aspects would you take into account?

2   The mother of a girl with severe learning disabilities who is now 13 years has asked you to assist in ensuring that she will be sterilised as soon as possible. What action would you take and what advice would you give the mother?

3   You are aware that one of your clients with learning disabilities, who lives in a community home and who has a private income from a family trust fund, is extremely generous with his money and is being exploited by the other residents. What action would you take and what is the law?

4   You have been asked to assist a charity which organises out of door activities for those with learning disabilities. You would like to help but are uncertain of the legal situation. What are the legal implications of accepting the invitation?

References

1 Shanley, E. & Starrs, T. (eds) (1993) *Learning Disabilities: A Handbook of Care*, 2nd edn. Churchill Livingstone, Edinburgh.

2 Hessler, I. & Kay, B. (1993) *Learning Disabilities: A Handbook of Care*. In: (eds E. Shanley & T. Starrs) 2nd edn. Churchill Livingstone, Edinburgh.

3 Fraser, R. Physiotherapy in Learning Disability. *ACPPLD Journal*, October 1994, 10–14.

4 Knapp, M.B. & Strade, C.L. (1984) Sexuality and the Developmentally Delayed Teenager In: *Human Sexuality* (ed. N. Fulgate-Woods) Mosby.

5 Grimmer, M. (1993) A bad case of housemaid's knee. *ACPPLD Journal* January 1993, 2.

6 *F* v. *West Berkshire Health Authority and Another* [1989] 2 All ER 545.

7 Papathanasiou, I. & Lyon-Maris, S.J. (1997) Outcome measurements and Case weightings in Physiotherapy Services for people with learning disabilities. *Physiotherapy* **83**, 12, 633–8.

8 Eastburn, J. (1990) Riding Course for people with a learning difficulty *ACPMH Journal* December 1990, 2–6.

9 *Taken from* Fraser, R. (1994) Physiotherapy in Learning Disability *ACPPLD Journal* October 1994, 10–14.

10 *F* v. *West Berkshire Health Authority and Another* [1989] 2 All ER 545.

11 Law Commission (1995) Report No. 231 *Mental Incapacity*. HMSO, London.

12 Lord Chancellor's Office (1997) *Who Decides?* HMSO, London.

13 *R* v. *Bournewood Community and Mental Health NHS Trust, ex parte L*. (HL) reported in *The Times* 30 June 1998, [1998] 3 All ER 289.

14 *F* v. *West Berkshire Health Authority and Another* [1989] 2 All ER 545.

15 Law Commission (1995) Report No. 231 *Mental Incapacity*. HMSO, London.

16 Law Commission (1995) Report No. 231 *Mental Incapacity*. HMSO, London.

17 *R* v. *Hudson Court of Criminal Appeal* [1965] 1 All ER 721.

18 Criminal Law Revision Committee (1984) Cmnd 9213 *15th Report: Sexual Offences*. HMSO, London.

19 Royal College of Nursing/Society of Mental Handicap (1991) *Nursing AIDS – a proactive approach to mental handicap*. Scutari Press, Harrow.

20 Dimond, B.C. (1988) *Ethical and Legal Issues raised by the sterilisation of the mentally handicapped*. MA thesis, University College Swansea.

21 *In Re D (a minor) (wardship: sterilisation)* [1976] 1 All ER 326.

22 *In Re B (a minor) (wardship: sterilisation)* [1987] 2 WLR 1213.

23 *F* v. *West Berkshire Health Authority and Another* [1989] 2 All ER 545.

24 Practice Note [1993] 3 All ER 222 (replaces previous Practice Note issued 1989).

25 Law Commission (1995) Report No. 231 *Mental Incapacity*. HMSO, London.

Chapter 23
Care of Children

The physiotherapist can make a considerable contribution to the care of children, from the special care baby unit to the child with special needs and working with the adolescent. Each division within a child care specialty requires its own procedures and protocols.

It is not possible in a work of this kind to cover all the many laws which relate to the care of the child and the physiotherapist may need to refer to some of the more specialist works on child law. The aim in this chapter is to give to the physiotherapist who works with children an overview of the main principles of law applying to the care and rights of the child[1]. The following topics will be covered:

- The Children Act 1989
- Child protection
- Education and training requirements
- Special educational needs
- Consent by children
- Confidentiality of child information
- Access of the child to health records
- Standards in the care of children
- Conclusions

Reference should also be made to Chapters 20, 21 and 22 which cover the law relating to the physically disabled, mentally ill and those with learning disabilities. Chapter 13 on giving evidence in court will also be useful for those who are involved in child protection issues. For the law in relation to the dying child reference should be made to Chapter 25.

The Children Act 1989

This Act set up a new framework for the protection and care of children and established clear principles to guide decision making in relation to their care. The principles which the court should take into account are shown in Figure 23.1. The overriding principle is that 'the child's welfare shall be the court's paramount consideration'.

Figure 23.1 **Principles of the Children Act 1989.**

(1) The welfare of the child is the paramount consideration in court proceedings.
(2) Wherever possible children should be brought up and cared for in their own families.
(3) Courts should ensure that delay is avoided, and may only make an order if to do so is better than making no order at all.
(4) Children should be kept informed about what happens to them, and should participate when decisions are made about their future.
(5) Parents continue to have parental responsibility for their children, even when their children are no longer living with them. They should be kept informed about their children and participate when decisions are made about their children's future.
(6) Parents with children in need should be helped to bring up their children themselves.
(7) This help should be provided as a service to the child and his family, and should:
  (a) be provided in partnership with parents;
  (b) meet each child's identified needs;
  (c) be appropriate to the child's race, culture, religion, and language;
  (d) be open to effective independent representations and complaints procedures; and
  (e) draw upon effective partnership between the local authority and other agencies including voluntary agencies.

The involvement of the child in the decision making is also a major principle and Figure 23.2 sets out the considerations which the court should take into account in making certain orders.

Figure 23.2 **Circumstances to be taken into account by the court under the Children Act 1989 – section 1(3).**

(a) the ascertainable wishes and feelings of the child concerned (considered in the light of his age and understanding);
(b) his physical, emotional and educational needs;
(c) the likely effect on him of any change in his circumstances;
(d) his age, sex, background and any characteristics of his which the court considers relevant;
(e) any harm which he has suffered or is at risk of suffering;
(f) how capable each of his parents, and any other person in relation to whom the court considers the question to be relevant, is of meeting his needs;
(g) the range of powers available to the court under this Act in the proceedings in question.

[Finally, in deciding whether or not to make an order, the court] shall not make the order or any of the orders unless it considers that doing so would be better for the child than making no order at all. (section 1(5) [i.e. whoever started the proceedings, there has to be a positive advantage to the child in moving away from the *status quo*]

Whilst the considerations set out in Figure 23.2 apply to specific decisions to be made under the Children Act 1989 there is good reason for the physiotherapist to follow these same considerations in her care of the child.

It is not possible to cover the full contents of the Children Act 1989 but Figure 23.3 sets out the parts of the Act and the main areas which the Act covers.

Figure 23.3 **Summary of main areas of the Children Act 1989.**

Part I	Introductory (general principles relating to the welfare of the child, 'parental responsibility' and the appointment of guardians)
Part II	Orders With respect to Children in Family Proceedings
Part III	Local Authority Support for Children and Families
Part IV	Care and Supervision
Part V	Protection of Children
Part VI	Community Homes
Part VII	Voluntary Homes and Voluntary Organisations
Part VIII	Registered Children's Homes
Part IX	Private Arrangements for Fostering Children
Part X	Child Minding and Day Care for Young Children
Part XI	Secretary of State's Supervisory Functions and Responsibilities
Part XII	Miscellaneous and General (including the duty to notify the local authority of children accommodated in different establishments, tests to establish paternity, criminal offences, search warrants, and the jurisdiction of the courts)

Child protection

Where a physiotherapist is concerned that a child in her care, or the sibling or child of one of her patients, is being abused, whether physically, sexually or mentally, she should take immediate action to ensure that this is drawn to the attention of the appropriate persons. This means that she must be familiar with the provisions for child protection and who are the persons to be contacted. It is not always easy to decide if action is necessary and the physiotherapist should see as her main priority the safety of the child. As the guidelines on inter agency co-operation state[2]

> 'The difficulties of assessing the risk of harm to a child should not be under-estimated. It is imperative that everyone who deals with allegations and suspicions of abuse maintains an open and inquiring mind.' (Paragraph 1.13)

Should the physiotherapist be wrong in her fears, and it appears that there is no abuse, her name could not be divulged to the parents[3].

Procedure for the management of child abuse

There should be in existence an agreed procedure for the management of child abuse cases and the physiotherapist should be acquainted with this. The procedure should specifically refer to the role of the physiotherapy department if child abuse is suspected. This would require any professional staff working in the department who suspect that there is a possibility of ill-treatment, serious neglect, or sexual or emotional abuse of a child to inform the senior physiotherapist in charge of the department who should contact a consultant paediatrician. If the consultant confirms the possibility of abuse, then the Social Services Department should be informed immediately.

Inter-agency co-operation

There should be in existence in each local authority area, a forum to ensure co-operation between all the agencies involved in the protection of children at risk. This forum is known as the Area Child Protection Committee (ACPC). On this committee there should be representatives of the medical and nursing services. This representation should be at a senior level and there should be a designated senior professional for child protection within the hospital or community unit.

The ACPC has the tasks set out in Figure 23.4.

Figure 23.4 **Tasks of the Area Child Protection Committee.**

- Establishing, maintaining and reviewing inter-agency guidelines on procedures to be followed in individual cases.
- Monitoring the implementation of legal procedures.
- Identifying significant issues arising from the handling of cases and reports from enquiries.
- Scrutinising arrangements to provide treatment, expert advice and inter-agency liaison, and making recommendations to the responsible agencies.
- Scrutinising progress on work to prevent child abuse and making recommendations to the responsible agencies.
- Scrutinising the work related to inter-agency training and making recommendations to the responsible agencies.
- Conducting reviews required under Part 8 of the Guide.
- Publishing an annual report about local child protection matters.

The role of the physiotherapist

What if the doctor disagrees with the physiotherapist?
The physiotherapist should ensure that her concerns are made known to a senior member of the physiotherapy department who should decide whether it is appropriate to bring the consultant in to see the child. It is important to ensure that the physiotherapist records in writing all the facts which have given rise to her suspicions and fears and keeps a copy of this document. If the consultant subsequently takes the view that there is no abuse, then the physiotherapist has to accept this, but she should remain vigilant about the safety of the child and continue to report any concerns.

What about the physiotherapist's duty of confidentiality?

Reference to the Rule III of the *Rules of Professional Conduct*[4] on confidentiality will show that the Rule recognises that certain apparent breaches of confidentiality are justified 'where it is necessary to protect the welfare of the patient or to prevent harm, or . . . (rarely) . . . in the public interest'. If the physiotherapist is in doubt, then she should seek advice. Any reasonable suspicion of child abuse should be notified to the appropriate agencies without fear of a successful action for breach of confidentiality by the parents (see Chapter 8).

If a suspected case is reported to the police, social services, or NSPCC and it turns out that the suspicions are unfounded, the parents have no right to be given the name of the person reporting them. The House of Lords has held that it is not in the public interest for such information to be disclosed to the parents[5].

The Child Protection Register

Each local authority must maintain a child protection register. The purpose of the Register is set out in Figure 23.5.

Figure 23.5 **Purpose of Child Protection Register.**

- To provide a record of all children in the area who are currently the subject of a Child Protection Plan and to ensure that the plans are formally reviewed at least every six months.
- To provide a central point of speedy enquiry for professional staff who are worried about a child and want to know whether the child is the subject of a Child Protection Plan.
- To provide statistical information about current trends in the area.

Access to this register would be permitted to an agreed list of personnel which would include senior medical staff or paediatric social workers in the local hospital departments. Difficulties can sometimes arise if the register is kept by the social services who do not arrange a 24 hour access service to it. This should be brought up at the ACPC and arrangements could be made for the register to be kept by the paediatric department or by the police.

■ What if the child is not on the register and abuse is not certain?

If the consultant was not able to confirm that this was a case of suspected child abuse and there were no medical grounds for requiring the child to be detained in hospital, then the parent could not be stopped from taking the child home. However there should be arrangements in place for all such concerns to be notified to the appropriate health visitor or school nurse, and also to the appropriate general practitioner.

When suspected child abuse is confirmed

If the consultant paediatrician confirms the suspected child abuse the agreed procedures and the inter-agency arrangements should be followed immediately.

The provisions of the Children Act 1989 enable the following orders to be made. For further details of these orders and the other provisions of the Children Act 1989 reference should be made to the Department of Health guides to the Children Act 1989[6].

Child assessment order – section 43
This is available where:

- the court is satisfied that the applicant has reasonable cause to suspect that the child is suffering or likely to suffer significant harm;
- an assessment is required to determine whether or not the child is suffering or is likely to suffer significant harm; and
- it is unlikely that an assessment can be carried out without an order being made.

Notice must be given of an application for a child assessment order to:

- the child's parents;
- any person, not the parent, but who has parental responsibility for the child;
- any other person caring for the child; and
- others who have a contact order.

The child assessment order cannot not be made if the court is satisfied that there are grounds for making an emergency protection order (see below) and that it ought to make that order rather than an assessment order.

The order must specify the date by which the assessment is to begin and have effect for a specified period not exceeding seven days beginning with that date. The effect of the order is to authorise any person carrying out the assessment, or any part of the assessment, to do so in accordance with the terms of the order (section 43(7)). The child has the right, if he is of sufficient understanding to make an informed decision, to refuse to submit to a medical or psychiatric examination or other assessment (section 43(8)).

Emergency protection order – section 44
If the court is satisfied that there is reasonable cause to believe (in the case of a personal application) that the child is likely to suffer significant harm if:

- he is not removed to accommodation provided by or on behalf of the applicant; or
- he does not remain in the place in which he is then being accommodated;

then the court can order that an emergency protection order be made.

Where the applicant is a local authority it must show that:

- enquiries are being made under section 47(1)(b) (the local authority's duty to investigate)
- these enquiries are being frustrated by access to the child being unreasonably refused;
- and the applicant has reasonable cause to believe that access to the child is required as a matter of urgency (section 44(1) (b)).

An application may also be made by the NSPCC as an authorised person.

Removal and accommodation of children by police in cases of emergency – section 46

This section enables the child to be taken in to police protection. Where a constable believes that a child would be likely to suffer significant harm he may remove the child to suitable accommodation and keep him there. He may also take reasonable steps to ensure that the child's removal from hospital, or any other place in which he is being accommodated, is prevented. The section, once invoked, lasts a maximum of 72 hours.

Education and training requirements

The physiotherapist who works with children should ensure that as far as possible arrangements are made for the child to receive education. She should therefore liaise with the local authority in whatever arrangements have been made and are appropriate for a specific child. Arrangements for the education of the sick child might include the following:

- The establishment of hospital special schools.
- Hospital teaching units/hospital classes which are not formally classified as hospital schools.
- Home tuition.

This following section considers the effect of the statutory duties upon home tuition and the next one looks at the law on assessing and meeting special educational needs.

Home tuition

The statutory duty

The Education Act 1993 (section 298(1) now consolidated in the Education Act 1996) placed a duty on local education authorities (LEAs) to provide suitable education for children out of school for reasons of illness or otherwise. The full subsection is set out in Figure 23.6.

Figure 23.6 **Education Act 1996.**

Each local education authority shall make arrangements for the provision of suitable full time or part time education at school or otherwise than at school for those children of compulsory school age who, by reason of illness, exclusion from school or otherwise, may not for any period receive suitable education unless such arrangements are made for them.

The duty set out in Figure 23.6 applies to children of compulsory school age and the duty is mandatory, i.e. the LEA *shall make arrangements*. In contrast the duty in relation to those above compulsory school age is permissive. This is set out in section 298(4) and is shown in Figure 23.7.

Figure 23.7   Education Act 1996.

The local education authority may make arrangements for the provision of suitable full time or part time education otherwise than at school for those young persons who, by reason of illness, exclusion from school of otherwise, may not for any period receive suitable education unless such arrangements are made for them.

Suitable provision is defined in relation to a child or young person in section 298(7) as 'efficient education suitable to his age, ability and aptitude and to any special educational needs he may have.'

Government guidance

Government guidance was issued in June 1993. Home tuition is not expected to be provided for very short absences from school. Four weeks or more away from school is considered to be the point at which home tuition can be provided. Below that length it would normally be expected that the school would itself provide home work to be done outside school. However it is a question of discretion and some LEAs provide home tuition for three weeks away from school if need exists. Calculation would obviously take into account the length of time that the child has already been in hospital with or without tuition.

The guidance recommends that the LEAs have a written policy on home tuition which covers the organisation and staffing of the service, the timing of provision and giving a named contact for parents, hospital teachers and others.

The contribution of the physiotherapist

With fewer children staying in hospital for long periods, and more caring and treatment taking place in the community, those children suffering from a chronic condition are more likely to benefit from home tuition. The physiotherapist should ensure that she works closely with the tutor in caring for the child.

The National Association for the Education of Sick Children has been set up to relieve the educational disadvantages suffered by sick children. It published the results of a survey on the provision by LEAs, the teaching available, home tuition, and the falling number of hospital schools[7]. The NAESC has a government grant to monitor the effects of implementing the new duty.

Special educational needs

Part IV of the Education Act 1996 (replacing Part III of the Education Act 1993) covers provision for children with special educational needs. A summary of its main provisions is shown in Figure 23.8.

Figure 23.8   Children with special educational needs.

- Meaning of 'special educational needs' and 'special educational provision' etc. – section 312
- Code of Practice – sections 313 to 314
- Special educational provision – sections 315 to 320
- Identification and Assessment of children with special educational needs – sections 321 to 332
- Special Educational Needs Tribunal (SENT) – sections 333 to 336
- Special Schools and Independent Schools – sections 337 to 348
- Variation of deeds (changing a school's constitution) – section 349

Definition of special educational needs

The definition given in section 312 is shown in Figure 23.9.

Figure 23.9   *Definition of special educational needs – section 312.*

(1) For the purposes of the Education Acts, a child has 'special educational needs' if he has a learning difficulty which calls for special educational provision to be made for him.

(2) For the purposes of this Act, subject to subsection (3) below, a child has a 'learning difficulty' if—
 (a)   he has a significantly greater difficulty in learning than the majority of children of his age;
 (b)   he has a disability which either prevents or hinders him from making use of educational facilities of a kind generally provided for children of his age in schools within the area of the local education authority; or
 (c)   he is under the age of five years and is, or would be if special educational provision were not made for him, likely to fall within paragraph (a) or (b) when over that age.

[The definition of child includes any person who has not attained the age of nineteen years and is a registered pupil at a school]

It has been decided by the courts that dyslexia can constitute a 'disability' for the purposes of Section 312 (2)(b).

Case: *R* v. *Hampshire County Council, ex parte J*[8]

The judge found that dyslexia which affected the capacity of a boy aged $13\frac{1}{2}$ for continuous reading, spelling, and essay writing, whilst not preventing him from making use of educational facilities, clearly hindered him.

The definition (under a previous Act) can extend to what might otherwise be regarded as medical treatment.

Case: *R* v. *Lancashire County Council, ex parte Moore*[9]

A child born in 1979 had hearing and speech problems and required speech therapy on an intensive basis. The dispute arose as to the definition of special educational needs and as to whether speech therapy could be regarded as educational provision rather than medical treatment. It was noted that in the Government's White Paper on Special Needs in Education[10] it was recognised that:

> 'for many children with special educational needs, a wide range of services needs to be made available by social services departments and health authorities ... Health authorities may have to provide a wide range of medical and nursing skills, including those of health visitors, district and school nurses, physiotherapists, and speech and occupational therapists, as well as providing personal aids and equipment.' (paragraph 69)

The Court of Appeal held that speech therapy could be regarded as special educational needs provision and the authority's appeal was dismissed.

The Education (Special Educational Needs) Regulations 1994

These regulations[11], which came into force on 1 September 1994, cover the following topics:

- Delegation of functions from head teacher to other qualified teachers.
- Service of Documents.
- Assessment – notices relating to assessments, advice to be sought, time limits.
- Statements – notices, form of the statement, time limits, review of the statement, transfer of statements, restriction on disclosure of statements (see below).

In a Schedule to the Regulations forms are provided under Regulations 12 and 13 for giving notice to a parent accompanying a statement of special educational needs (Part A) and the format for the statement itself (Part B). This format has the following sections:

- Introduction (name and address of child and parent or person responsible)
- Special Educational Needs: in terms of the child's learning difficulties which call for special educational provision
- Special Educational Provision: objectives, educational provision to meet needs and objectives, monitoring
- Placement
- Non-Educational Needs
- Non-Educational Provision.

The appendices cover written representations and other statutory requirements for advice as follows:

- Parental representation
- Parental evidence
- Advice from the child's parent
- Educational advice
- Medical advice
- Psychological advice

- Advice from the social services authority
- Other advice obtained by the authority.

The Code of Practice

The Secretary of State has a statutory duty, following consultation, to issue and from time to time to revise and publish, a Code of Practice giving practical guidance on the carrying out of the duties by the local education authorities under Part IV of the 1996 Act. They and the relevant governing bodies must have regard to the Code and, on any appeal, the Tribunal must have regard to any provision of the code which appears to it to be relevant. Any draft code must be placed before both Houses of Parliament for approval before it is issued.

The Code of Practice[12] issued in 1994 (under the provisions of the 1993 Act but still applicable) covers the areas shown in Figure 23.10.

Figure 23.10 **Code of Practice on special educational needs and assessment.**

(1) Introduction: Principles and Procedures
(2) School-based Stages of Assessment and Provision
(3) Statutory Assessment of Special Educational Needs
(4) Statement of Special Educational Needs
(5) Assessments and Statements for Under Fives
(6) Annual Review
(7) Appendix: Transitional Arrangements
(8) Glossary

The fundamental principles identified in the Code are shown in Figure 23.11.

Figure 23.11 **Fundamental principles in the Code of Practice.**

(1) The needs of all pupils who may have special educational needs either throughout, or at any time during, their school careers must be addressed; the Code recognises that there is a continuum of needs and a continuum of provision, which may be made in a wide variety of different forms.

(2) Children with special educational needs require the greatest possible access to a broad and balanced education, including the National Curriculum.

(3) The needs of most pupils will be met in mainstream, and without a statutory assessment or statement of special educational needs. Children with special educational needs, including children with statements of special educational needs, should, where appropriate and taking into account the wishes of their parents, be educated alongside their peers in mainstream schools.

(4) Even before he or she reaches compulsory school age a child may have special educational needs requiring the intervention of the LEA as well as the health services.

(5) The knowledge, views and experience of parents are vital. Effective assessment and provision will be secured where there is the greatest possible degree of partnership between parents and their children and schools, LEAs and other agencies.

Any physiotherapist who is involved in the assessment of special educational needs and the preparation of a statement on a child should ensure that she obtains a copy of the Code of Practice. There is also guidance from the Association of Paediatric Chartered Physiotherapists, which has published a document entitled *Statutory Assessment of Children with Special Educational Needs*[13].

Duty to secure the education of children with special educational needs in ordinary schools

Section 316 requires those responsible under the Act to ensure that a child with special educational needs is educated in an ordinary school if certain conditions are satisfied, unless this is incompatible with the wishes of his parent. The conditions are:

- his receiving the special educational provision which his learning difficulty calls for;
- the provision of efficient education for the children with whom he will be educated; and
- the efficient use of resources.

Involvement of health authority

Section 322 places a duty upon the health authority or local authority to help the local education authority and specifies the action which they should take in specific circumstances.

Assessment of special educational needs

Bringing about an assessment

The parents can request an assessment of educational needs under section 329 of the 1996 Act and the governing body of a grant-maintained school under section 330.

The health authority or an NHS Trust has a duty to notify parents if they form the opinion in providing services for a child under five years that he has special educational needs (section 332). After giving the parent an opportunity to discuss that opinion with an officer of the health authority or Trust, they have a duty to bring it to the attention of the appropriate LEA. In addition, if the health authority or NHS Trust are of the opinion that a particular voluntary organisation is likely to be able to give the parent advice or assistance with any special educational needs that the child may have, they have a duty to inform the parent.

Carrying out the assessment

Where a local educational authority considers that a child has special educational needs and it is necessary for the authority to determine the special educational provision which any learning difficulty he has may call for, then the LEA must carry out an assessment. They must serve notice on the parents covering the following information:

- their intention to make an assessment;
- the procedure to be followed;
- the name of the officer from whom further information may be obtained; and
- the parents' right to make representations, and submit written evidence to the authority.

A Schedule of the Act covers the making of the assessments and enables regulations to be made and also requires the LEA to seek medical, psychological and educational advice in connection with the assessment.

Statement of special educational needs

If, in the light of the assessment, it is necessary for the LEA to determine the special educational provision which any learning difficulty the child may have calls for, the authority must make and maintain a statement of his special educational needs. The statement must set out the facts required. Schedule 27 sets out the details of the parents' right to make representations and further regulations on statementing.

Copy to the hospital school

The local education authority should give or provide on request a copy of the statement specifying certain special educational or non-educational provision to the hospital school or service. The LEA may have to make an amendment to the statement in order to name the hospital school where a child with special educational needs is likely to be a long-stay pupil. The parents have the right to comment on any such amendment in accordance with the provisions set out in Schedule 27 to the Education Act 1960 (replacing Schedule 10 of the Education Act 1993).

Parents' right of appeal

The parents can appeal both against an LEA decision not to make a statement and also against the description in the statement of the authority's assessment of the child's special educational needs (section 326 of the 1996 Act), the special educational provision specified in the statement, or, if no school is named in the statement, that fact. The appeal is made to a Special Educational Needs Tribunal (SENT).

Special Educational Needs Tribunals

These were established following the implementation of the Education Act 1993 (now consolidated in the Education Act 1996).

The constitution of the SENT is set out in sections 333 to 336 of the Education Act 1996. The chairman must be someone with a seven year general qualification within the meaning of section 71 of the Courts and Legal Services Act 1990 (i.e. a solicitor or barrister holding a right of audience, granted by the authorised body). Regulations cover the procedure to be followed and who can be panel members.

Powers

When an appeal is made to a SENT under section 326, it has the following powers:

- to dismiss the appeal;
- to order the authority to amend the statement, so far as it describes the authority's assessment of the child's special educational needs or specifies the special educational provision, (and to make such other consequential amendments as the SENT thinks fit); or
- to order the authority to cease to maintain the statement.

The SENT cannot order the LEA to specify the name of any school in the statement unless the parent has expressed a preference or, in the proceedings, the parent, the LEA or both have proposed the school.

The local education authority cannot be obliged by a ruling in the Special Needs Tribunal to provide educational services which were surplus to meeting the special educational needs of the child[14].

SENTs and the physiotherapist

The physiotherapist may be involved in providing reports for special education purposes and may consequently be called as a witness to hearings including the Special Educational Needs Tribunal. Reference should be made to Chapter 13 on giving evidence in court.

Consent by children

Chapter 7 covers the basic principles relating to trespass to the person and the importance of obtaining the consent of the patient. This section deals with the specific laws relating to consent by or on behalf of the child (i.e. a person under 18 years of age).

The child of 16 and 17

A child of 16 or 17 has the right to give consent to treatment under section 8 of the Family Law Reform Act 1969. This is shown in Figure 23.12.

Figure 23.12   **Family Law Reform Act 1969 – section 8.**

(1) The consent of a minor who has attained the age of 16 years, to any surgical, medical or dental treatment, which in the absence of consent, would constitute a trespass to the person, shall be as effective as it would be if he were of full age; and where a minor has by virtue of this section given an effective consent to any treatment it shall not be necessary to obtain any consent for it from his parent or guardian.

(2) In the section 'surgical, medical or dental treatment' includes any procedure undertaken for the purposes of diagnosis and this section applies to any procedures (including, in particular, the administration of an anaesthetic) which is ancillary to any treatment as it applies to that treatment.

(3) Nothing in the section shall be construed as making ineffective any consent which would have been effective if this section had not been enacted.

The definition of treatment under section 8(2) would probably cover most treatments given by a physiotherapist where these are under the aegis of a doctor.

Section 8(3) has been interpreted as covering two situations – the giving of consent by a parent on behalf of the child of 16 or 17 and the giving of consent of a Gillick competent child (see below) under 16 years.

It does not, therefore, follow that a child of 16 or 17 cannot be compelled to have treatment and the Court of Appeal in the case of *Re W*[15] upheld the decision of the High Court judge to order a child of 16 years who was suffering from anorexia nervosa to undergo medical treatment against her will.

The child under 16

The parent has a right at common law to give consent on behalf of the child. In addition, as a result of the House of Lords ruling in the *Gillick* case[16], children under 16 years who have sufficient understanding and intelligence to be capable of making up their own minds can give a valid consent to treatment. As a result of this case we now have the term 'Gillick competent' which signifies a child who has the maturity and competence to make a decision in the specific circumstances arising.

In life saving situations, however, it is unlikely that the child under 16 years would be able to make a decision contrary to his or her best interests. Even where the child and parents both agree that treatment should not be given, as in the case of a Jehovah's Witness family, the court can order treatment to proceed if it is considered to be in the best interests of the child (case of *Re E* (1993))[17].

Disputes between parents

Even when parents are divorced or separated, under the Children Act 1989 section 2(1) both parents retain parental responsibility for their children. Under section 2(7) where more than one person has parental responsibility for a child each of them may act alone and without the other (or others) in meeting that responsibility. Even where one parent has a residence order in his or her favour, the other still retains parental responsibility and can exercise this to the full. One parent does not, therefore, have the right of veto over the other's actions. If, however, there has been a specific order by the court relating to a decision affecting the care or treatment of the child, then a single parent cannot change this or take any action which is incompatible with this order unless the approval of the court is obtained.

It therefore follows that if there is a dispute between parents over treatment decisions in respect of the child, either can go to court for a specific issue or prohibited steps order to be made.

Prohibited steps order

Where one parent wishes to prevent the other taking action which he or she does not consider is in the interests of the child, he or she may seek a prohibited steps order. This can be made under section 8 of the Children Act 1989 and means that no step which could be taken by a parent in meeting his or her parental responsibility for a child and which is of a kind specified in the order shall be taken without the consent of the court. Thus if one parent feared, for example, that the other was likely to agree to a mentally impaired daughter being sterilised, then that parent could obtain a prohibited steps order preventing consent being given without the consent of the court.

If the child is considered to be 'Gillick competent' and disagreed with actions which the parents were intending, he or she could seek the leave of the court to obtain a prohibited steps order. The child would have to apply to the High Court[18]. The court must be satisfied that the child has sufficient understanding to make the proposed application (section 10(8)).

The health professional's first duty is to the interests of the child client and, while these would be in no way served by promoting discord between child and parent(s), it is possible that the health professional may become aware of situations where the Gillick competent child is in fundamental disagreement with how his or her parents are planning to proceed. This might be particularly so in carrying out treatments such as physiotherapy where talk and confidences are easily forthcoming. In such circumstances the physiotherapist should be aware of the help that is available and be able to steer her client in the right direction for legal assistance.

Specific issue order

This is the procedure where action is to be taken rather than prevented, for example in a dispute between parents over adaptations for a disabled child. A situation could arise where adaptations are required for a child under the Housing Acts (see Chapter 20); the parents live in different houses but the local authority is only prepared to pay for adaptations to one house. How is such a dispute resolved?

Either parent could take the case to court for a specific issue order and for a declaration from the court as to which parent was entitled to have the adaptations in his or her house. Obviously account would be taken of where the child was likely to want to spend most time and which parent, if any, had a residence order. (It would of course be possible, funds permitting, for an individual parent to pay for the second house to be adapted as well.)

Confidentiality of child information

The same principles apply in relation to maintaining the confidentiality of information provided by the child patient as apply to information provided by the adult patient (see Chapter 8). However there may be situations where the interests of the child require confidential information to be passed on to an appropriate authority.

If possible the consent of the child should be obtained to the disclosure. However where the child refuses consent, or where the child lacks the capacity to give consent, the physiotherapist should notify the child of her view that the information should be passed on in the best interests of the child.

She should not make a commitment to the child that the confidential information will never be passed on. She should, however, ensure that she takes advice before breaching confidentiality. She should record the action she has taken and the reasons for it, and be prepared to justify her actions if subsequently challenged.

Confidentiality and the statement of special educational needs

There are specific statutory provisions regulating the disclosure of the statement prepared on the special educational needs of the child[19]. Paragraph 19 of the 1994 regulations restricts disclosure of the statement without the parent's consent except in specific circumstances set down in the Regulations or the Act. These exceptions include disclosure:

- To persons to whom, in the opinion of the authority concerned, the statement should be disclosed in the interests of the child.
- For the purposes of any appeal under the Act.
- For the purposes of educational research which, in the opinion of the authority, may advance the education of children with special educational needs. This may be done if, but only if, confidentiality is preserved by the person doing the research undertaking not to publish anything unless in a form which does not identify any individual concerned, especially the child and his or her parents.
- On the order of any court or for the purpose of any criminal proceedings.
- For the purposes of any investigation under the Local Government Act 1974 Part III.
- To the Secretary of State when he requests disclosure to decide whether to give directions or make an order under Section 68 or 99 of the Education Act 1944.
- For the purposes of an assessment of the needs of the child with respect to the provision of any statutory services for him being carried out by officers of a social services authority under section 5(5) of the Disabled Persons (Services, Consultation and Representation) Act 1986.
- For the purposes of a local authority performing its duties under the Children Act 1989.
- To Her Majesty's Inspectors.

Access of the child to health records

Chapter 9 covers the basic principles which apply to access to records. Here we are concerned with access to records about children.

Access by child to computerised records

Where the child has the capacity he can apply for access to his personal health data kept in computerised form under the Data Protection Act 1984. The Department of Health recommends[20] that a certificate should be signed in which a responsible adult certifies that the child understands the nature of the application. The procedure under the Data Protection Access provisions is considered in Chapter 9.

Access by child to non-computerised personal health records

Section 3(1)(a) of the Access to Health Records Act 1990 gives the right of access to the patient. However where in the case of a record held in England and Wales, the patient is a child (i.e. someone under 16 years) access shall not be given under subsection (2) of section 3 unless the holder of the record is satisfied that the patient is capable of understanding the nature of the application.

No definition of the capability of the child is given in the Act but it is submitted that the Gillick test of competence (see above) adapted to the specific conditions of access to records would be applied.

Right of the parent

Under section 3(1)(c) where, in England and Wales, the patient is a child, a person having parental responsibility for the patient has a right of access. However this is qualified by section 4(2), which prevents access unless the holder of the record is satisfied either:

- that the patient has consented to the making of the application; or
- that the patient is incapable of understanding the nature of the application and the giving of access would be in his or her best interests.

Exclusion of access

Whether the records are held in computerised or manual form, the application for access can be refused if serious harm would be caused to the physical or mental health of the patient or another person or would identify a third person (not being a health professional involved in the care of the child) who did not wish to be identified.

Standards in the care of children

Chapter 10 sets out the principles of law which apply in ensuring that reasonable standards of professional care are provided. This will include multi-disciplinary team working and the rational determination of priorities. Physiotherapists must ensure that they maintain their competence and that they keep up to date with developments in their field of specialisation. The APCP has prepared a document on *Standards of Practice for Paediatric Physiotherapists* which is available from the CSP[21].

Unorthodox treatments

Multi-disciplinary care of the child may involve the use of unorthodox treatments. The physiotherapist must be aware that there is no legal concept of team liability, and if she acts contrary to the standards of professional competence of a reasonable physiotherapist, she could not use as a defence that she was carrying out the instructions of the team. If, therefore, a team member proposes an unorthodox treatment in the care of a child, she must be assured that this complies with the reasonable standards of care and that the parents/and or the child have given informed consent to the treatment, in the full knowledge that the proposed treatment is not of the usual kind but is in the circumstances justifiable.

Working with parents and others

It is clear that physiotherapists are unlikely to achieve major progress in the treatment of children unless they are able to secure and develop a partnership with parents and other health care professionals and other agencies such as schools. For example in the care and treatment of dyspraxia Michele Lee and Graham Smith[22] were able to show through the use of outcome measures that physiotherapy had a positive effect on dyspraxia over three months. They hoped that, by giving parents and children a long-term management programme, the improved gain in muscle strength and skill abilities would be maintained. The authors emphasise the need for close liaison between physiotherapists, parents and schools. The programme involved the setting of goals by parents and child which they hoped to achieve by the review date.

The effectiveness of care in the community is often dependent upon the involvement of parents in the treatment of the child. The role of a domiciliary physiotherapist in the treatment of children with cystic fibrosis was reviewed by Diane Rogers and Mary Goodchild[23]. They show that the provision of a domiciliary physiotherapy service for CF has been a major development, allowing patients and their families increased access to physiotherapy both in the clinic and at home. Compliance with physiotherapy has been improved by discussion and demonstration in the home. They conclude that there is room for improvement in the service, but more detailed feedback is required from patients and their families.

Contributory negligence and the child

In Chapter 10 the defence of contributory negligence was discussed. This means that if the client is partly to blame for the harm which has occurred then there may still be liability on the part of the professional but the compensation payable might be reduced in proportion to the client's fault. However where a child has been harmed, any defence of contributory negligence must take into account the fact that children are less capable than adults of taking care of themselves. The courts have been reluctant to find contributory negligence by a child, where an adult is at fault. The following case illustrates the law on contributory negligence in relation to children.

Case: *Gough* v. *Thorne*[24]

On 13 June 1962 a group of children were crossing the New Kings Road, Chelsea, London. They were Malcolm Gough who was 17, his brother John who was 10, and his sister Elizabeth, the plaintiff, who was $13\frac{1}{2}$. They were coming from the Wandsworth Bridge Road, crossing the New Kings Road, and going to a swimming pool on the other side. They waited on the pavement for some little time to see if it was safe to cross. Then a lorry came up, coming up the Wandsworth Bridge Road and turning left into New Kings Road. The lorry driver had got pretty well half-way across the road, towards the bollards, and he stopped at about five feet from the bollards. He put his right hand out to warn the traffic which was coming up the road. He saw the children waiting he beckoned to them to cross, and they did. They had got across just beyond the lorry when a 'bubble' car, driven by the defendant, came through the gap between the front of the lorry and the bollard, about five feet, just missed the eldest boy, and struck the young boy of 10, but ran into and seriously injured the plaintiff, Elizabeth, aged $13\frac{1}{2}$. The judge held that the 'bubble' car was going too fast in the circumstances, and that the driver did not keep a proper look-out because he ought to have seen the lorry driver's signal but did not see it. On the issue of contributory negligence, the trial judge found that she was 33% to blame for the accident. The plaintiff appealed.

Lord Denning in the Court of Appeal disagreed with the finding of contributory negligence:

'I am afraid that I cannot agree with the judge. A very young child cannot be guilty of contributory negligence. An older child may be; but it depends on the circumstances. A judge should only find a child guilty of contributory negligence if he or she is of such an age as reasonably to be expected to take precautions for his or her own safety: and then he or she is only to be found guilty if blame should be attached to him or her. A child has not the road sense or the experience of his or her elders. He or she is not to be found guilty unless he or she is blameworthy.'

Lord Salmon expressed the situation in the following words:

'The question as to whether the plaintiff can be said to have been guilty of contributory negligence depends on whether any ordinary child of $13\frac{1}{2}$ could be expected to have done any more that this child did. I say, "any ordinary child" I do not mean a paragon of prudence, nor do I mean a scatter-brained child, but the ordinary girl of $13\frac{1}{2}$.'

Occupier's liability and a child

Case: *J (a minor)* v. *Staffordshire County Council*[25]

A 13 year old pupil was injured when she pushed open the right hand door of double doors comprising glass panes. Her hand slipped from the push plate onto the adjacent panel of glass. The glass shattered causing severe injuries to her right hand and wrist. The County Council was found liable under the Occupier's Liability Act 1957 and at common law in failing to fulfil its duty of care. It had failed to comply with the BS standards for glass in doors. There was no finding of contributory negligence.

Where a child is allowed onto premises the duty of the occupier to ensure that the visitor is reasonably safe takes into account the fact that children will require a higher standard of care than an adult. Thus the Occupier's Liability Act 1957, section 2(3) as set out in Figure 23.13 states the position explicitly.

> ***Figure 23.13*** **Occupier's Liability Act 1957 – section 2(3).**
>
> The circumstances relevant for the present purpose include the degree of care, and of want of care, which would ordinarily be looked for in such a visitor, so that (for example) in proper cases ... an occupier must be prepared for children to be less careful than adults ...

Physiotherapists must therefore take into account any reasonably foreseeable harm which could arise if children come into their departments or onto their premises. Children would also include those who may not be their patients, but are the offspring of the patients. They would also come under the definition of visitors.

Conclusions

Paediatric care can present considerable challenges to the physiotherapist. Many lessons can be learnt from a clear and consistent monitoring of the service provided and a willingness to learn from weaknesses. Lynne Howard,[26] writing in the *Occupational Therapist's Journal*, has researched multi-disciplinary quality assessment in relation to the child development team and concludes that quality assessment requires a judicious combination of both consumer satisfaction and professional standard setting, and that the biggest stumbling block is outcome assessment. This may also be true of physiotherapy and must be remedied if the physiotherapist is to play her full role in the care of the child.

 Questions and exercises

1　A parent brings to the out-patients department a child whom you suspect is subject to abuse. Outline the procedure which you would follow.

2　You are involved in the assessment of the special needs of a child, prior to his being statemented. You then discover that your recommendations are likely to be overruled by the local authority on resource grounds. What is the legal position?

3　You are involved in the care of a girl with learning disabilities and learn that her mother wishes her to be sterilised. You are of the view that her disability is not severe. What action would you take? (See also Chapter 22)

4　A child that you are caring for tells you in confidence that she is being abused by her father. She emphasises that she does not want you to take any action. What is the legal situation? Does the age of the child make any difference and if so how?

References

1 Dimond, B.C. (1996) *The Legal Aspects of Child Health Care.* Mosby, London (provides an overview of child health law for all health professionals).

2 Home Office, Department of Health, Department of Education and Science & Welsh Office (1991) *Working Together Under the Children Act 1989: a guide to arrangements for inter-agency co-operation for the protection of children from abuse.* HMSO, London.

3 *D* v. *National Society for the Prevention of Cruelty to Children* [1977] 1 All ER 589.

4 Chartered Society of Physiotherapy (1996) *Rules of Professional Conduct.* CSP, London.

5 *D* v. *National Society for the Prevention of Cruelty to Children* [1977] 1 All ER 589.

6 DoH (1989) *An introductory guide to the Children Act for the NHS.* HMSO, London.

7 Housby Smith, N. (1994) A new era in education. *Paediatric Nursing* **6**, 9, 6 and 14. (Author public relations officer for the NAESC)

8 *R* v. *Hampshire County Council, ex parte J* (1985) 84 LGR 547.

9 *R* v. *Lancashire County Council, ex parte Moore* (CA) (1985) 87 LGR 567.

10 White Paper *Special Needs in Education.* (Cmnd 7996) August 1980, HMSO, London.

11 The Education (Special Educational Needs) Regulations 1994. SI No. 1047, HMSO, London.

12 Department of Education (1994) *Code of Practice on the identification and assessment of special educational needs.* Department for Education, London.

13 Association of Paediatric Chartered Physiotherapists *Statutory assessment of Children with Special Educational Needs.*

14 *Hereford and Worcester County Council* v. *Lane* (CA) The Times Law Report, 10 April 1998; and reaffirmed in *Hackney London Borough Council* v. *Silyadin* The Times Law Report, 17 September 1998.

15 *Re W (a minor) (Medical Treatment)* [1992] 4 All ER 627.

16 *Gillick* v. *West Norfolk and Wisbech Area Health Authority* [1986] 1 AC 112.

17 *Re E (a Minor) (Wardship: Medical Treatment)* [1993] 1 FLR 386.

18 See further the rights of the child as applicant in Wyld, N. (1994) *When Parents Separate.* Children's Legal Centre, Colchester.

19 The Education (Special Educational Needs) Regulations 1994. Paragraph 19, SI No. 1047, HMSO, London.

20 HC(89)29 paragraph 4.

21 Association of Paediatric Chartered Physiotherapists *Standards of Practice for Paediatric Physiotherapists.* CSP, London.

22 Lee, M.G. & Smith, G.N. (1998) The Effectiveness of Physiotherapy for Dyspraxia. *Physiotherapy* **84**, 6, 276–84.

23 Rogers, D. & Goodchild, M.C. (1996) Role of a Domiciliary Physiotherapist in the treatment of Children with Cystic Fibrosis. *Physiotherapy* **82**, 7, 396–402.

24 *Gough* v. *Thorne* [1966] 3 All ER 398.

25 *J (a Minor)* v. *Staffordshire County Council* (1997) 2 CLR 3783.

26 Howard, L.M. (1994) Multidisciplinary Quality assessment: The case of the child development team. Parts 1, 2 and 3 *British Journal of Occupational Therapy.* 1994 **57**, 9, 10 and 11, 345–8, 393–6 and 437–40.

Chapter 24
Care of the Elderly

It would be a mistake to see the elderly as a clear client group. From a legal perspective there are no differences between the health care rights which apply to those over 75 or 85 or any other age level. However from a clinical perspective the older people become the more likely it is that they have multiple health needs, and that these are likely to be exacerbated by economic and social problems. It is clear that the physiotherapist has a major role to play in the care of the elderly patient and that they are likely to form an increasing proportion of her case load. A study in 1993 suggested that there were inadequate resources in terms of occupational therapists which led to reduced efficiency and quality in the care of elderly patients[1]. Patients waited on average 3.9 days for home visits by occupational therapists to take place. Similar research is necessary to determine the availability of physiotherapists.

The basic principles of the law relating to patients' rights and to accountability and professional conduct cover adults of all ages. However there are specific issues which can arise in the care of the elderly because:

- they may lack the competence to make decisions;
- they may require greater protection from risks; and
- their economic and social situation may cause concerns for the physiotherapist.

The topics to be covered in this chapter are given below but reference should also be made to the basic principles of law covered in other chapters and in particular to Chapter 25 on the law relating to death and dying.

- Rights of the elderly – ageism
- Issues on consent and capacity
- Risk taking
- Restraint – the wanderer
- Exploitation by relatives and others
- Abuse of the elderly
- Use of volunteers
- Inter-agency co-operation
- Health and safety and manual handling
- Resources
- Conclusion

Rights of the elderly – ageism

There is a tendency for elderly clients to be treated differently because of their age. Thus it is more likely that relatives will be told the diagnosis and prognosis before the patient, it is more likely that relatives will be asked for their consent for treatments to proceed and there is a danger that arbitrary age limits will be set, above which certain treatments will not take place. However in law the basic principles of law of consent and confidentiality and rights to treatment do not change because a person is elderly. If the clients are competent then they alone are able to give consent and should be informed of any diagnosis, and they should have the right to decide whether or not they wish this information to be given to the relatives.

Similarly there should be no cut-off points at which certain treatments are not made available. The criteria should be the physical ability of the patient to benefit from the specific treatment being discussed, whether that would be in her best interests and, if she is mentally competent, whether she gives consent.

A private member's Bill was introduced into the House of Commons by MP David Winnick on 9 February 1996. If passed it would have made discrimination against the aged in employment unlawful. However it failed to get Government support and therefore a second reading. In the absence of any legislation against discrimination the aged have no remedies against employers although they may be able to rely upon the Disability Discrimination Act 1995 (see Chapter 17). However where they are refused medical treatment, where the duty of confidentiality is broken and where consent is not obtained, the elderly have all the rights which the young adult has and which are described in earlier chapters in this book.

It is important that research on the care of the elderly is given a high profile. For example Dawn Skelton and Ann McLaughlin[2] examined the feasibility and acceptability of an exercise class run by health care professionals, and whether an eight week period of moderate intensity exercise could effect improvements in women aged 74 years and over. They concluded that repeated moderate intensity exercise which involves the practice of functional tasks and mobility can produce substantial increases in strength, balance, flexibility and selected functional abilities.

Issues on consent and capacity

Autonomy and intermittent incompetence

If the elderly client is competent then he or she has the right to give or withhold consent to treatment. The right of a mentally competent adult to refuse treatment has been reiterated by the Court of Appeal[3]. The court stated that it was the duty of the professional to ensure that the refusal was valid, i.e. that the adult had the requisite mental competence and was not under the undue influence of another nor suffering from any disability which impaired his or her capacity to give consent (see Chapter 7).

One of the difficulties facing the physiotherapist is the possibility that the client is suffering from intermittent mental incapacity. This may be a feature of

Alzheimer's Disease. In such situations the physiotherapist would be advised to seek the assistance of others who could help to determine the mental capacity of the patient.

Situation: Refusal to accept residential care

> A physiotherapist visits a patient at home for treatment following a stroke. She was extremely concerned about the patient's condition. It appeared that she was not able to care for herself properly and no one was helping her. The physiotherapist formed the view that the patient did not have the physical or mental competence to live on her own. What should the physiotherapist do?

This is not an unfamiliar situation to many physiotherapists. The physiotherapist would have to contact social services and arrange for a community care assessment to be made with interim assistance being provided until a residential placement could be arranged. Such a plan is of course dependent upon persuading the patient to leave home in her best interests. There are statutory powers under the Mental Health Act 1983 to remove the person to a place of safety but very specific conditions must be shown (see Chapter 21).

Powers under the National Assistance Act 1948

There are also statutory powers under the National Assistance Act 1948 for persons to be removed to a place of safety. The purpose of these powers is set out in Figure 24.1.

Figure 24.1 **The National Assistance Act 1948 – section 47.**

The following provisions of this section shall have effect for the purposes of securing the necessary care and attention for persons who—

(a) are suffering from grave chronic disease or, being aged, infirm or physically incapacitated, are living in insanitary conditions; and

(b) are unable to devote to themselves, and are not receiving from other persons, proper care and attention.

Such persons can be removed to a place of safety on an application by the community medical specialist (replacing the medical officer of health) who is required to give seven days notice to a magistrates court. Because of the problems which could arise from this delay an amending Act was passed in 1951 which enables an order to be made without notice in an emergency.

These provisions have been the subject of review by the Law Commission. The Law Commission in its Consultation Paper 130[4] has suggested that section 47 of the National Assistance Act 1948 and the National Assistance (Amendment) Act 1951 should be repealed and replaced by a new scheme giving clearer and more appropriate powers to local social services authorities to intervene to protect incapacitated, mentally disordered or vulnerable people. Draft legislation was included in the final report of the Law Commission[5] but the Government has not at present indicated its intentions. A further consultation paper on mental incapacity was issued by the Lord Chancellor in 1997[6].

Where consent is refused

Where the client refuses to give consent to treatment and care, whatever the reason, the physiotherapist cannot usually compel the client to participate in therapy. Many therapies require the intentional involvement of the client. Where this is not so it would be advisable for the physiotherapist to obtain the services of another health professional to determine the competence of the client to give consent. Forms are provided by the NHS Management Executive to cover the situation where treatment is given without consent in the case of a mentally incompetent person, who is not under the Mental Health Act 1983[7]. There are also suggested forms for completion where the health professional giving the treatment and care is neither doctor nor dentist.

Situation: Refusal of treatment

> An elderly patient is admitted to hospital with confusion, secondary to an infection. Treatment with antibiotics is implemented. The patient makes a good recovery and the physiotherapist is asked to get her mobile. The patient refuses to even attempt to stand. The physiotherapist knows the importance of starting mobilisation as soon as possible to prevent loss of postural awareness, weakness and muscle and joint stiffness. What can the physiotherapist do in the face of such opposition?

This common situation requires all the physiotherapist's interpersonal skills. A good ploy would be for the physiotherapist to be on the ward when the patient is moved from bed to chair or when he needs the toilet, so that he is in a weight bearing situation, and develop mobilisation from that point. If such tactics fail, then taking the patient off the ward to the physiotherapy department to unfamiliar surroundings, might assist in persuading the patient to commence mobilisation.

The mentally incompetent patient

Where the client is incompetent and unable to give consent, the physiotherapist can continue to provide care and treatment on the basis of the ruling in the case of *Re F*[8]. In this case the House of Lords established that treatment and care can be given out of necessity to a person who does not have the capacity to give a valid consent. The treatment must be given in the best interests of the person and the health professional must follow the reasonable standard of care as defined by the Bolam test. The House of Lords confirmed this common law (i.e. judge made law) power to act out of necessity on behalf of a mentally incapacitated adult in the Bournewood case[9].

The proposals of the Law Commission[10] for powers of decision making on behalf of the mentally incapacitated adult to be recognised would fill the gap which currently exists in the law.

Living wills or advance refusals of treatment are considered in the next chapter on death and dying. If a physiotherapist is aware that an elderly patient wishes to make a living will, she should ensure that the mental competence of the patient to do so is established and that care is taken in recording their wishes.

Risk taking

It is recognised that if vulnerable clients are to lead lives with a reasonable quality then certain risks must be faced. Thus it would be less risky keeping clients in an institution rather than taking them out for walks or other activities.

Counsel and Care has produced advice and guidance to staff who care for older people on risk taking in residential and nursing homes[11] and the same principles would apply to the care of an elderly person in his or her own home or in hospital.

The law would require that reasonable care should be taken to prevent the harm arising from reasonably foreseeable risks. This would necessitate a risk assessment not unlike that which would be required under the health and safety regulations (see Chapter 11).

In the event of harm actually arising to the client or another person, the health professional caring for the client would have to show:

- what risks were reasonably foreseeable;
- what reasonable action was taken to meet those risks; and
- that this was in accordance with the reasonable standards of professional practice.

It follows that it is essential that records are kept of the basis of the decision making and any instructions given to others who are to care for the clients. This is a difficult area for the physiotherapist who may feel that she is squeezed between two principles of law – the right of the mentally competent adult to autonomy and the duty of care owed by the health professional to the client.

The risk of a fall and its consequences

A simple example of risk assessment and management can be seen in the risk of an elderly person falling. Thus Adele Reece and Janet Simpson[12] discuss the need to teach older people how to cope after a fall. They suggest that older people are slightly more likely to learn successfully how to get up from the floor by the backward chairing method. Those who cannot learn to get up from the floor, should be helped by developing alternative strategies for summoning help and for preventing the consequences of the long lie.

In a subsequent article, Janet Simpson and others describe guidelines which have been developed for the collaborative rehabilitative management of elderly people who have fallen[13]. These guidelines are an example of multi-disciplinary planning and working. They set out four aims:

- to improve elderly people's ability to withstand threats to their balance;
- to improve the safety of elderly people's surroundings;
- to prevent elderly people suffering the consequences of a long lie;

- to optimise elderly people's confidence and, whenever relevant, their carers' confidence, in their ability to move about as safely and as independently as possible.

At the heart of the philosophy of such guidelines are the basic principles of risk management – a fall is reasonably foreseeable, therefore simple measures can be introduced to minimise the risks.

Sometimes the patient might insist on walking unaided in spite of being advised against it. The physiotherapist would have to use all her persuasive powers to curb the patient's eagerness and to take all the reasonable means she can to protect the patient.

The risks of inactivity

The risk of wasting muscle power and loss of balance is also reasonably foreseeable amongst the immobile elderly. Rosemary Oddy describes how the gymnastic ball offers excellent opportunities for strengthening muscle power and improving balance of elderly patients. When used with a retaining cuff, even those with dementia can sit on it and derive benefit from it[14].

All areas of clinical practice benefit from the adoption of the same principles of risk management which apply in health and safety situations (see Chapter 11).

Situation: risks in rehabilitation

> A physiotherapist attempts to assist an elderly person to walk following a stroke. As she moves him from the chair he lets go his hold on her and falls to the floor, fracturing his pelvis. What is the legal situation of the physiotherapist?

The first question which must be asked is, what is the reasonable standard of the physiotherapist in this situation? Would any competent physiotherapist have acted as she did? Would a simple risk assessment not have suggested that a second person should be at hand to assist in the first steps of mobilisation? The physiotherapist is unlikely to face litigation personally, since her employer would be vicariously liable for her actions (see Chapter 10).

During the process of stroke rehabilitation the physiotherapist would try slowly to withdraw the level of support. The patient may progress from standing between two people, walking between two people, walking with one person, walking with an aid, and walking unaided. This progress is based on the clinical judgment of the physiotherapist. It has to be accepted that many patients never reach the point of walking unaided. Central to the clinical judgment at each stage in the progress is a risk assessment and management process.

Risk to others

Situation: Too risky

> A stroke patient, previously active with a full social life, is discharged having made a good recovery. He has been advised that he must contact the DVLA and his insurance company before thinking about driving again. He admits to the physiotherapist during a

Day Hospital visit that he has driven but 'only around the village'. What is the physiotherapist's legal duty?

The physiotherapist should make it clear to the patient that in driving contrary to clinical advice he is breaking the law as well as putting at risk his own safety and that of others. Where she has considerable concerns about his mental and physical capacity to drive safely, there may well be justification in warning the patient that if he fails to notify the DVLA then she may feel obliged as part of her duty of care, to inform them herself. (See Chapter 8 on the exceptions to the duty of confidentiality.)

Restraint – the wanderer

Some elderly people can present special problems because of their disregard for their own health and safety and their inability to make rational decisions. In residential and nursing homes and also hospitals there is a temptation to lock doors or use forms of restraint to prevent the client wandering off into harm. Such forms of restraint are not good practice and ideally there should be sufficient staff to prevent the need for doors to be locked or patients held under restraint.

Guidance is given in the *Code of Practice*[15] on the Mental Health Act 1983 on the care of informal patients who are likely to wander off causing harm to themselves and the use of a policy and clear documentation on locking doors. Advice is also given by Counsel and Care on the uses and abuses of restraint in residential and nursing homes for older people[16]. The Royal College of Nursing has also given guidance to its members on alternatives to the use of restraint[17] and this advice would be of value for other health professionals. The RCN emphasises that there are many procedures and practices which could prevent the need for restraint arising.

Situation: Wanderers

A physiotherapist visits a nursing home where a stroke patient is being cared for. She notes that many of the residents are sitting in seats with tables in front of them or with seats sloping down to the rear so that the resident is effectively trapped in them. She queries this with the home manager who tells her that that is the safest way of preventing them wandering off from the home, because they have been told they cannot lock the doors. The physiotherapist wonders if this is lawful.

Restraint can be a form of imprisonment. It may be justified if it is reasonable, of short duration and in the best interests of a mentally incompetent person. However permanent on-going restraint through clothing or design of furniture is not best practice and could, if brought to court, be held unlawful. The physiotherapist should discuss alternative systems of keeping the elderly person safe. If the managers of the home are not prepared to consider changes, then this may be raised with the registration body (which for a nursing home would be the local health authority). If the social services purchase places in the home they will also be concerned with standards of care and can issue notice if there appears to be a breach in the contract. Contractual conditions can be more demanding than the provisions of the Registered Homes Act 1984.

Exploitation by relatives and others

The physiotherapist may occasionally encounter situations where it is apparent that an elderly client is being exploited financially. If the draft legislation proposed by the Law Commission is enacted, there would be a legal framework where protection could be provided for the victim[18]. At the present moment the physiotherapist would have to ensure that the Department of Social Security were notified if the exploitation relates to the use of social security funds. For larger amounts the Court of Protection has a procedure for protecting the property of the mentally incompetent, but this is cumbersome and expensive in itself and legislation is urgently needed as recommended by the Law Commission.

Abuse of the elderly

'Granny bashing' and other forms of physical and mental abuse have only been recently recognised as a danger of which all health and social services professionals should be aware. Should a physiotherapist suspect that her client is the victim of such action, she should take such care as is reasonable in all the circumstances to ensure that the elderly person is safe. This will probably necessitate referring the client to the community health services such as the health visitor and also informing social services.

The Social Services Inspectorate has provided a report on confronting abuse of the elderly[19]. This sets out the ways in the social services departments respond to and manage cases of elder abuse which arise in domestic settings. It suggests ways in which practice might be improved through clearer policies and guidelines.

Use of volunteers

One of the principal philosophies of the community care policy is that provision of services for those in need should be based on a partnership between the statutory services, the private sector (including the voluntary sector) and the family. The physiotherapist should be aware of the contribution which voluntary groups and individual volunteers can make towards the care and quality of life of the patient/client, whether at home or in the hospital. She should, however, be alert to the legal implications of delegating tasks to volunteers and ensure that the principles set out in Chapter 10 on delegation and supervision are observed. A physiotherapist who delegated tasks to a volunteer who lacked the knowledge and experience to undertake that activity with reasonable safety could be liable for any harm which was caused.

Situation: Volunteers

A volunteer borrows a wheel chair from the physiotherapy department to take a patient into the grounds for some fresh air (or a smoke!). He does not put the patient's foot securely onto the footrest of the chair and the foot is twisted back and injured when the chair is pushed forward. Who is liable?

There has clearly been negligence in the care of this patient. A duty of care is owed to the patient, reasonable care has not been taken and as a consequence the patient suffers harm. In order to assess who is responsible, the initial questions to be asked are

- Who was responsible for delegating activities to the volunteer?
- Had the volunteer been taught how to ensure a patient was safe in a wheel chair?
- Had the volunteer been given clearly defined boundaries?

If faults can be shown in the delegation to and supervision of the volunteer, then that person delegating is liable and the employer would be vicariously liable for those failures. If the volunteer has had appropriate training, instructions and supervision, but disobeyed the rules, then he is liable. Although the volunteer is not an employee and so in strict law there is no employer to be vicariously liable for the volunteer, the NHS trust or other employer would probably accept liability, in accordance with Department of Health expectations, since it is directly liable for the patient's safety.

Inter-agency cooperation

Statutory provisions require health authorities and local authorities to work closely together and with the private/voluntary sector in the performance of their statutory functions. Other organisations with which the physiotherapist may be involved include local authority housing departments, housing associations, care organisations, and many companies and firms which provide services for the elderly.

Physiotherapists should be aware of the resources available for the care of the elderly and from whom further information may be obtained. In October 1998 Kings Fund published a guide to the choice of residential care[20]. It is designed to give guidance to the resident or carer on what to look for in choosing a home. Physiotherapists might find the check list useful in helping patients make this momentous decision.

Day hospitals

The physiotherapist should have a major role to play in the functioning of a day hospital and the assessment of clients. Jane Sword and Rod Lambert provided a useful procedure and documentation for the assessment of domestic function in a day hospital for elderly mentally ill people[21]. The form covers:

- comprehensive assessment of all areas of domestic function;
- a format which is easy to use and administer;
- information from which a consistent report format can be established;
- a high degree of correlation in the results obtained in the use of the form by a number of therapists; and

- the highlighting of areas of ability and deficit, thereby enabling specific recommendations to be made and facilitating subsequent programme planning.

The value of multi-disciplinary assessment is shown in the evaluation of the uniform data system for medical rehabilitation described by Arthur Peter[22].

There is a danger that professionals in a day hospital are too over protective to a patient, providing the same level of physical support that they would give to a patient in hospital. It should be remembered that the patient is managing for herself at home and too much assistance in the hospital might undermine her confidence.

Health and safety and manual handling

The physiotherapist who cares for the elderly should ensure that she follows the principles set out in Chapter 11 in relation to manual handling and other health and safety regulations. Even though she may see some manual handling in the care of her elderly clients as therapeutic, it still comes under the Manual Handling Regulations and she would be expected to carry out an appropriate risk assessment. She must also ensure that she receives regular updating of her training.

Situation: Teaching the carers

> A physiotherapist watches a husband demonstrate how he gets his wife out of a chair. The patient puts her arm around her husband's neck and pulls, putting him at considerable risk. The physiotherapist warns the husband of the dangers, but he says that he has always done it this way and sees no problem with it. Where does the physiotherapist stand if he later suffers harm?

It is quite likely in this situation that the husband will ignore the advice of the physiotherapist to introduce a different method of lifting his wife. If she arranges for the delivery of a hoist, he may well not use it. However the physiotherapist has a duty to ensure that she gives the appropriate advice in such a way that he can see the serious dangers in his present method, and that she arranges the supply of any necessary equipment. If, having fulfilled her duty of care, the husband ignores her advice and does not use the equipment, then any harm which he suffers is at his own risk and he could not successfully hold the physiotherapist or her employers liable for it.

Resources

The elderly have not always received the priority in the allocation of resources which their needs require. Physiotherapists should beware of the dangers of using arbitrary age levels to deny services on a blanket basis, rather than assessing patients individually. It may be that a person in her 90s requires treatment which could be contra-indicated in a person much younger, because her physical condition is much better.

Because of the mismatch between the demand for services and the resources available, physiotherapists have a duty to ensure that resources are used reasonably.

Situation: Enough is enough

A physiotherapist considers that a stroke patient has reached her full potential and would now benefit from feeling 'in charge of her life'. The patient's husband disagrees and wants his wife to continue with regular rehabilitation. Should the physiotherapist provide further sessions?

No physiotherapist should accept instructions which are contrary to her professional judgment. This applies whoever is giving the instructions – patients, relatives or other professional colleagues. In this situation, it is a matter of professional judgement whether further sessions are clinically justified and if the physiotherapist has formed the view that progress will not be made, then she must make this clear to the patient and her husband. The latter has no legal right to enforce treatment which is not clinically indicated. The physiotherapist should explain this sensitively, since the sessions may be seen by the relative as a necessary support, emotional as well as practical, and the physiotherapist may offer to review the situation after a specified time. She should, of course, ensure that her record keeping is above reproach and should be prepared for the possibility of a complaint arising from the situation.

The Community Care (Residential Accommodation) Act 1998 requires local authorities to assist residents in the payment of fees for residential accommodation without undue delay, as soon as their capital resources fall below £16 000. If the resources fall below £10 000 the council is obliged to pay all the fees. The Act reinforces the decision of the court in a case brought against Sefton Council by a resident who had had to contribute to the fees even though her resources were well below £10 000. Sefton Council were following a policy of requiring the elderly to pay their own fees until all they had left was £1500, about the price of a funeral. The court declared Sefton's actions illegal and this decision is incorporated in the 1998 Act[23].

Conclusion

The demographic changes show that those over 65 will increase as a proportion of society and that the number of elderly over 80 and 90 is increasing significantly. The resource implications for the provision of health and social care, as well as pensions and social security, are now coming onto the agenda of every political party. It can no longer be assumed that public expenditure can be the main source of assistance. A Royal Commission[24] has been established to consider the funding of long-term care for the elderly and reported in March 1999. Its recommendations include the payment for some elements of care from public funds, and the establishment of a National Care Commission. The care of the elderly will continue to be one of the principal responsibilities and challenges for the physiotherapist.

Questions and exercises _____

1 A physiotherapist is concerned that an elderly person living on her own is refusing to accept any assistance and is neglecting herself. What legal powers exist in this situation?

2 An elderly person visiting a day hospital refuses to have post stroke exercises. What is the legal situation?

3 In a residential home, a physiotherapist discovers that all the doors are kept locked. When she enquires about this she is told that this is the only way in which the residents can be prevented from going out on to the main road. What action, if any, should she take?

References

1 King, D., Jones, M., Barrett, J.A. & Lorraine, J.W. (1993) Are elderly patients getting enough occupational therapy? *British Journal of Occupational Therapy* **65**, 11, 412–14.

2 Skelton, D.A. & McLaughlin, A.W. (1996) Training Functional Ability in Old Age. *Physiotherapy* **82**, 3, 159–67.

3 *Re T (Adult: Refusal of Medical Treatment)* [1992] 4 All ER 649.

4 Law Commission (1993) *Mentally Incapacitated and Other Vulnerable Adults: Public Law Protection*, (the third paper dealing with decision making and the mentally incapacitated adult) HMSO, London.

5 Law Commission (1995) Report No. 231 *Mental Incapacity*. HMSO, London.

6 Lord Chancellor's Department (1997) *Who Decides?* LCD, London.

7 NHS Management Executive (1990) *A Guide to consent for examination and treatment* (HC(90)22) DoH, London.

8 *F* v. *West Berkshire Health Authority and Another* [1989] 2 All ER 545.

9 *R* v. *Bournewood Community and Mental Health NHS Trust* (HL) [1998] 3 All ER 289.

10 Law Commission (1995) Report No. 231 *Mental Incapacity*. HMSO, London.

11 Counsel and Care (1993) *The Right to Take Risks*. Counsel and Care, London. (see list of addresses).

12 Reece, A.C. & Simpson, J.M. (1996) Preparing Older People to Cope after a Fall. *Physiotherapy* **82**, 4, 227–35.

13 Simpson, J., Harrington, R. & Marsh, N. (1998) Guidelines for Managing Falls Among Elderly People. *Physiotherapy* **84**, 4, 173–7.

14 Odd, R. (1996) Taming the Gymnastic Ball. *Physiotherapy* **82**, 8, 477–9.

15 Department of Health (1993) *Code of Practice on the Mental Health Act 1983*. 2nd edn. DoH, London.

16 Counsel and Care (January 1992) *What if they hurt themselves?* Counsel and Care, London.

17 Royal College of Nursing (1992) *Focus on Restraint*. 2nd edn. RCN, London.

18 Law Commission (1995) Report No. 231 *Mental Incapacity*. HMSO, London.

19 Social Services Inspectorate (1992) *Confronting Elder Abuse*. DoH and HMSO, London.

20 Kings Fund (1998) *Home from Home*. Kings Fund, London.

21 Sword, J. & Lambert, R. (1989) Assessment of Domestic Function within a day hospital for elderly mentally ill people. *British Journal of Occupational Therapy* **52**, 1, 16–17.

22   Peter, A. (1994) Evaluation of the Uniform Data System for medical Rehabilitation (including the functional independence measure) by Glenrothes geriatric day hospital team. *British Journal of Occupational Therapy* **57**, 3, 91–4.

23   *R* v. *Sefton Metropolitan Borough Council ex parte Help the Aged* [1997] 4 All ER 532.

24   Royal Commission on Long Term Care (1999) *With Respect to Old Age.* Cm 4192–1 1999, The Stationery Office, London.

Chapter 25
Death and the Dying

It is an inevitable fact that physiotherapists across all specialisms will be involved in the care of dying patients. It is important that at such difficult times the physiotherapist has confidence in her knowledge of the law which applies. This chapter discusses the law relating to the following topics:

- The extent of the duty to maintain life
- Involvement of the court
- Living wills
- Can the court order doctors to provide treatment?
- 'Not for resuscitation' orders
- Parents' refusal to consent to treatment
- Care of the dying patient
- Registration of death and the role of the coroner
- Organ transplants
- Conclusions

The extent of the duty to maintain life

Health care professionals can be faced with the problem of whether there is a duty in law to carry out every possible procedure known to science in order to save the life of the patient or whether the law enables a person to be allowed to die. The law draws a distinction between withholding care and taking positive action to end life. The former may or may not be legally permissible depending upon the prognosis of the patient. The latter will always be illegal. It is not therefore the duty of the health professional to continue to provide high technology care when the patient's prognosis is considered hopeless; and the patient can be allowed to die.

Murder and manslaughter

To kill a patient may be murder or manslaughter.

'Murder is when a man of sound memory, and of the age of discretion, unlawfully killeth within any country of the realm any reasonable creature *in rerum natura* under the King's peace, with malice aforethought, either expressed by the party or implied by law, so as the party wounded, or hurt, etc. die of the wound or hurt etc. (within a year and a day after the same).' (Coke)

This definition of murder was given in a court case in the 17th century. In 1996 the limitation of time was removed, so that it is not now required that the person dies within a year and a day of the act which caused the death.

Manslaughter is divided into two categories – voluntary and involuntary. Voluntary covers the situation where there is the mental intention to kill or complete indifference to the possibility that death could arise from one's actions (i.e. the mental requirement of a crime (*mens rea*) but there are extenuating factors:

- Provocation
- Death in pursuance of a suicide pact
- Diminished responsibility.

The effect of these extenuating factors is that a murder verdict would not be obtained but the defendant could be guilty of voluntary manslaughter.

Involuntary manslaughter exists when the *mens rea* for murder is absent. Such circumstances would include:

- gross negligence;
- killing recklessly where the recklessness may be insufficient for it to be murder;
- an intention to escape from lawful arrest.

Defences to a charge of murder or manslaughter include:

- killing in the course of preventing crime or arresting offenders;
- killing in the defence of one's own person or that of another;
- killing in defence of property.

Use of excessive force will negate these defences.

Where the accused is convicted of manslaughter the judge has complete discretion over sentencing. In contrast, where there is a murder conviction at present the sentence is a mandatory one of life imprisonment although this is being reviewed by the Law Commission.

Voluntary euthanasia

By this is meant the killing of a person with that person's consent. This is unlawful. It could amount to murder, punishable on conviction by life imprisonment, or it could be seen as manslaughter with the discretion over sentencing. Alternatively, if the act amounts to assistance in a suicide bid, then it is illegal under section 2(1) of the Suicide Act 1961 which is shown in Figure 25.1.

Figure 25.1 **The Suicide Act 1961 – section 2(1).**

A person who aids, abets, counsels or procures the suicide of another or an attempt by another to commit suicide, shall be liable on conviction on indictment to imprisonment. [up to 14 years]

Situation: Asking for help

> The wife of a patient who was in the terminal stages of a respiratory disease was concerned that the patient found breathing difficult in spite of constant oxygen and no longer wished to carry on living. She asked the physiotherapist if she would provide her with some medicines to help her husband out of his misery. What right of action does the physiotherapist have?

There is no grey area of law here. Any action on the part of the physiotherapist to assist the wife in ending her husband's misery would constitute a criminal wrong and they could both face murder or manslaughter proceedings.

Even where the parents wish a grossly handicapped baby to die, any professional who intentionally speeds up the process of death could be guilty of causing the death of the child.

Case: *R* v. *Arthur*[1]

> A paediatrician was prosecuted for attempting to cause the death of a grossly handicapped baby who was suffering from Down's Syndrome and who had other disabilities when he prescribed dihydrocodeine and nursing care only.

The judge had stated that:

> 'There is no special law in this country that places doctors in a separate category and gives them extra protection over the rest of us ... Neither in law is there any special power, facility or license to kill children who are handicapped or seriously disadvantaged in an irreversible way.'

Dr Arthur was however acquitted by the jury

In contrast, at the other end of life, Dr Nigel Cox[2] was convicted when he prescribed potassium chloride to a terminally ill patient and was sentenced to a year's imprisonment which was suspended for a year. He also had to appear before disciplinary proceedings of the Regional Health Authority, his employers and before the General Medical Council.

The Select Committee of the House of Lords[3] has reported that there should be no change in the law to permit euthanasia. This is also the view put forward by the Law Commission in a recent report[4].

Letting die

Do these cases mean that it is never lawful to permit patients to die whatever the circumstances of their condition? The answer is that the law does not expect constant medical intervention whatever the prognosis and, in certain circumstances, it is legally permissible to let a patient die. A distinction is however drawn between letting die and killing.

Adults

Where an adult wishes to die and refuses treatment, then crucial to the decision making and withholding treatment is their mental capacity to make a decision or the existence of a living will (see below).

Situation: Coming off a ventilator

> A tetraplegic patient attended by the physiotherapist told her that he wished to be allowed to die and come off the ventilator. What is the legal situation?

This is the situation which arose in the Karen Quinlan case in the USA where an extremely long court case resulted in a decision being made that she could come off the ventilator. Once off, ironically, she survived for several years.

A mentally competent person has the right to refuse treatment. However in this situation the physiotherapist should be careful not to undertake any action which could be interpreted as aiding or abetting a suicide attempt. She should also obtain independent advice on the mental competence of the patient to refuse treatment (see Chapter 7 and the law relating to consent).

Children

The following is an example of the court permitting a child to be allowed to die.

Case: *Re C*[5]

> In this case a baby was born suffering from congenital hydrocephalus and had been made a ward of court for reasons unconnected with her medical condition. The local authority sought the court's determination as to the appropriate manner in which she should be treated in the event of her contracting a serious infection or her existing feeding regimes becoming unviable. A specialist paediatrician assessed C's condition as severely and irreversibly brain-damaged, the prognosis of which was hopeless. He recommended that the objective of any treatment should therefore be to ease suffering rather than prolong life. While not specifying the adoption or discontinuance of any particular procedures, he further advised consultation with C's carers as to the appropriate method of achieving that objective. The judge accepted this report and approved the recommendations as being in her best interests. However, he made a very restrictive order to treat the child 'to die'.
>
> The official solicitor who had been appointed *guardian ad litem* (see glossary) of the child, appealed to the Court of Appeal on the ground that the judge had not jurisdiction and was plainly wrong in the exercise of his discretion to make an order that the hospital be at liberty to treat the minor to die.

The Court of Appeal varied the judge's order and the words 'to die' were changed to 'to allow her life to come to an end peacefully and with dignity'. The court emphasised that the decisions on treatment rested with the medical professionals:

> 'The hospital do continue to treat the minor within the parameters of the opinion expressed by [the specialist paediatrician] in his report of 13.4.1989 which report is not to be disclosed to any person other than the health authority.'

In *Re J*[6] (1990) the baby was a ward of court and in contrast with the case of *Re C* the baby was not at the point of death.

Case: *Re J* (1990)

J's prognosis was not good and, although he was expected to survive a few years, he was likely to be blind, deaf, unable to speak and have serious spastic quadriplegia. The judge made an order that he should be treated with antibiotics if he developed a chest infection but if he were to stop breathing he should not receive artificial ventilation. The official solicitor on behalf of the child appealed against the order on the grounds that unless the situation was one of terminal illness or it was certain that the child's life would be intolerable, the court was not justified in approving the withholding of life saving treatment.

The Court of Appeal held that the court can never sanction positive steps to terminate the life of a person. However the court could direct that treatment without which death would ensue need not be given to prolong life, even though the child was neither on the point of death nor dying. The court had to undertake a balancing exercise in assessing the course to be adopted in the best interests of the child, looked at from his point of view and giving the fullest possible weight to his desire, if he were in a position to make a sound judgment, to survive, but also taking into account the pain and suffering and quality of life which he would experience if life were prolonged and the pain and suffering involved in the proposed treatment.

The parents do not have the final say, though their wishes must be taken into account in determining the outcome for the child. Ultimately the courts, as is seen in the case of *Re J* (1992) (see below), have made it clear that the decision should be in the hands of the health professionals i.e. the doctors.

The Royal College of Paediatrics and Child Health (RCPCH)[7] has published a framework for practice in determining whether life saving treatment should be withheld or withdrawn. These proposals cover the following situations.

Situations where withholding or withdrawal of treatment could be considered:

- Brain dead
- Persistent vegetative state
- The 'no chance' situation
- The 'no purpose' situation
- The 'unbearable' situation.

The principles to be applied are set out in Figure 25.2.

Figure 25.2 **Principles set by the Royal College of Paediatrics and Child Health.**

(1) To act always in the child's best interests.
(2) It is unrealistic to expect a complete consensus – aim to seek as much ethical common ground as possible.
(3) Seek court intervention if disputes between the health care team, the child, the parents and carers cannot be resolved.
(4) Consider each situation on its merits.
(5) There is no ethical difference between the withdrawal and the withholding of treatment.

Continued

***Figure 25.2* Continued.**

(6)   The duty of care is not absolute.
(7)   Redirection of care from life sustaining to palliation is not withdrawal of care.
(8)   It is never permissible to withdraw pain relief or contact.
(9)   Treatments the primary aim of which is the relief of suffering, but which may incidentally hasten death, may be justified.

Involvement of the court

When should the consent of the court should be obtained to taking action? There are probably many occasions in practice when a patient is allowed to die without court approval being obtained. If a patient refuses treatment and it is determined that the patient has the capacity to refuse to give consent, then the patient's refusal cannot be overruled (see Chapter 7 and the case of *Re C*).

Where the patient lacks mental competence, if the doctors, the parents and the rest of the multi-disciplinary team are agreed that the prognosis of the patient is extremely poor and that aggressive treatment is inappropriate there is unlikely to be a court hearing. The patient will be allowed to die and 'nature to take its course'.

The Tony Bland case

However, where the patient is mentally incompetent and there is no living will, then the withholding of artificial feeding is a matter for court intervention as the Tony Bland case shows.

Case: *Airedale NHS Trust* v. *Bland*[8]

The patient was a victim of the football stadium crush at Hillsborough and it was established that, although he could breathe and digest food independently, he could not see, hear, taste, smell or communicate in any way and it appeared that there was no hope of recovery or improvement. Given the importance of the issues involved the matter was referred to the House of Lords which had to decide if it was lawful to permit artificial feeding to be discontinued in the case of a patient in a persistent vegetative state.

The House of Lords held that it would be in the best interests of the patient to discontinue the nasal gastric feed and he was later reported as having died. It specifically recommended that if any similar decisions were required to be made in the future there should be application before the courts and a court in Bristol gave consent in a similar case[9] a few months after the House of Lords decision on Tony Bland.

Court guidance

A practice note has now been issued by the Official Solicitor[10] for such situations. It is summarised in Figure 25.3.

Figure 25.3 **Practice note on withdrawal of medical treatment from a patient in a persistent vegetative state (PVS) (summarised).**

(1) The termination of artificial feeding and hydration for patients in PVS will in virtually all cases require the prior sanction of a High Court Judge.

(2) The diagnosis of PVS should be made in accordance with the most up-to-date generally accepted guidelines for the medical profession. (Note that Royal College of Physicians advised in March 1996 that diagnosis of PVS is not absolute but based on probabilities.) Such a diagnosis should not be considered confirmed until the patient has been in a continuing PVS for at least 12 months (following head injury) or at least 6 months (following other kinds of brain damage). Before then, as soon as the patient's condition has stabilised, rehabilitative measure such as coma arousal programmes should be instituted. It is not appropriate to apply to court to end artificial feeding until the condition is judged permanent.

(3) Applications to court should be by originating summons issued in the Family Division of the High Court seeking a declaration in a specified form. The application should follow the procedure laid down for sterilisation cases in *F.* v. *West Berkshire Health Authority*[11] and in the practice note of May 1993[12].

(4) Applications in relation to minors should be made within wardship proceedings and leave sought rather than a declaration.

(5) Sets out the specific wording of the originating summons, 'may ... furnish such treatment and nursing care ... as may be appropriate to ensure X suffers the least distress and retains the greatest dignity' until he dies.

(6) The case should normally be heard in open court, but anonymity will be preserved.

(7) The applicants may be either the next of kin or other individual closely associated or the relevant Health Authority or NHS Trust (which in any event ought to be a party). The views of the next of kin are very important and should be made known to the court in every case.

(8) The Official Solicitor should be invited to act as guardian ad litem (see glossary) of the patient.

(9) There should be at least two neurological reports on the patient, one of which will be commissioned by the Official Solicitor. Other medical evidence, such as evidence about rehabilitation or nursing care, may be necessary.

(10) The Official Solicitor will interview the next of kin and others close to the patient as well as seeing the patient and those caring for him. The views of the patient may have been previously expressed, either in writing or otherwise. The High Court exercising its inherent jurisdiction may determine the effect of a purported advance directive as to future medical treatment. The patient's previously expressed views, if any, will always be an important component in the decisions of the doctors and the court.

(11) Members of the Official Solicitor's legal staff are prepared to discuss PVS cases before proceedings have been issued. Contact with the Official Solicitor may be made by telephoning 0171-911 7127 during office hours.

The future

The referral of a case of a dying patient to court is not necessarily the most appropriate forum for such decisions to be made. Legislation may follow the Law Commission's recommendations[13] on decision making and the mentally incapacitated adult. There needs to be clarification on when the court's intervention should be sought in the care of a terminally ill child or adult. The BMA at its conference in Cardiff in July 1998 has asked for guidance to be provided for doctors on when to keep people alive. It notes that there are widespread differences across the country and seeks greater uniformity. The BMA issued a consultation document on withholding and withdrawing treatment[14], the consultation period ending on 16 October 1998.

Living wills

A living will (also known as an advance refusal of treatment or an advance directive) is a statement, made when a person is mentally competent, over what treatments and care they would wish to refuse at a later time, when they no longer have the mental capacity to make decisions. There is at the time of writing no statutory provision (i.e. by Act of Parliament) for the recognition of a living will. However the House of Lords in the Tony Bland case stated that, had Tony Bland when competent expressed any refusal of treatment, then that would have been binding upon the health professionals caring for him (i.e. at common law living wills will be recognised). The Law Commission[15] has put forward recommendations relating to advance refusals of treatment but these are still to be given statutory force.

The BMA has prepared guidelines[16] for the preparation of a living will. It suggests that, as a minimum, the following information is included:

- Full name
- Address
- Name and address of general practitioner
- A clear statement of your wishes, either general or specific
- Whether advice was sought from health professionals
- The name, address and telephone number of your nominated person, if you have one.
- Signature
- Witness signature
- Date drafted and reviewed

If a health professional withholds treatment on the basis of a refusal of a patient contained in an advance directive and there is no reason to believe that it is invalid, then the health professional should not be held liable for a breach of the duty of care. The Law Commission recommended that an advance refusal of treatment should not include the refusal of basic care. This it defined as 'care to maintain bodily cleanliness and to alleviate severe pain and the provision of direct oral nutrition and hydration'. Thus the existence of an advance statement of refusal would not prevent a health professional from providing basic care. This may make the concept of a living will more acceptable to professionals. However there are some, such as Buddhists, who would consider that giving people pain relief against their will is an unacceptable limitation on their autonomy.

Situation: Refusing treatment

A patient, on hearing that he was suffering from Motor Neurone Disease, wrote an advanced refusal of treatment indicating that he would not wish to receive any artificial feeding. He is now finding it more and more difficult to swallow and artificial feeding is seen as the only option. The consultant has stated that this should be commenced and refuses to accept that the living will has any significance to his clinical judgment. What is the law?

If there is no reason to doubt the validity of the living will and if there is no reason to believe that the patient changed his mind, then it is valid in law. There is therefore an obligation upon all health professionals to respect the wishes of the patient. If the consultant treats the patient contrary to the wishes expressed in a valid living will, then he is guilty of trespass to the person (see Chapter 7) and those acting on behalf of the patient could instigate an action against him.

Can the court order doctors to provide treatment?

Case: *Re J (1992)*[17]

J was born in January 1991 and suffered an accidental fall when he was a month old with the result that he was profoundly handicapped both mentally and physically. He was severely microcephalic, his brain not having grown sufficiently following the injury. He also had severe cerebral palsy, cortical blindness and severe epilepsy. He was in general fed by a nasal gastric tube.

Medical opinion was unanimous that J was unlikely to develop much beyond his present functioning, that that level might deteriorate and that his expectation of life, although uncertain, would be short. The paediatrician's report stated that, given J's condition, it would not be medically appropriate to intervene with intensive procedures such as artificial ventilation if he were to suffer a life-threatening event.

The baby was in the care of foster parents with whom the local authority shared responsibility. The local authority applied to the court under section 100 of the Children Act 1989 to determine whether ventilation should be given to the child. The mother supported the requirement that the hospital and doctors should be forced to put the baby on a life support machine.

The judge regarded J's best interests as well as the interests of justice in preserving his life as both pointing in favour of the grant of an interim injunction requiring such treatment to take place. The hospital appealed.

In the Court of Appeal Lord Donaldson, Master of the Rolls, stated that he could not at present conceive of any circumstances in which requiring a medical practitioner (or a health authority acting by a medical practitioner) to adopt a course of treatment, which in the *bona fide* clinical judgement of the practitioner was contra-indicated as not being in the patient's best interests, would be other than an abuse of power, as directly or indirectly requiring the practitioner to act contrary to the fundamental duty he owed to his patient.

Lord Donaldson said that the order of the judge, ordering specific treatment to take place, was wholly inconsistent with the law as stated in *Re J*[18] (see above) and in *Re R*[19] and could not be justified on the basis of any known authority. It was also erroneous on two other substantial grounds:

- its lack of certainty as to what was required of the health authority; and
- its failure adequately to take account of the sad fact of life that health authorities might on occasion find that they had too few resources, either human or material or both, to treat all the patients whom they would like to treat in the way they would like to treat them.

It was the health authority's duty to make choices. The court would have no knowledge of competing claims to resources and was in no position to express any view on their deployment of these resources.

The Court of Appeal thus held that where a paediatrician caring for a severely handicapped baby considered that mechanical ventilation procedures would not be appropriate the court would not grant an injunction requiring such treatment to take place.

The effect of the Court's decision to set aside the judge's ruling was to leave the health authority and its medical staff free, subject to consent not being withdrawn, to treat J in accordance with their best clinical judgement. That did not mean that in no circumstances should J be subjected to mechanical ventilation.

The reluctance of the court to interfere with the decision making of the doctors in the interests of the patient was seen in a recent case in very different circumstances. In a case[20] where the father of a girl of ten suffering from leukaemia brought an action against the health authority for its refusal to fund a course of chemotherapy followed by a second bone marrow transplant operation, the Court of Appeal took the view that the courts should not intervene in such a decision but that the health authority should follow medical advice as to what was in the best interests of the child. (See Chapter 6 for a fuller discussion of the case.)

On the other hand the courts have made it clear that decisions relating to the sterilisation of a mentally incompetent adult[21] and the cessation of artificial feeding do require the involvement of a court and it is likely that the need for reference in other cases may be made explicit.

'Not for resuscitation' orders

The legal aspects of such orders are considered elsewhere by the author[22] and the Royal College of Nursing has issued a paper for guidance[23].

What is the legal significance of such orders?

Competent adults
If patients have the mental competence to understand the situation they are entitled to refuse to give consent to any treatment, even though the treatment is life saving (see Chapter 7).

Children

Whilst a child of 16 or 17 has a statutory right to give consent to treatment, a recent case has decided that children cannot refuse treatment which is in their best interests. In the case of *Re W*[24] a girl of 16 years refused to be treated for anorexia nervosa, but her refusal was overruled by the court (see Chapter 23). If, however, the decision made by the minor is considered to be in his or her best interests, then it would be valid for all professional carers of that patient to accept that refusal of care and the instructions that the patient is not to be resuscitated.

Mental incapacity

Where the patient is mentally incapacitated and the decision has been made by the consultant in charge of the care of the patient, that the patient should not be resuscitated, then the legality of such a decision depends upon the prognosis of the patient and, in dubious cases, there are advantages in a declaration from the court being obtained.

Relatives and carers

■ Could the relatives give 'Not For Resuscitation' or 'Do Not Resuscitate' instructions?

Relatives do not have any right to make decisions on behalf of a mentally incapacitated adult. It is clear that, whilst the relatives should be fully consulted in the decision making, they do not have the right to refuse treatment.

An NFR matrix

Figure 25.4 provides a matrix showing how the factors of mental competence and prognosis impact on each other in NFR decisions.

Figure 25.4   A matrix for 'Not for Resuscitation'.

Is the patient competent?	No	Yes – and the patient asks for treatment	Yes – but the patient refuses treatment
Good Prognosis	**resuscitate**	**resuscitate**	**NFR**
Bad Prognosis	**NFR**	**???**	**NFR**

The question marks in the middle box on the bottom line, where the mentally competent patient is asking for treatment when the prognosis is bad, show the uncertainty about the legal situation. A mentally competent patient does not have an absolute right to insist on treatment when it is not clinically indicated. However it depends upon the detailed circumstances – resuscitation may or may not be clinically indicated and if it is not clinically indicated, a mentally competent person cannot compel such treatment to be given.

Parents' refusal to consent to treatment

An example of where the courts refused to uphold the parents' wish to allow the child to die is seen in the following case.

Case: *Re B*[25]

In *Re B* a child was born suffering from Down's syndrome and an intestinal blockage. She required an operation to relieve the obstruction if she was to live more than a few days. If the operation were performed, the child might die within a few months but it was probable that her life expectancy would be 20 to 30 years. Her parents, having decided that it would be kinder to allow her to die rather than live as a physically and mentally handicapped person, refused to consent to the operation. The local authority made the child a ward of court and, when a surgeon decided that the wishes of the parents should be respected, they sought an order authorising the operation to be performed by other named surgeons.

The judge decided that the parents' wishes should be respected and refused to make the order.

The local authority appealed to the Court of Appeal which allowed the appeal. It stated that:

(1) The question for the court was whether it was in the best interests of the child that she should have the operation and not whether the parents' wishes should be respected.
(2) Since the effect of the operation might be that the child would have the normal span of life of a Down's syndrome person; and
(3) Since it had not been demonstrated that the life of a person with Down's syndrome was of such a nature that the child should be condemned to die;
(4) The court would make an order that the operation be performed.

Crucial to the decision in this case was the prognosis of the child. In a contrasting case the parents' refusal was upheld by the courts.

Case: *Re T (a minor) (wardship: medical treatment)*[26]

A child was born with a life-threatening liver defect. After unsuccessful treatment, the prognosis was that he would not live beyond two and a half years without a liver transplant. The mother refused to give consent to the operation because she was not willing to permit the child to undergo the pain and distress of invasive surgery. She later moved out of the country. The Local Authority, at the consultants' instigation, applied to the court for permission to carry out the operation and for the child to be returned to the jurisdiction in order that the operation could be carried out. The High Court judge held that the mother's refusal was unreasonable and it was in the child's best interests to undergo the liver transplant. The mother appealed.

The Court of Appeal upheld that appeal. The paramount consideration was the welfare of the child and not the reasonableness of the parent's refusal of consent. However since the welfare of the child depended upon the mother, her views were relevant. The judge had failed to assess the relevance or the weight of the mother's concern as to the benefits to her child of the surgery and post-operative treatment, the dangers of failure both long term as well as short term, the possibility of the need for further transplants, the likely length of life and the effect on her child of all those concerns, together with the strong reservations expressed by one of the consultants about coercing the mother into playing a crucial part in the aftermath of the operation and thereafter.

It must be stressed, however, that *Re T* is an unusual case and there were very special circumstances which led to the court upholding the wishes of the parents over those of the doctors.

The right to insist on treatment

Parents
Parents do not have the right to insist upon care or treatment which the doctors consider is not in the best interests of the child. As has been discussed above, the court would not order the doctors to carry out treatment on a child, which the doctors considered was not in the best interests of the child. (See also the case of Jamie Bowen discussed in Chapter 6.)

Mentally competent adults
Nor do any adults have an absolute right to insist upon treatment. A health professional would be failing in her obligations if she provided treatment, on the patient's insistence, knowing that it was professionally contra-indicated, or even just of no effect. If a patient purported in a living will to direct that treatment be given rather than just refusing treatment in anticipation, this direction is likely to be of little effect if it is not supported by professional judgment as to its appropriateness (see Figure 25.4 above and also Chapter 6).

Care of the dying patient

Children

The Association for children with life-threatening or terminal conditions and their families has been active in developing a Charter for their care. Its clauses are set out in Figure 25.5.

Figure 25.5 **The ACT charter for children with life-threatening conditions and their families.**

(1) Every child shall be treated with dignity and respect and shall be afforded privacy whatever the child's physical or intellectual ability.

(2) Parents shall be acknowledged as the primary carers and shall be centrally involved as partners in all care and decisions involving their child.

(3) Every child shall be given the opportunity to participate in decisions affecting his or her care, according to age and understanding.

(4) Every family shall be given the opportunity of a consultation with a paediatric specialist who has particular knowledge of the child's condition.

(5) Information shall be provided for the parents, and for the child and the siblings according to age and understanding. The needs of other relatives shall also be addressed.

(6) An honest and open approach shall be the basis of all communications which shall be sensitive and appropriate to age and understanding.

(7) The family home shall remain the centre of the caring whenever possible. All other care shall be provided by paediatric trained staff in a child-centred environment.

(8) Every child shall have access to education. Efforts shall be made to enable the child to engage in other childhood activities.

(9) Every family shall be entitled to a named key worker who will enable the family to build up and maintain an appropriate support system.

(10) Every family shall have access to flexible respite care in their own home and in a home-from-hospital setting for the whole family with appropriate paediatric nursing and medical support.

(11) Every family shall have access to paediatric nursing support in the home when required.

(12) Every family shall have access to expert, sensitive advice in procuring practical aids and financial support.

(13) Every family shall have access to domestic help at times of stress at home.

(14) Bereavement support shall be offered to the whole family and be available for as long as required.

A report was prepared by a working party on the care of dying children and their families by the British Paediatric Association, King Edward's Hospital Fund for London and the National Association of Health Authorities in 1988[27]. The aim of the report is to guide health authority members, managers and practitioners. This is discussed in more detail in the author's work on the legal aspects of childhealth care[28].

General application

Many of the books covering specific illnesses provide valuable advice on caring for the dying patient, which can be useful for physiotherapists. Thus *Motor Neurone Disease* by Sue Beresford provides helpful advice on terminal care[29]. She emphasises the importance of honesty – 'honesty is vital but should never be brutal'.

Situation: Am I dying?

> A community physiotherapist was asked by a patient suffering in the terminal stages of MND 'How much longer do I have?' The physiotherapist knew that he was dying but found it difficult to answer since the patient's wife refused to acknowledge to the patient the true position.

The answer to the question may require all the physiotherapist's skills and sensitivity. On the one hand she cannot lie to the patient, although in fact she would probably not know the exact answer to the question. Nor should she collude with the spouse in keeping information from the patient. On the other hand she needs to attempt to create some understanding between patient and spouse and should be aware of organisations which could assist in this dilemma.

Registration of death and the role of the coroner

The doctor who attended the patient during the last illness must certify the death and give the cause unless the circumstances are such that the death should be reported to the coroner. These would include the following[30]:

- Where the deceased was not attended in his last illness by a doctor.
- Where the deceased was not seen by a doctor either after death or within the 14 days prior to death.
- Where the cause of death is unknown.
- Where death appears to be due to industrial disease or poisoning.
- Where death may have been unnatural or caused by violence or neglect or abortion or attended by suspicious circumstances.
- Where death has occurred during an operation or before recovery from an anaesthetic.

The following causes of death would therefore be reportable to the coroner:

- deaths following from a criminal offence such as murder, manslaughter or causing death by dangerous driving;
- suicide;
- deaths arising from road traffic accidents, industrial accidents, domestic accidents, etc.;
- death in custody – prison or police custody;
- deaths associated with medical treatment;
- sudden death;
- deaths following abortion, drug dependence or alcoholism;
- infant deaths where no midwife or doctor was present, cot deaths.

Usually the individual coroners will make known their requirements in respect of the notification of deaths occurring in hospital. Some, for example, may require reporting of all deaths occurring within 24 hours of emergency admission[31].

Until the coroner has formally notified the doctor of his decision in relation to the deceased, the body remains under the control of the coroner, i.e. under his jurisdiction. He has the right to request a post mortem and there can be no action taken in respect of the body without his consent.

Situation: Unnatural death

> A physiotherapist visits a patient who is terminally ill. When she arrives, she is met by a distraught partner who says that he has just found the patient unconscious in bed with empty bottles of painkillers beside her. He does not know whether the doctor should be called.

It would appear from the few facts given here that the patient has made a suicide attempt. The duty of care owed to the patient would require the physiotherapist to ensure that a doctor was called. The doctor would have to decide the value in summoning emergency medical care to save the patient's life and this would relate to the prognosis of the patient. Were the patient to die, the doctor might be unable to certify the cause of death and would need to notify the coroner.

■ Can relatives view the body?

Once the coroner has jurisdiction over the body, his or her consent must be obtained before the body can be viewed by the relatives[32].

Post mortem

If the coroner orders a post mortem, the relatives have no right to refuse this. This is so even when the religious views of the deceased would be against a post mortem[33]. On the other hand if the doctor requests a post mortem where the body is not under the jurisdiction of the coroner the person in charge of the body, usually a spouse or relative, could refuse to give consent. In any event the requirements of the Human Tissue Act 1961 and the Anatomy Act 1984 must be followed.

Inquest

Where a death has been reported to the coroner he will decide whether or not an inquest will be held. He is obliged by law to hold an inquest:

- where there are reasons to suspect a criminal offence has caused the death
- in cases of industrial accidents and diseases, and
- on deaths in prison or police custody.

The existence of a general discretion to hold an inquest has been doubted[34]. The purpose of the inquest is to ascertain:

(1) who the deceased was; and
(2) how, when and where the deceased came by his death[35].

Possible verdicts are:

- natural causes
- unlawful killing
- killed lawfully
- suicide
- accidental death
- misadventure
- dependence upon a drug
- non-dependent abuse of drugs
- industrial disease
- neglect
- want of attention at birth
- attempted/self-induced abortion

An open verdict indicates that there is insufficient evidence to determine the nature of the death, i.e. the evidence did not further or fully disclose the means whereby the cause of death arose. Once completed the inquest cannot be resumed but the High Court has the power under section 13(1)(b) of the Coroners Act 1988 to order another inquest to be held.

The physiotherapist and the coroner's court

A physiotherapist might be required to give evidence at an inquest on the events which preceded death. She should be alert to this possibility – for example the physiotherapist may know that a child who has died in an apparent cot death suffered from certain symptoms prior to his death. This information from the physiotherapist may be vital at any inquest.

It is essential that the physiotherapist obtains assistance from a senior manager or lawyer on the preparation of a statement which the coroner's office will require from her. If she is subsequently asked to attend the inquest she should have assistance in preparation for giving evidence. One means of preparation is for the physiotherapist to attend a different inquest so that she can have an understanding of the geography of the court, the procedure which is followed and the level of formality required at a time when she is not personally involved (see Chapter 13 on giving evidence).

She should note that the coroner's court is known as an 'inquisitorial' one. This means that, unlike the magistrates', crown courts and civil courts where an action is brought by one person or organisation against another and the judge controls the proceedings – an 'adversarial' system – the coroner determines the witnesses who will give evidence, the course of the proceedings and he will disallow any question which in his opinion is not relevant or otherwise not a proper one. He can himself examine the witnesses often asking leading questions where information is not disputed to speed up the hearing. Hence the words 'inquisitorial' and 'inquest' (see glossary).

Where the death has been reported to the coroner, no certificate can be issued or registration take place until he has made his decision. If he decides that a post mortem should be carried out, but no inquest is needed, he will issue Form B which is sent or taken to the Registrar. The Registrar will then issue the death certificate and the certificate for disposal which is required by the undertaker before burial can take place. Authorisation for cremation requires an additional medical certificate or the certificate issued by the coroner.

Death and miscarriage

Born alive
If a baby is born alive and then dies, there must be a registration of both the birth and the death.

Stillbirth
A stillbirth is defined as:

'Where a child issues forth from its mother after the 24th week of pregnancy, and which did not at any time after being completely expelled from its mother breathe or show any signs of life' (Section 41 of the Births and Deaths Registration Act 1953, as amended by section 1 of the Still Birth Act 1992).

The stillbirth has to be registered as such and the informant has to deliver to the Registrar a written certificate that the child was not born alive. This must be signed by the registered medical practitioner or the registered midwife who was in attendance at the birth or who has examined the body. The certificate must state, to the best of the knowledge and belief of the person signing it, the cause of death and the estimated duration of the pregnancy (section 11(1)(a)). Alternatively a declaration in the prescribed form giving the reasons for the absence of a certificate and that the child was not born alive could be made (section 11(1)(b)).

A stillbirth should be disposed of by burial in a burial ground or church yard or by cremation at an authorised crematorium. A health authority should not dispose of a stillbirth without the consent of the parents.

Foetus of less than 24 weeks

If the foetus was delivered without any signs of life, then no registration is necessary. The foetus may be disposed of without formality in any way which does not constitute a nuisance or an affront to public decency. If the foetus, after expulsion, shows signs of life and then dies, it would have to be treated as both a birth and a death.

Health professionals should be sensitive to the fact that parents may suffer the same feelings of bereavement what ever the period of gestation and should therefore arrange for counselling and support as they would if the baby were full term.

Organ transplants

The donation of organs from a deceased person and from a living person are both regulated by law. The Human Tissue Act 1961 and the Corneal Tissue Act 1986 cover the use of organs of a deceased person and the Human Organ Transplants Act 1989 covers the transplant of organs from a live donor.

Human Tissue Act 1961 (as amended by the Corneal Tissue Act 1986)

This Act covers two separate situations:

(1) Where the donor, before death, has agreed in writing (or by word of mouth expressed during his last illness in the presence of two witnesses) a request that his body be used after his death. It would be necessary to check with relatives to ascertain whether there is evidence that the deceased withdrew this request.
(2) Where the deceased has made no request, but the person lawfully in possession of the body has no reason to believe that the deceased had expressed an objection to the donation or that the surviving spouse or any surviving relative objects to the body being so dealt with.

The patient must be certified dead and the removal of the organs or tissue must be by a registered medical practitioner. The eye or part of any eye can also be removed by an NHS employee who is not a doctor provided that it is carried out on the instructions of a registered medical practitioner.

Human Organ Transplants Act 1989

Section 1 of this Act prohibits commercial dealings in human organs, both purchaser and seller would be guilty of an offence as is anyone who acts as a broker of organs.

The Act also established the Unrelated Live Transplant Regulatory Authority (ULTRA) whose authorisation is required before an organ can be removed from a live donor for use by a non-blood relative. ULTRA must be satisfied that no payment is involved and that the donor (except in cases where the primary purpose is the medical treatment of the donor) has been given full information about the procedure, understands this information, and has given a valid consent (knowing that it can be withdrawn at any time). The Act does not affect the validity of transplants from a live donor to natural parents and children, sisters, brothers, uncles, aunts, nephews and nieces and first cousins. The doctors have to check that this relationship exists. Nor does the Act cover the donation of regenerative tissue such as bone marrow and blood.

Situation: Live donation

> A physiotherapist cares for a renal patient aged 23 years. She has been on dialysis for a number of years but has been advised that a kidney transplant is urgently required. Her mother has offered to be a donor and seeks the advice of the physiotherapist over whether such an offer would be accepted.

It is important that the physiotherapist knows who is the appropriate person to give advice and information to the mother. It may be essential to involve an independent person to ensure that the mother has the mental capacity to make the decision and that she is not under any duress. Regulations specify how the checking of the relationship between donor and recipient is to be carried out[36]. Otherwise there would be an offence under the Human Organs Transplants Act 1989.

Conclusions

In their care of terminally ill patients, physiotherapists need to be confident in their knowledge about the laws which apply. They may, for example, feel great empathy for a tetraplegic patient who no longer has the desire to live. They must be aware, however, that to assist in the death would be to commit a crime under the Suicide Act. Similarly in the care of patients suffering from motor neurone disease they must keep a clear distinction between the right of the mentally capacitated patient to refuse to be treated, including the right of the patient to make a living will, and the criminal act of killing the patient.

Questions and exercises

1 In what circumstances could a patient facing a terminal illness refuse treatment? (See also Chapter 7.)
2 Draw up the requirements for a valid living will.
3 Parents of a child suffering from cystic fibrosis have suggested to you that physiotherapy and antibiotic treatment should be stopped. What are the legal considerations in this request and what action would you take?
4 Following the death of a patient in hospital who had been receiving physiotherapy treatment you are asked to provide a statement for the coroner. What principles would you bear in mind in preparing the statement? (See also Chapter 13.)

References

1   *R* v. *Arthur* reported in *The Times* 6 November 1981.
2   *R* v. *Cox* [1993] 2 All ER 19.
3   House of Lords: Committee on Medical Ethics, Session 1993–4 (31 January 1994) HMSO, London.
4   Law Commission (1995) Report No. 231 *Mental Incapacity*. HMSO, London.
5   *Re C (a minor) (Wardship; medical treatment)* [1989] 2 All ER 782.
6   *Re J (a minor) (wardship; medical treatment)* [1990] 3 All ER 930.
7   Royal College of Paediatrics and Child Health (September 1997) *Withholding or Withdrawing Life Saving Treatment in Children. A Framework for Practice.* RCPCH, London.
8   *Airedale NHS Trust* v. *Bland* [1993] 1 All ER 821.
9   *Frenchay Healthcare NHS Trust* v. *S* [1994] 2 All ER 403.
10 Practice Note [1996] 4 All ER 766.
11 *F* v. *West Berkshire Health Auhtority* [1989] 2 All ER 545.
12 Practice Note [1993] 3 All ER 222.
13 Law Commission (1995) Report No. 231 *Mental Incapacity*. HMSO, London.
14 British Medical Association (1998) *Withdrawing and Withholding Treatment: A consultation paper from the BMA's Medical Ethics Committee.* BMA, London.
15 Law Commission (1995) Report No. 231 *Mental Incapacity*. HMSO, London.
16 British Medical Association (1995) *Advance Statements about medical treatment: Code of Practice* (April 1995) BMA, London.
17 *Re J* [1992] 4 All ER 614; The Times Law Report, 12 June 1992.
18 *Re J (a minor) (wardship; medical treatment)* [1990] 3 All ER 930.
19 *Re R* [1991] 4 All ER 177.
20 *R* v. *Cambridge and Huntingdon Health Authority ex parte B* The Times Law Report, 15 March 1995. [1995] 2 All ER 129.
21 *F* v. *West Berkshire Health Authority* [1989] 2 All ER 525.
22 Dimond, B.C. (1992) Not for resuscitative treatment *British Journal of Nursing* **1**, 2 (14–27 May), 93–4.
23 Royal College of Nursing *Resuscitation: Right or Wrong.* Paper No 000 163.
24 *Re W (a minor) (medical treatment)* [1992] 4 All ER 206.
25 *Re B (a minor) (wardship; medical treatment)* [1981] 1 WLR 1421.
26 *Re T (a minor) (wardship: medical treatment)* [1997] 1 All ER 906; *Re C (sic) (a minor; refusal of parental consent)* [1997] 8 Med LR 166.
27 Thornes, R. (1988) *The care of dying children and their families from guidelines*

prepared by the British Paediatric Association, King Edward's Hospital Fund for London and the National Association of Health Authorities in 1988. Birmingham National Association of Health Authorities, Birmingham.

28   Dimond, B.C. (1996) *The Legal Aspects of Childhealth care.* Mosby, London.

29   Beresford, S. (1995) *Motor Neurone Disease.* Chapman & Hall, London.

30   List taken from The Registration of Births and Deaths Regulations 1987 SI No. 2088; *see further* Knight, B. (1992) *Legal Aspects of Medical Practice.* 5th edn. pp 95–102, Churchill Livingstone, Edinburgh.

31   Knight, B. (1992) *Legal Aspects of Medical Practice.* 5th edn. p 96, Churchill Livingstone, Edinburgh.

32   Dimond, B.C. (1995) Death in the Accident and Emergency Department. *Accident and Emergency Nursing* **3**, 1, 38–41 (further details of the coroner's jurisdiction).

33   *R* v. *Westminster City Coroner, ex parte Rainer* (1968) 112 *Solicitors Journal* 883.

34   *R* v. *Poplar Coroner, ex parte Thomas* (CA) (1993) 2 WLR 547.

35   Coroners Act 1988 section 11(5)(b).

36   Human Organ Transplants (Establishment of Relationships) Regulations 1989. SI No. 2107 of 1989.

Section F
Specialist Topics

Chapter 26
Teaching and Research

This chapter looks at the specific problems which face the physiotherapist who is involved in teaching and research. Reference should also be made to Chapter 5 which considers the educational issues and the role of the Physiotherapy Board, the Council for Professions Supplementary to Medicine and the Chartered Society of Physiotherapy.

The following topics will be considered:

- Liability in connection with education and training
- Legal issues arising from the conduct of research
- Conclusions

Liability in connection with education and training

Failure to maintain professional competence

Every physiotherapist has a duty to maintain her professional competence; failure to do so could lead to being called to account in several different forums:

- civil proceedings for negligence if a person is harmed as a result of this failure;
- professional conduct proceedings which could result in the physiotherapist being struck off the register;
- disciplinary proceedings if the physiotherapist is an employee.

An example of the problems which can be faced by inadequate post-registration training can be seen from the survey carried out by Lesley Silcox[1] on training for wheelchair prescribing. The results of the survey showed that the situation on training had only slightly improved since the McColl Report[2] which criticised the number of people in unsuitable wheelchairs showing inadequate standards of wheelchair assessment, prescription and advice. If harm arose to a client as the result of a physiotherapist failing to ensure that her competence to practice was maintained and that she was up to date with relevant information, she or her employer could be liable for that harm.

Liability of the instructor

Failures in teaching

This duty to maintain competence applies equally to the physiotherapist lecturer/ tutor as it does to the practitioner. Even an instructor could be held liable in negligence for failures as a teacher. It would have to be proved that a student, in reliance on negligent advice from the instructor, caused harm to a colleague or client and that this harm could be seen as a reasonably foreseeable result of that negligent advice. The causation element (see Chapter 10) may be difficult to establish, since the instructor could argue that there are many sources of advice for the student who should not rely entirely upon the instructor.

Administrative failures

However if the instructor were to give the student the wrong information about the syllabus which was being studied or the timetable or place of the examinations, and as a result the student failed the examination, then liability of the instructor and her employer could be established. In addition, if students pay the fees for the tuition themselves, there could be liability in contract law for any failure to provide tuition in accordance with the contract stipulations.

For developments in the law of negligence relating to the giving of references see Chapter 10.

Lecturers and other educationalists should be aware that administrative weaknesses or inefficiencies could give rise to court hearings and complaints. Thus in one case a would-be physiotherapy student was wrongly informed through the admissions system by the University of Salford that he was being offered a place. He wrote accepting the offer, and then learnt later that a mistake had been made and there had never been a place for him. His application for specific performance of the contract and a mandatory injunction compelling the University to give a place was dismissed. He appealed to the Court of Appeal[3] which held that there probably was a binding agreement that the University would accept him for the degree course in physiotherapy, but it was not prepared to order an injunction on the grounds that it was not just to compel the university to provide a place for a student whose academic record was not good enough. His appeal was therefore dismissed. Even though the prospective student failed on the facts in this case, the fact remains that a contract is created between student and institution with obligations on both sides.

Teaching intimate procedures

Teachers on post-graduate training courses should be particularly diligent to follow the guidelines issued by the CSP when providing instruction in intimate examinations, such as pelvic floor and vaginal assessment. The CSP has issued guidance[4] on instruction to post-graduate physiotherapists in these assessments. Where fellow students are used to practise such examinations it recommends that

- full information should be given to the students in advance;
- students should be given the option to opt in or out; and
- consent forms should be used which would include information as to what would be involved in such a practical session.

Teaching manipulation

The CSP has also issued guidance on the safe teaching of manipulation to undergraduates[5]. It emphasises the importance of undertaking an assessment of the student who is to be used as a model and the facilities available. It also sets out the principles for safe teaching and practice, stressing the importance of obtaining consent from the student and ethical approval from the institution.

Supervision of students in clinical placements

The same principle would apply in the supervision of students in clinical placements. The student is entitled to receive a reasonable standard of care from the clinical instructor, and, if harm were to occur to the student or to others in the failure to provide the appropriate level of supervision or in delegating inappropriate activities to the student, the instructor and her employer would be liable in negligence.

Reference should be made to Chapter 10 on negligence and in particular the section on supervision and delegation.

One interesting initiative is the use of learning contracts in physiotherapy clinical education. Vinette Cross[6] describes the approach used with one group of undergraduates and the relevance of learning contracts to Chartered Society of Physiotherapy initiatives on continuing professional development. The approach is based on three key requirements. Learning contracts should:

- provide a structure for clinical education experiences;
- foster a supportive learning climate for both students and clinical educators; and
- facilitate reflective practice.

Legal responsibility for the clinical education remains with the clinical instructors who define the boundaries of the learning decisions and decide on non-negotiable aspects of the learning process.

Liability for harm to students or harm caused by students

If harm arises to the student, then the student would have to show that a reasonable standard of care was not provided. The student would not be an employee and could not therefore point to the duty of care owed by employer to employee at common law (see Chapter 11). Instead the student could rely upon the duty of care owed in the law of negligence or upon statutory duties set out in the Health and Safety Regulations or the Occupier's Liability Act 1957.

If the student caused harm to another person, it depends upon the facts as to whether there was negligence and who was at fault. Thus the tutor might assess the student as competent to carry out a particular activity and ensure that she was receiving the appropriate supervision. However in spite of this appropriate delegation and supervision, the student might still act negligently and therefore be to blame for causing harm to another person. In such an event, compensation would be paid out by the college or the Trust, depending on the memorandum of agreement between the college and those offering the clinical placement. This agreement should lay down provisions as to which party is responsible vicariously for the negligence of the student.

Duty of employer to provide facilities for post-registration training

It could be argued that, since the health care employer has a duty of care at common law to its patients and/or clients it must therefore as part of this duty ensure that its staff are competent. In addition, as part of the contractual duty that it owes to its employees, it must provide competent fellow staff. Should the employer fail to fulfil this duty, and harm befall a patient/client or employee as a result, then the employer could be directly liable in negligence. Thus one can assume that the employer's duty includes the duty to ensure that staff are kept competent and that therefore paid study leave should be made available as an implied condition of the contract of employment.

This logic has not, however, so far been categorically established in the courts. The uncertainty has meant that there is wide variation across the country as to the rights of employees in obtaining paid study leave. Practitioners registered with the UKCC now have to prove that they have undertaken at least five study days (or comparable training) every three years in order that they can be re-registered. However there is no agreement that NHS Trusts will automatically fund this activity and practice varies from Trust to Trust.

Physiotherapists do not have a comparable statutory obligation to maintain competence, though this would be implied at common law as part of ensuring that they practice according to the accepted approved practice of reasonable practitioners in that field (the Bolam test). It is clearly of interest to physiotherapists to use local collective bargaining to ensure that provision is made in their contracts for paid study leave, secondment and other forms of post-registration training and education. At present, the demand for physiotherapists exceeds the supply and, in order to retain or attract their services, NHS Trusts may be prepared (or forced) to compile attractive packages.

If and when the government implements the recommendations following the review organised by JM Consulting of the 1960 Act, there may well be a statutory obligation for physiotherapists to undergo a specified number of training days to be entitled to be remain on the register.

Training of assistants

It must not be forgotten that as the dependence on assistants increases so resources must be allocated to ensure that they are appropriately trained. There appears little doubt that the skill-mix ratio in physiotherapy will change as there are increasing numbers of assistants being employed in comparison to registered physiotherapists.

In Chapter 10 the legal issues relating to delegation and supervision are discussed. A prior requirement of delegation is that the assistant should be properly trained. Ruth Parry and Catherine Vase[7] discuss the training and assessment of physiotherapy assistants. They note that the physiotherapists interviewed considered that the assistants' potential was under-used but also that they were undertrained.

Legal issues arising from the conduct of research

The CSP's continuing professional development (CPD) strategy was produced in December 1994 and recognised the importance of research as a component of continuing professional development. All physiotherapists, whether they work in a clinical, management, research or academic setting have a responsibility to be involved in research. A consultation paper was issued by the CSP research development group in January 1996[8]. It emphasises the importance of clinical effectiveness research and suggests a model of CPD which encompasses research activity.

The debate was taken further by a paper prepared on behalf of the CSP research group by Tracy Bury[9]. Its main conclusions drawn from the consultation process are shown in Figure 26.1.

Figure 26.1 **Conclusions from CSP research development group 1996.**

- Research and evaluation are integral rather than peripheral to practice.
- Familiarity with research enhances confidence in addressing evidence-based practice and clinical effectiveness issues.
- Activities with which many physiotherapists are familiar, such as clinical audit and guidelines, offer a basis for developing research.
- In-service education opportunities to discuss, evaluate and disseminate research findings will benefit practice.
- Resources such as staff skills, time and money are required to underpin the commitment to integrate research.
- Satisfying immediate demands should not be at the expense of long-term goals, i.e. developing an evidence-based profession.

In 1996 it was proposed that a central register should be created between the CSP, the College of OTs and the Royal College of Speech and Language Therapists researchers. The aims include:

- to provide a comprehensive national register which could be accessed by NHS bodies and research councils etc.;
- to facilitate multi-professional collaboration in research; and
- to provide details of therapy expertise in clinical, educational and methodological aspects of research.

The questionnaire and application was contained in the August 1996 issue of *Physiotherapy*[10]. Legal issues arising from research are likely to affect the physiotherapist in three ways:

(1) Their practice must, where possible, be research based so that they should be aware of the need to ensure that recent supported research findings are incorporated into their practice and that they maintain their competence.
(2) They may be caring for clients who are the research subjects of research undertaken by physiotherapy colleagues or other health or social services professionals and they should ensure that the rights of the clients are respected.
(3) They may be carrying out their own research or supervising the research of

others in which case they should ensure that the research is properly approved and the client is appropriately protected.

Research based practice

The Bolam test (which is discussed in Chapter 10) is the accepted test for defining acceptable professional practice. As was discussed, what a reasonable body of responsible practitioners would accept as appropriate practice will change as standards of care improve and develop. The findings from substantiated research will therefore eventually become integrated into accepted practice and it is essential that the professional keeps abreast of changes in recommended practice. Should she fail to do so and harm occurs to the client as a result, then she or her employer could face an action for negligence (see Chapter 10).

Further, with pressures on resourcing, physiotherapists need to justify their activities in terms of clinical effectiveness. Only research can establish that the service they can provide in different clinical situations justifies its use (see Chapter 17).

Protecting the patient from the researcher

Consent

Consent must be obtained from adult mentally competent patients/clients or the Gillick competent child (see Chapter 23) or from parents of children before research is carried out. It is also essential that all relevant information should be given about any risks of harm from the research.

A distinction should, however, be made between therapeutic and non-therapeutic research in the discussion of consent in relation to research. Where the patient/client stands to benefit personally from the research, then it could be argued that the research on adults incapable of giving consent could be conducted as part of their treatment plan. However if the individual has no personal benefit it, research to which any risks, however slight, were attached would not be justified. This would also apply to research on children. Reference should be made to Chapter 23 and the law relating to consent by a child (i.e. a person under 18 years).

The information which is given to the patient/client and the consent form to be signed should be approved by the Local Research Ethics Committee (see below) before the research commences.

Confidentiality

Exactly the same principles of confidentiality apply in relation to the personal information obtained from undertaking research as apply to information obtained in respect of treatment. It is probable, however, that the exceptions to the duty to maintain confidentiality recognised by the law in relation to personal information obtained in the course of caring for patients (see Chapter 8) would also apply to information obtained through research.

In 1996 three doctors were brought before professional conduct proceedings of the General Medical Council as a result of the publication of a case study on a patient which she claimed was recognised as being about her and which she alleged to have been published without her consent. The doctors were not struck off the Register. It was emphasised, however, that the rules were now that it is necessary to get the specific consent of the patient to the publication of a case study.

The physiotherapist as researcher

Local Research Ethics Committees

The Department of Health has requested each health authority to ensure that an LREC[11] is set up to examine research proposals. Any NHS body asked to agree a research proposal falling within its sphere of responsibility should ensure that it has been submitted to the appropriate LREC for research ethics approval. A Manual for research ethics committees provides guidance on every aspect of their work, including the special procedures for multi-centre research[12].

The role of the LREC is defined in the Manual as being 'to consider the ethics of proposed research projects which will involve human subjects' and to advise the NHS body concerned. It is the NHS body which has the responsibility of deciding whether or not the project should go ahead, taking into account the ethical advice of the LREC. They are not 'in any sense management arms of the District Health Authority'. The LREC is comprised of multi-disciplinary members including lay persons.

The guidelines require the LREC to be consulted for any proposal which involves:

- NHS patients including those private sector patients treated under contract
- Foetal material and IVF involving NHS patients
- The recently dead, in NHS premises
- Access to the records of past or present NHS patients
- The use of, or potential access to, NHS premises or facilities.

The LREC *must* be consulted but the NHS body should also give permission before the project can proceed.

The LREC could also advise other non NHS bodies such as private sector companies, the Medical Research Council or universities. It would therefore be possible for physiotherapists in private practice who wish to undertake research to arrange for the LREC of an NHS Trust to review and monitor their proposals and ensure that patients' rights were protected. It would also be possible for a physiotherapist who was interested in research and patients' rights to enquire about being appointed to an LREC.

Obtaining the approval of an LREC should ensure that the patient/client is reasonably protected from zealous researchers. However particular difficulties can arise where the researcher is also the health professional concerned with the treatment of the patient. In such cases, it is not easy to ensure that treatment concerns remain paramount and that patients are assured that they can opt out of the research at any time without suffering any sanction from the health professional.

Publication

As indicated above, it is now the policy of the GMC that publication of individual case studies requires the prior consent of the patient and it may be prudent for other health professionals to work on this basis too.

It is also extremely wise for researchers to discuss and agree arrangements for possible publication of the research before it is undertaken in order to prevent disputes arising over censorship and control once the outcome is known. Some funding bodies who have sponsored the research may require that they see the findings before they permit publication. This may be seen, however, as an unjustified restraint on the dissemination of the results.

Often research results are publicised at conferences by way of poster displays. An extremely useful article in *Physiotherapy* gives guidance on the preparation of posters for display[13].

Accuracy

It is possible that if research is published which contains errors of design and interpretation and persons suffer harm as a result of dependence upon the conclusions drawn, then there could be liability in negligence. A centre for cancer treatment in women in Bristol suffered financial loss as the result of a research report which suggested that the centre achieved worse results than other treatment centres. It was later learnt that the researchers had failed to take account of the fact that the Bristol centre took patients at a much later stage in their illness compared with other centres and therefore like was not being compared with like.

Physiotherapists who knowingly take part in research which is not sound could face professional conduct proceedings. There is a useful chapter on the sources of error in research in Carolyn Hicks' book *Research for Physiotherapists*[14].

Intellectual property and copyright

Sometimes research projects can lead to lucrative rewards – the design of a new piece of equipment or an innovative idea for supporting disabled persons.

■ If a physiotherapist is fortunate enough to have a commercially valuable idea, who should get the rewards?

The answer depends upon the circumstances in which the project was conceived. Thus if the physiotherapist is undertaking research and development as part of her work as a full-time employee, then the employer would be seen as the owner of the research, though a generous employer may well develop an income sharing scheme with the employee. If, on the other hand, the research has been developed by the physiotherapist entirely on her own, with no involvement from the employer or its resources, she would be the owner of the intellectual property. She should take advice on patenting the design so that her ownership is legally recognised[15].

Involvement of users in research

Carol Thomas and Anne Perry[16] reported on research to examine the health needs of persons with strokes and the place of the user's views in health care planning. They conclude that in order to give users more opportunity to direct knowledge that is generated, there should be more partnership at every stage – before the design of any research project is agreed, in validating the results of the research, and also in identifying how the results can be disseminated to users as well as purchasers and providers.

Another means of using consumers in research is by means of the focus group. Julius Sim and Jackie Snell[17] point out the advantages of using focus group techniques in comparison with other methods of data collection in physiotherapy research. However there are dangers: for example the moderator can unconsciously or subconsciously lead the group to endorse a preconceived hypothesis and careful planning is necessary before the focus group convenes.

Conclusions

Physiotherapy practice must be based on knowledge obtained through research. Evidence based practice will be essential in the 21st century. Ultimately the Bolam test (see Chapter 10) as to what is the accepted approved practice of the reasonable physiotherapist should be supported by clinical evidence. The initiatives set out in the White Paper[18] the National Institute of Clinical Excellence, National framework standards and the Commission for Health Improvement should lead to standards being developed across all health specialities and professions. Research should be encouraged to underpin practice. Professor Newham in his Founders' Lecture in 1996 set out the importance of ensuring that physiotherapy practice was based on research and that external and internal challenges to physiotherapy research were explored[19].

 Questions and exercises _____

1 A physiotherapy student reports to you, her tutor, that she was aware that a client in a home for those with learning disabilities was being abused by a member of staff. What action would you take and what action would you advise her to take?

2 Obtain a copy of the memorandum of agreement between your college and the NHS Trust which takes your students on placements. To what extent does it determine responsibility for the negligence of the student or responsibility for harm to the student whilst on clinical placement?

3 You are wishing to carry out a research project. Draw up a schedule setting out the initial tasks you should undertake before you actually begin the data collection.

References

1 Silcox, L. (1995) Assessment for the Prescription of Wheelchairs: What training is available to therapists. *British Journal of Occupational Therapy* **58**, 3, 115–18.

2 McColl, I. (1986) *Review of the artificial limb and appliance centres*. HMSO, London.

3   *Moran* v. *University of Salford* (CA) reported in *The Times* 23 November 1993; 12 November 1993, Lexis Transcript.

4   CSP Pelvic Floor and Vaginal Assessment Information paper No. PA 19 1996, CSP, London.

5   CSP Professional Affairs Department Information Paper No 40 Guidance on the safe teaching of manipulation to undergraduates. September 1997, CSP, London.

6   Cross, V. (1996) Introducing learning contracts into physiotherapy clinical education. *Physiotherapy* **82**, 1, 21–27.

7   Parry, R. & Vase, C. (1997) Training and Assessment of Physiotherapy Assistants. *Physiotherapy* **83**, 1, 33–40.

8   Bury, T. (1996) Physiotherapy Research and Continuing Professional Development. *Physiotherapy* **82**, 1, 58–62.

9   Bury, T. (1996) Physiotherapy Research and Continuing Professional Development: The way forwards. *Physiotherapy* **82**, 9, 504–6.

10   August 1996 *Physiotherapy* **82**, 8 445–6.

11   HSG(91)5.

12   Centre for Medical Law and Ethics (1997) *King's College Manual for Research Ethics Committees.* King's College, London.

13   Murray, R., Thaw, M. & Strachan, R. (1998) Visual Literacy: Designing and Presenting a Poster. *Physiotherapy* **84**, 7, 319–27.

14   Hicks, C. (1995) *Research for Physiotherapists: project design and analysis.* Churchill Livingstone, Edinburgh.

15   McKeough, J. (1996) Intellectual Property and scientific research. *Australian Journal of Physiotherapy* **42**, 3, 235–42.

16   Thomas, C. & Perry, A. (1996) Research on Users' Views about Stroke Services. *Physiotherapy* **82**, 1, 6–12.

17   Sim, J. & Snell, J. (1996) Focus Groups in Physiotherapy Evaluation and Research. *Physiotherapy* **82**, 3, 189–198.

18   DoH (1997) *The New NHS: Modern, Dependable.* Command Paper 3807, HMSO, London.

19   Newham, D.J. (1997) Physiotherapy for Best Effect. *Physiotherapy* **83**, 1, 5–11.

Chapter 27
Complementary Medicine

There is no doubt about the interest which now exists in complementary or alternative therapies[1]. It is estimated that a third of the population have tried its remedies or visited its practitioners[2]. The Health Education Authority has published an *A to Z Guide* which covers 60 therapies[3]. Much research needs to be done on the efficacy of these therapies and the Health Authority Council has approved a research project to be undertaken by the National Association of Health Authorities and Trusts (NAHAT) into the prevalence of complementary therapies and their services for patients, purchasers and providers. The Health Authority Council has appointed a steering and working group to co-ordinate the project which is being undertaken by Blueprint Consultancy[4].

The Prince of Wales suggested the setting up of a group to consider the current positions of orthodox, complementary and alternative medicine in the UK and how far it would be appropriate and possible for them to work more closely together. Four working groups looking at

- research and development;
- education and training;
- regulation; and
- delivery mechanisms

were established under a steering group chaired by Dr Manon Williams, Assistant Private Secretary to HRH the Prince of Wales. It reported in 1997 and made extensive recommendations[5]. These include:

- encouraging more research and the dissemination of its results;
- emphasising the common elements in the core curriculum of all health care workers, both orthodox and in complementary or alternative medicine;
- establishing statutory self-regulatory bodies for those professions which could endanger patient safety; and
- identifying areas of conventional medicine and nursing which are not meeting patients' needs at present.

It also recommended the establishment of an Independent Standards Commission for Complementary and Alternative Medicine.

Physiotherapists are affected by this development in two ways. The physiotherapist may be aware that patients are consulting practitioners in complementary medicine therapies and may be taking medicines, or other treatment, for the same conditions for which the physiotherapist herself is giving advice. Conversely some physiotherapists are themselves undertaking training in a therapy regarded as complementary to conventional medicine.

This chapter therefore looks at the definition of complementary therapy and at the following topics:

- Definition of complementary therapies
- The clients receiving complementary therapy
  - disclosure to the physiotherapist
  - ignorance on the part of the physiotherapist
- The physiotherapist as complementary therapist
  - Agreement of employer
  - Consent of patient
  - Defining standards
- Examples of therapies undertaken by physiotherapists

Definition of complementary therapies

'Complementary is defined as: completing: together making up a whole, ... of medical treatment, therapies, etc. ... (1. Complementum – *com-*, intens. and *plere* to fill).' (Pamphlet of the British Complementary Medicine Association (BCMA))[6]

It is thus seen to work in parallel with orthodox medicine. The BCMA therefore states that therapy groups which are represented by the BCMA should advise and encourage patients to see their doctor wherever appropriate.

The client receiving complementary therapy

Disclosure to the physiotherapist

When a patient is referred to a physiotherapist in the NHS, then information relating to that person's care within the NHS would also be given. In addition where there is a referral within social services, then the person referring, whether general practitioner or social worker, would provide the physiotherapist with the information required in order to determine priorities. Thus the physiotherapist should have basic information about the client in order to determine the care which is required by the client. In addition the physiotherapist would usually have access to health records kept on the patient, to ensure that her care is compatible with other treatment the patient is receiving.

In contrast, where the patient is receiving treatment from a complementary therapist, there is usually no official way in which this information can be made known to the physiotherapist other than through the patient. The physiotherapist therefore relies upon the openness of the patient in disclosing information which may be relevant to the treatment and care which the physiotherapist is offering.

Clearly the importance of this communication between patient and physiotherapist will depend upon the relevance of the complementary therapy to the treatment and care which the physiotherapist provides. Some therapies may have little effect; others, such as acupuncture, may have a significant effect on the recommendations the physiotherapist may make.

The CSP has given guidance on patients who seek treatment both within and outside the NHS[7] emphasising the importance of good communication between the practitioners. If there is a conflict between the two treatments, then the therapists need to discuss this with the patient who should be given the choice over which course to pursue, with a reassurance that they can return to the other, when the chosen course has ended.

Ignorance on the part of the physiotherapist

■ Does it matter that the physiotherapist has no knowledge of the complementary therapy which the patient is undergoing?

The answer is that it may have an important effect and, had the physiotherapist been aware of certain information about the therapy, she may have advised the patient differently.

Situation: Complementary therapy

A physiotherapist employed by an NHS Trust is caring for a patient with chronic back pain. The physiotherapist is not aware that the patient is also visiting an acupuncturist for his condition and is also considering consulting a chiropractor or osteopath. If harm occurs to the patient, how can the physiotherapist show that it was not her treatment which caused the harm?

In this situation it would have been of value to the client if the work of the physiotherapist had been undertaken in the light of the methods, effects and intentions used by the acupuncturist, so that her work complemented this rather than possibly conflicted with it. Unless, however, the physiotherapist has a basic understanding of the practice of acupuncture, she would be unable to work in parallel.

Where harm has occurred, expert evidence on causation would be required to show whether anything the physiotherapist had done could have caused that harm. It is hoped that, in reviewing the practice of the physiotherapist, it would be revealed that the patient had been receiving treatment from other persons. In the light of this any liability on the part of each of these persons could be analysed.

Situation: Working together

A patient informs the physiotherapist that she is also receiving treatment from an osteopath. The physiotherapist recommends that the patient gives her the details so that she can contact the osteopath with a view to working in tandem. The patient refuses to give that information.

The patient's attitude makes it very difficult for the physiotherapist to ensure that there is harmony in the practice of the two therapists. It may be that the physiotherapist would find it difficult to provide appropriate treatment not knowing what the other therapist is doing. However she should not automatically refuse the patient NHS physiotherapy care. She should seek advice and discuss further with the patient her objections to her having contact with the osteopath.

Osteopathy and chiropractic have now received state registered status and the popularity and availability of their services within the NHS might increase. It is important for physiotherapists to understand the benefits and limits of the treatments which they offer, so that they can understand how their practice as physiotherapists fits into the service which they provide.

The physiotherapist as complementary medicine therapist.

Agreement of employer

It is recognised that many physiotherapists are considering the use of complementary therapies in the treatment of clients. If a physiotherapist obtains a training in a complementary therapy, she should ensure that she obtains the agreement of the employer before she uses this skill as part of her practice as a physiotherapist. If she fails to do this and causes harm to the patient whilst using her complementary therapy skills, then her employer could argue that she was not acting in course of employment when she caused the harm. The employer is therefore not vicariously liable (see glossary) the physiotherapist must accept personal liability for the harm which has been caused. The following example explains the legal position.

Situation: Acupuncture

A physiotherapist following her basic training developed skills in acupuncture. One of her NHS patients was suffering from considerable pain and the physiotherapist offered to provide acupuncture to relieve the pain. It was arranged that the patient would come to the hospital at the end of the day's clinic. Unfortunately, the physiotherapist placed the needle in a nerve and caused permanent damage to the patient. The patient is claiming compensation.

If the NHS trust gave expressed or implied consent to this work by the physiotherapist then her work as an acupuncturist could be seen as being in the course of employment. In this case the NHS Trust would be vicariously liable for the harm which has been caused and pay any compensation due. On the other hand if the NHS Trust was unaware of the work as an acupuncturist then it may refuse to accept vicarious liability for her work as an acupuncturist, arguing that the work was not performed in the course of her employment as a physiotherapist (see Chapter 10 on vicarious liability). In this case the physiotherapist would have to accept personal liability for the harm done and be responsible for payment of the compensation due. It is therefore crucial that the physiotherapist ensures that she has her own insurance cover for such work.

It is also essential for the physiotherapist to obtain the consent of the employer if she intends to practice privately during working hours. In the case of *Watling* v. *Gloucester County Council*[8] (the full facts are discussed in Chapter 17) an occupational therapist was dismissed when he saw private patients for alternative therapy during working hours. His application for compensation for unfair dismissal failed.

Consent of the patient

It is also essential that the patient should explicitly give consent before the physiotherapist is allowed to use any complementary therapies on him. The basic principles of obtaining consent apply (see Chapter 7) but, since a patient would not normally expect a physiotherapist to be providing complementary therapies, it is imperative that the physiotherapist gives full details of all that is involved and makes it absolutely clear that the patient is fully entitled to receive the treatment usually provided by the physiotherapist even though he or she refuses the complementary therapy and care. It is preferable to obtain the consent in writing and to put in a leaflet the information which the patient should be told about the treatment.

Gill Westland notes in her articles on massage[9] that:

'permission should always be sought before massaging a client and the practitioner should observe for indicators of inconsistency between agreeing verbally to be massaged and non-verbally saying 'no' to the touch. These indicators would include breathing more rapidly, breath holding and tensing parts of the body.'

Clearly in such a situation, the practitioner should verify that the client is giving a real consent.

Defining standards

One of the difficulties of some complementary therapies is that there may not be a clear definition of the expected standard of care. If harm were to occur, to succeed in a claim for compensation the patient would have to establish that the therapist failed to use the reasonable standard of care which he, the patient, was entitled to expect. This may not be easy to prove.

In her two articles on massage as a therapeutic tool[10] Gill Westland notes that (at the time of writing in 1993)

'there are no legal requirements for massage therapists practising privately and outside statutory agencies. Some local authorities issue licences and inspect premises, essentially to protect against prostitution and the spread of infection. However, it is possible for anyone to set up in practice with minimal or no training.'

She goes on to explain the work of the British Complementary Medicine Association, the Institute for Complementary Medicine, the Council for Complementary and Alternative Medicine, the UK Council for Psychotherapy, and other bodies and the teaching institutions in the development of training, codes of ethics and practice and ways of maintaining standards and registering complaints.

Examples of therapies undertaken by physiotherapists

Aromatherapy

A sub-group of the Association for Chartered Physiotherapists with an Interest in Massage (ACPIM) is the aromatherapy group, i.e. physiotherapists who have trained in aromatherapy. At the present time this activity is seen as beyond the scope of the professional practice of a chartered physiotherapist and the CSP does not consider that a Chartered Physiotherapist working in aromatherapy is covered by the professional protection of the CSP or by its insurers.

This is a serious issue for Chartered Physiotherapists practising in this area. If they do not have confirmation in writing that they are covered by the CSP, then they must ensure that they obtain personal insurance cover from an aromatherapy organisation or one of the umbrella groups for complementary therapies[11]. If they are using aromatherapy during their employment, they should also ensure that they have the approval (preferably in writing) of their employer/ senior manager for that activity.

Acupuncture

The Acupuncture Association of Chartered Physiotherapists (AACP) gives advice and guidance to members on the practice of acupuncture by physiotherapists and acts as a forum for the interchange of information. The CSP has issued guidance on the licensing of acupuncture[12] explaining the provisions of the Local Government (Miscellaneous Provisions) Act 1982 in relation to the licensing of premises in England and Wales but outside of London.

Val Hopwood and George Lewith[13] discuss how acupuncture can be used in the motor recovery of the upper limb after a stroke, but emphasise the importance of additional case studies to confirm their results.

Healing energy

A physiotherapist, Steve Gibbs, has set up the British Healing Energy Therapy Association (BHETA). It aims to focus upon the theories regarding Healing Energy Therapy (HET) and will take a multi-disciplinary approach. He hopes to see healing energy accepted from the scientific angle, so that it can be incorporated into mainstream practice[14]. BHETA is conducting two pilot studies into the use of HET to aid recovery from chronic fatigue syndrome and for pain relief in arachnoiditis and is putting forward theories based on scientific research to suggest how the mechanisms behind traditional 'laying on of hands' may work[15].

Craniosacral therapy

This is described by Susan Hollenbery[16] as

'about the ability to perceive, acknowledge, allow, enhance and facilitate the patient's own healing process without the necessity to judge, intervene or perform. Treatment is the art of being, not of doing.'

In contrast to physiotherapy which seeks to treat the symptoms that the patient is complaining about, craniosacral therapy looks at the patient as a whole.

'Any attempt to treat only the local disorder with localised treatments, may shift the problem, sooner or later, to another part of the body.'

Chinese Medicine, physiotherapy and psychiatry

John Tindall examined Traditional Chinese Medicine (TCM) and Natural Medicine in *Psychiatry*[17] and concluded that physiotherapists are in a good position to use various natural health care models within psychiatry, but that it is important to receive full and comprehensive training in those particular areas. In his clinic they were developing a Chinese herbal medicine pharmacy and wrote more than 3000 prescriptions a year for various ailments from substance abuse, to HIV, mental health problems, dermatology, etc.

Conclusions

There is every likelihood that the interest in and demand for complementary therapy will continue to grow and patients will demand that these therapies should be provided within the NHS. In the past some GP fundholders have used their purchasing power to buy such therapies for their patients. In remains to be seen what effect the abolition of GP fundholding and the establishment of primary health care groups will have on the availability of complementary therapies within the NHS. It seems likely, however, that more and more physiotherapists will acquire double qualifications and/or will be caring for clients who are recipients of alternative therapies.

The greater the use by and training of physiotherapists in additional therapies, the more likely that they are to become concerned at the meaning and direction of physiotherapy itself. It is possible that eventually some of the therapies at present seen as complementary could become an integral part of physiotherapy practice.

✍ Questions and exercises

1 You have decided that you would like to undertake a training in aromatherapy and eventually use it as part of your practice as a physiotherapist. What actions would you take to ensure that your plans are compatible with your role as a physiotherapist?

2 You are visiting a patient in the community and become concerned that she appears to be paying a lot of money to a chiropractor and her condition does not seem to be improving, in fact you consider that it is deteriorating. What action, if any, would you take?

3 Do you consider that those complementary therapies which so wished, should be permitted to have registered status under the Council for Professions Supplementary to Medicine? (Refer also to Chapter 3.) If not, what criteria would you lay down for a profession to receive registered status?

References

1 Dimond, B.C. (1998) *The Legal Aspects of Complementary Therapy Practice.* Churchill Livingstone, Edinburgh.

2 Jeremy Laurance, 'Alternative Health: An honest alternative or just magic?' *The Times* 5 February 1996, page 11.

3 Health Education Authority (1995) *A-Z guide on complementary therapies.*

4 For further details contact the Regional Development Manager, NHS Confederation (see address list).

5 Foundation for Integrated Medicine (1997) *Integrated Healthcare: A Way Forward for the Next Five years.*

6 Further information can be obtained from the BCMA at Exmoor Street, London W10 6DZ (Tel 0181 964 1205 & Fax 0181 964 1207).

7 CSP Professional Affairs Department (1994) No. PA 5 (November 1994) *Patients Seeking Treatment in the Public & Private Sector.* CSP, London.

8 *Watling* v. *Gloucester County Council.* EAT/868/94, 17 March 1995, 23 November 1994, Lexis transcript.

9 Westland, G. (1993) Massage as a therapeutic tool. *British Journal of Occupational Therapy* **56**, 4, 129–134 and 5, 177–180.

10 Westland, G. (1993) Massage as a therapeutic tool. *British Journal of Occupational Therapy* **56**, 4, 129–134 and 5, 177–180.

11 For further information on this aspect see Dimond, B.C. (1998) *The Legal Aspects of Complementary Therapy Practice.* Churchill Livingstone, Edinburgh.

12 CSP Professional Affairs Department (1995) No. PA 24 (January 1995) *Licensing of Acupuncture.* CSP, London.

13 Hopwood, V. & Lewith, G. (1997) The Effect of Acupuncture on the Motor Recovery of the Upper Limb after Stroke. *Physiotherapist* **83**, 12, 614–9.

14 Gibbs, S. (1996) The British Healing Energy Therapy Association. *In Touch.* Autumn Issue 1996, 81, 24.

15 Gibbs, S. (1997) Healing Energy Therapy. *Physiotherapy* **83**, 2, 73–4.

16 Hollenbery, S. (1995) Touching is Believing: Treatment with Craniosacral Therapy. *In Touch* Winter 1995, 74, 12–3.

17 Tindall, J. (1994) Traditional Chinese Medicine (TCM) and Natural Medicine in Psychiatry. *Journal of the Association of Chartered Physiotherapists in Psychiatry.* September 1994, XI, 8–13.

Conclusion

Chapter 28
The Future

The 21st century will bring major changes and challenges to the role of the physiotherapist. There are significant changes taking place in the organisational structure of the NHS. The internal market is being abolished, but there is no doubt that the pressures on funding will continue. Clearly the community care changes brought about by the NHS and Community Care Act 1990 have brought in their wake more problems than solutions. Demand for residential and nursing home places often outstrips the resources of social services to meet the needs. A Royal Commission which reported in March 1999 has made significant and expensive recommendations for the funding of the long term care of the elderly.

The NHS White Paper introduced a National Institute of Clinical Excellence, a Commission for Health Improvement, the National Standards Framework, and Clinical Governance. All these initiatives present challenges for the physiotherapist. Clinically effective treatments and research based practice will be a requirement of any physiotherapist who practices according to the reasonable standard of care which the patient is entitled to expect. Physiotherapists will continue to have to justify the treatments which they provide in terms of the 'value added' which they can bring to the quality of life of the patient.

These major developments together with changes within the professional framework by which the profession is regulated and the rules set for educational standards mean that the physiotherapist must keep aware of the changing context within which she practices.

Also we can no longer look only at physiotherapy as practised within the United Kingdom. With the advent of free movement within the European Union, the need to ensure that we are part of the developments across Europe is essential. Reference to *Practice of Physiotherapy in the European Union*, published by the Standing Liaison Committee of Physiotherapists within the EU in September 1996, provides a comprehensive guide to the regulation and professional status of physiotherapists, to quality assurance and to fields of activity and categories of procedures across the EU.

The legal context within which physiotherapy is practised also changes – new Acts of Parliament and new decisions in the courts redefine the constraints and the opportunities which are placed upon or given to the physiotherapist.

This book is therefore the beginning of a necessary awareness of the legal context within which the physiotherapist practises and every effort should be made to ensure that she maintains and updates her knowledge in the light of the many changes with which she is now faced and with which she will be challenged in the future.

Appendix
Schedule 1 to Human Rights Act 1998

SCHEDULE 1

THE ARTICLES

PART I

THE CONVENTION

RIGHTS AND FREEDOMS

Article 2

Right to life

1. Everyone's right to life shall be protected by law. No one shall be deprived of his life intentionally save in the execution of a sentence of a court following his conviction of a crime for which this penalty is provided by law.

2. Deprivation of life shall not be regarded as inflicted in contravention of this Article when it results from the use of force which is no more than absolutely necessary:

   (a) in defence of any person from unlawful violence;

   (b) in order to effect a lawful arrest or to prevent the escape of a person lawfully detained;

   (c) in action lawfully taken for the purpose of quelling a riot or insurrection.

Article 3

Prohibition of torture

No one shall be subjected to torture or to inhuman or degrading treatment or punishment.

Article 4

Prohibition of slavery and forced labour

1. No one shall be held in slavery or servitude.

2. No one shall be required to perform forced or compulsory labour.

3. For the purpose of this Article the term "forced or compulsory labour" shall not include:

(a) any work required to be done in the ordinary course of detention imposed according to the provisions of Article 5 of this Convention or during conditional release from such detention;

(b) any service of a military character or, in case of conscientious objectors in countries where they are recognised, service exacted instead of compulsory military service;

(c) any service exacted in case of an emergency or calamity threatening the life or well-being of the community;

(d) any work or service which forms part of normal civic obligations.

Article 5

Right to liberty and security

1. Everyone has the right to liberty and security of person. No one shall be deprived of his liberty save in the following cases and in accordance with a procedure prescribed by law:

(a) the lawful detention of a person after conviction by a competent court;

(b) the lawful arrest or detention of a person for non-compliance with the lawful order of a court or in order to secure the fulfilment of any obligation prescribed by law;

(c) the lawful arrest or detention of a person effected for the purpose of bringing him before the competent legal authority on reasonable suspicion of having committed an offence or when it is reasonably considered necessary to prevent his committing an offence or fleeing after having done so;

(d) the detentioon of a minor by lawful order for the purpose of educational supervision or his lawful detention for the purpose of bringing him before the competent legal authority;

(e) the lawful detention of persons for the prevention of the spreading of infectious diseases, of persons of unsound mind, alcoholics or drug addicts or vagrants;

(f) the lawful arrest or detention of a person to prevent his effecting an unauthorised entry into the country or of a person against whom action is being taken with a view to deportation or extradition.

2. Everyone who is arrested shall be informed promptly, in a language which he understands, of the reasons for his arrest and of any charge against him.

3. Everyone arrested or detained in accordance with the provisions of paragraph 1(c) of this Article shall be brought promptly before a judge or other officer authorised by law to exercise judicial power and shall be entitled to trial within a reasonable time or to release pending trial. Release may be conditioned by guarantees to appear for trial.

4. Everyone who is deprived of his liberty by arrest or detention shall be entitled to take proceedings by which the lawfulness of his detention shall be decided speedily by a court and his release ordered if the detention is not lawful.

5. Everyone who has been the victim of arrest or detention in contravention of the provisions of this Article shall have an enforceable right to compensation.

Article 6

Right to a fair trial

1. In the determination of his civil rights and obligations or of any criminal charge against him, everyone is entitled to a fair and public hearing within a reasonable time by an independent and impartial tribunal established by law. Judgment shall be pronounced publicly but the press and public may be excluded from all or part of the trial in the interest of morals, public order or national security in a democratic society, where the interests of juveniles or the protection of the private life of the parties so require, or to the extent strictly necessary in the opinion of the court in special circumstances where publicity would prejudice the interests of justice.

2. Everyone charged with a criminal offence shall be presumed innocent until proved guilty according to law.

3. Everyone charged with a criminal offence has the following minimum rights:
   (a) to be informed promptly, in a language which he understands and in detail, of the nature and cause of the accusation against him;
   (b) to have adequate time and facilities for the preparation of his defence;
   (c) to defend himself in person or through legal assistance of his own choosing or, if he has not sufficient means to pay for legal assistance, to be given it free when the interests of justice so require;
   (d) to examine or have examined witnesses against him and to obtain the attendance and examination of witnesses on his behalf under the same conditions as witnesses against him;
   (e) to have the free assistance of an interpreter if he cannot understand or speak the language used in court.

Article 7

No punishment without law

1. No one shall be held guilty of any criminal offence on account of any act or omission which did not constitute a criminal offence under national or international law at the time when it was committed. Nor shall a heavier penalty be imposed than the one that was applicable at the time the criminal offence was committed.

2. This Article shall not prejudice the trial and punishment of any person for any act or omission which, at the time when it was committed, was criminal according to the general principles of law recognised by civilised nations.

Article 8

Right to respect for private and family life

1. Everyone has the right to respect for his private and family life, his home and his correspondence.

2. There shall be no interference by a public authority with the exercise of this right expect such as is in accordance with the law and is necessary in a democratic society in the interests of national security, public safety or the economic well-being of the country, for the prevention of disorder or crime, for the protection of health or morals, or for the protection of the rights and freedoms of others.

Article 9

Freedom of thought, conscience and religion

1. Everyone has the right to freedom of thought, conscience and religion; this right includes freedom to change his religion or belief and freedom, either alone or in community with others and in public or private, to manifest his religion or belief, in worship, teaching, practice and observance.

2. Freedom to manifest one's religion or beliefs shall be subject only to such limitations as are prescribed by law and are necessary in a democratic society in the interests of public safety, for the protection of public order, health or morals, or for the protection of the rights and freedoms of others.

Article 10

Freedom of expression

1. Everyone has the right to freedom of expression. This right shall include freedom to hold opinions and to receive and impart information and ideas without interference by public authority and regardless of frontiers. This Article shall not prevent States from requiring the licensing of broadcasting, television or cinema enterprises.

2. The exercise of these freedoms, since it carries with it duties and responsibilities, may be subject to such formalities, conditions, restrictions or penalties as are prescribed by law and are necessary in a democratic society, in the interests of national security, territorial integrity or public safety, for the prevention of disorder or crime, for the protection of health or morals, for the protection of the reputation or rights of others, for preventing the disclosure of information received in confidence, or for maintaining the authority and impartiality of the judiciary.

Article 11

Freedom of assembly and association

1. Everyone has the right to freedom of peaceful assembly and to freedom of association with others, including the right to form and to join trade unions for the protection of his interests.

2. No restrictions shall be placed on the exercise of these rights other than such as are prescribed by law and are necessary in a democratic society in the interests of national security or public safety, for the prevention of disorder or crime, for the protection of health or morals or for the protection of the rights and freedoms of others. This Article shall not prevent the imposition of lawful restrictions on the exercise of these rights by members of the armed forces, of the police or of the administration of the State.

Article 12

Right to marry

Men and women of marriageable age have the right to marry and to found a family, according to the national laws governing the exercise of this right.

Article 14

Prohibition of discrimination

The enjoyment of the rights and freedoms set forth in this Convention shall be secured without discrimination on any ground such as sex, race, colour, language, religion, political or other opinion, national or social origin, association with a national minority, property, birth or other status.

Article 16

Restrictions on political activity of aliens

Nothing in Articles 10, 11 and 14 shall be regarded as preventing the High Contracting Parties from imposing restrictions on the political activity of aliens.

Article 17

Prohibition of abuse of rights

Nothing in this Convention may be interpreted as implying for any State, group or person any right to engage in any activity or perform any act aimed at the destruction of any of the rights and freedoms set forth herein or at their limitation to a greater extent than is provided for in the Convention.

Article 18

Limitation on use of restrictions on rights

The restrictions permitted under this Convention to the said rights and freedoms shall not be applied for any purpose other than those for which they have been prescribed.

PART II

THE FIRST PROTOCOL

Article 1

Protection of property

Every natural or legal person is entitled to the peaceful enjoyment of his possessions. No one shall be deprived of his possessions except in the public interest and subject to the conditions provided for by law and by the general principles of international law.

The preceding provisions shall not, however, in any way impair the right of a State to enforce such laws as it deems necessary to control the use of property in accordance with the general interest or to secure the payment of taxes or other contributions or penalties.

Article 2

Right to education

No person shall be denied the right to education. In the exercise of any functions which it assumes in relation to education and to teaching, the State shall respect the right of parents to ensure such education and teaching in conformity with their own religious and philosophical convictions.

Article 3

Right to free elections

The High Contracting Parties undertake to hold free elections at reasonable intervals by secret ballot, under conditions which will ensure the free expression of the opinion of the people in the choice of the legislature.

PART III

THE SIXTH PROTOCOL

Article 1

Abolition of the death penalty

The death penalty shall be abolished. No one shall be condemned to such penalty or executed.

Article 2

Death penalty in time of war

A State may make provision in its law for the death penalty in respect of acts committed in time of war or of imminent threat of war; such penalty shall be applied only in the instances laid down in the law and in accordance with its provisions. The State shall communicate to the Secretary General of the Council of Europe the relevant provisions of that law.

Table of Cases

Table of Statutes

Glossary

acceptance	An agreement to the terms of an offer which leads to a binding legal obligation, i.e. a contract.
accusatorial	A system of court proceedings where the two sides contest the issues (contrast with *inquisitorial*).
Act	Of Parliament, statute.
actionable 'per se'	A court action where the plaintiff does not have to show loss, damage or harm to obtain compensation, e.g. an action for trespass to the person.
'actus reus'	The essential element of a crime which must be proved to secure a conviction (as opposed to the mental state of the accused (*mens rea*)).
adversarial	The approach adopted in an *accusatorial* system (see above).
advocate	A person who pleads for another – it could be paid and professional (such as a barrister or solicitor) or it could be a lay advocate, either paid or unpaid.
affidavit	A statement given under oath.
approved social worker (ASW)	A social worker who is qualified for the purposes of the Mental Health Act.
arrestable offence	An offence defined in section 24 of the Police and Criminal Evidence Act 1984 which gives to the citizen the power of arrest in certain circumstances without a warrant.
assault	A threat of unlawful contact (see *trespass to the person*).
bailee	A person to whom goods have been formally handed over, e.g. for safe-keeping or repair.
balance of probabilities	The standard of proof in civil proceedings.
barrister (counsel)	A lawyer qualified to take a case in court and who also gives specialist advice.
battery	An unlawful touching (see *trespass to the person*).
Bench	Magistrates, Justices of the Peace.
Bolam test	The test applied by the courts (taking its name from the case of *Bolam* v. *Friern Hospital Management Committee*) on the standard of care expected of a professional in cases of alleged negligence, i.e. that of 'the ordinary skilled man exercising and professing to have that special skill'.
burden of proof	The duty of a party to litigation, usually the plaintiff, to establish the facts (or in criminal proceedings the duty of the prosecution to establish both the *actus reus* and

	the *mens rea*). In special circumstances it can shift so that the defendant has to disprove the facts alleged.
cause of action	The facts that entitle a person to sue.
'certiorari'	An action taken to challenge an administrative or judicial decision (literally – to make more certain).
civil action	Proceedings brought in the civil courts.
civil wrong	An act or omission which can be pursued in the civil courts by the person who has suffered the wrong (see *torts*).
claim form	See *writ*.
claimant	See *plaintiff*.
committal proceedings	Initial hearings before the magistrates to decide if a person should be tried in the Crown court.
common law	Law derived from the decisions of judges – case law, judge made law.
conditional fee system	A system whereby client and lawyer can agree that payment of fees is dependent upon the outcome of the court action.
conditions	Terms of a contract (see *warranties*).
consideration	The money or money's worth in other goods or services offered and given as one side of the bargain in a contract.
constructive knowledge	Knowledge which is deemed to be deduced from the circumstances.
continuous service	The length of time which an employee must have worked with the employer in order to be entitled to receive certain statutory or contractual rights.
contract	An agreement enforceable in law.
*contract **for** services*	An agreement, enforceable in law, whereby one party provides services (not being employment) in return for payment or other consideration from the other.
*contract **of** service*	A contract of employment.
coroner	A person appointed to hold an inquiry (inquest) into a death in unexpected or unusual circumstances.
counter-offer	A response to an offer which suggests different terms and is therefore counted as a new offer not an acceptance.
criminal wrong	An act or omission which can be pursued in the criminal courts.
damages	A sum of money awarded by a court as compensation for a *tort* or breach of *contract*.
declaration	A ruling by the court, setting out the legal situation.
discovery	The process in a civil action whereby the parties each disclose to the other side all the relevant documents in their possession, whether or not they are prejudicial to their own case.
dissenting judgment	A judge who disagrees with the decision of the majority of his or her fellow judges hearing the case.
distinguished (of cases)	The rules of *precedent* require judges to follow decisions of judges in previous cases. However in some circumstances it is possible to come to a different decision because the facts of the earlier case are not comparable

	to the case now being heard, and therefore the earlier decision can be 'distinguished'.
'ex gratia'	Of payment offered to a claimant – given as a matter of favour, i.e. without admission of liability.
'ex parte'	An application made to the court (usually on an urgent matter) without the other side being present or represented.
expert witness	Evidence given by a person whose general opinion based on training or experience is relevant to issues in dispute.
frustration (of contracts)	The ending of a contract by operation of law, because of the existence of an event not contemplated by the parties when they made the contract, e.g. imprisonment, death, blindness.
'Re F' ruling	When professionals act in the best interests of an incompetent person who is incapable of giving consent, they do not act unlawfully if they follow the accepted standard of care according to the *Bolam test*.
guardian 'ad litem'	A person with a social work and child care background who is appointed to ensure that the court is fully informed of the relevant facts which relate to a child or mentally incompetent adult, and that the wishes and feelings of the child are clearly established. The appointment is made from a panel set up by the local authority.
'habeas corpus'	The proceedings commenced by a writ whereby an organisation or official who has another person in their custody is required to produce that person.
hearsay	Evidence of facts which have been learnt from another person rather than observed directly.
hierarchy	The recognised status of courts, which results in lower courts following the decisions of higher courts (see *precedent*). Thus decisions of the House of Lords must be followed by all lower courts, unless they can be *distinguished* (see above).
indictment	A written accusation against a person, charging him with a serious crime, triable by jury.
informal	Of a patient who has entered hospital without any statutory requirements.
injunction	An order of the court restraining a person from taking a specified action or (more rarely) requiring them to take action.
inquest	The procedure whereby the *coroner* investigates an unexpected or unusual death to establish its cause.
inquisitorial	A system of justice whereby the truth is revealed by an inquiry into the facts conducted by the judge, e.g. coroner's court hearings.
invitation to treat	The early stages in negotiating a contract, e.g. an advertisement, displayed goods or a letter expressing interest. An invitation to treat will often precede an *offer* which when accepted leads to the formation of an agreement which, if there is *consideration* and an

	intention to create legal relations will be a binding *contract*.
judicial review	An application to the High Court for a judicial or administrative decision to be reviewed and an appropriate order made: e.g. a *declaration* or '*certiorari*'.
Justice of the Peace	A lay *magistrate*, i.e. not legally qualified, who hears summary (minor) offences and sometimes indictable (serious) offences in the Magistrates' Courts, sitting in a group of three (*The Bench*).
litigation	Civil proceedings.
magistrate	A person who hears summary (minor) offences or indictable offences which can be heard in the Magistrates' Court.
'mens rea'	The mental element in a crime (contrasted with '*actus reus*').
next friend	A person who brings a court action on behalf of a minor.
offer	A proposal made by a party which if accepted can lead to a *contract*. It often follows an *invitation to treat*.
ombudsman	A Commissioner (e.g. health, Local Government, etc.) appointed by the Government to hear complaints.
pedagogic	Of the science of teaching.
personal representative	The person, usually appointed in the deceased's will, who deals with their affairs after death.
plaintiff	One who brings an action in the civil courts; claimant.
plea in mitigation	A formal statement to the court aimed at reducing the sentence to be pronounced by the judge.
practice directions	Guidance issued by the head of the court to which they relate on the procedure to be followed.
precedent	A decision which may have to be followed in a subsequent court hearing (see also *hierarchy*).
'prima facie'	At first sight, or sufficient evidence brought by one part to require the other party to provide a defence.
privilege	In relation to evidence – being able to refuse to disclose it to the court.
privity of contract	The relationship which exists between parties as the result of a legal agreement.
proof	Evidence which secures the establishment of a plaintiff's or prosecution's (or the defendant's) case.
prosecution	The pursuing of criminal offences in court.
'quantum'	The amount of compensation, or the monetary value of a claim.
reasonable doubt	To secure a conviction in criminal proceedings the prosecution must establish the guilt of the accused beyond reasonable doubt (see *balance of probabilities*).
rescission	Where a contract is ended by the order of a court, or by the cancellation of the contract by one party entitled in law to do so.
solicitor	A lawyer who is qualified and on the register held by the Law Society.
statute law (statutory)	Law made by Acts of Parliament.
stipendiary magistrate	A legally qualified magistrate who is paid (i.e. has a stipend) (see *Justice of the Peace*).

strict liability	Liability for a criminal act where the mental element (*mens rea*) does not have to be proved and in civil proceedings liability without establishing negligence.
'subpoena'	An order of the court requiring a person to appear as a witness (*subpoena ad testificandum*) or to bring records/documents to the court (*subpoena duces tecum*).
summary offence	A lesser offence which can only be heard by magistrates.
summary judgment	A procedure whereby when the facts are obvious, e.g. a bounced cheque, the plaintiff can obtain judgment without the defendant being permitted to defend the action.
tort	A civil wrong excluding breach of contract. It covers negligence, trespass (to the person, goods or land), nuisance, breach of statutory duty and defamation.
trespass to the person	A wrongful direct interference with another person. Harm does not have to be proved.
'ultra vires'	Outside the powers given by law (e.g. of a statutory body or company).
vicarious liability	The liability of an employer for the wrongful acts of an employee committed whilst in the course of employment.
'volenti non fit injuria'	To the willing there is no wrong – the voluntary assumption of risk.
ward of court	A minor is placed under the protection of the High Court, which assumes responsibility for him or her, and all decisions relating to his or her care must be made in accordance with the directions of the court.
warranties	Terms of a contract which are considered to be less important than the terms described as *conditions*. Breach of a condition entitles the innocent party to see the contract as ended, i.e. repudiated by the other party, breach of warranty only entitles the innocent party to claim damages.
without prejudice	Without detracting from or without disadvantage to. The use of the phrase prevents the other party using the information to the prejudice of the one providing it.
writ	A form of written command, e.g. the document which commences civil proceedings. After 26 April 1999 this will be known as a claim form.

Further Reading

Physiotherapy books

Bell, Lesley *Carefully: A Guide for Home Care Assistants* Age Concern (1993)

Beresford, Sue *Motor Neurone Disease* Chapman and Hall (1995)

Bobarth, Berta *Adult Hemiplegia: Evaluation and Treatment* 2nd edn. Heinemann Medical Books (1987)

Compton, Ann & Ashwin, Mary *Community Care for Health Professionals* Butterworth-Heinemann (1992)

Everett, Tina, Dennis, Maureen & Ricketts, Eirian (eds.) *Physiotherapy in Mental Health* Butterworth-Heinemann (1995)

Forster, Angeal & Palastanga, Nigel *Clayton's Electrotherapy Theory and Practice* 8th edn. Baillière Tindall (1981)

Hicks, Carolyn *Research for Physiotherapists: project design and analysis* Churchill Livingstone (1995)

Higgs, Joy & Jones, Mark (eds.) *Clinical Reasoning in the Health Professions* Butterworth-Heinemann (1995)

Hutson, Michael A. *Back Pain Recognition and Management* Butterworth-Heinemann (1993)

Hutson, Michael A. *Work Related Upper Limb Disorders: Recognition and Management* Butterworth-Heinemann (1997)

Jones, Robert J. (ed) *Management in Physiotherapy* Radcliffe Medical Press in conjunction with CSP (1991)

Lynch, Mary & Grisogono, ? *Strokes and Head Injuries* John Murray (1991)

Manelstam, Michael (compiler) *Equipment for Disability* 3rd edn. Disabled Living Foundation and Jessica Kingsley Publishers Ltd (1993)

Sagar, Harvey *Parkinson's Disease* Macdonald Optima (1991)

Sim, Julius *Ethical Decision Making in Therapy Practice* Butterworth-Heinemann Oxford (1997)

Law books

Note: *Most law books are regularly re-written – always ask for the most recent edition*

Clarkson, C.M.V. & Keating, H.M. *Criminal Law Text and Materials* Sweet and Maxwell

Dimond, B.C. *Legal Aspects of Nursing* Prentice Hall

Dimond, B.C. *Legal Aspects of Occupational Therapy* Blackwell Science

Dimond, B.C. *Legal Aspects of Child Health Care* Mosby

Dimond, B.C. *Patients Rights, Responsibilities and the Nurse* Central Health Studies Quay Publishing

Dimond, B.C. *Legal Aspects of Midwifery* Books for Midwives Press

Dimond, B.D. & Barker, F. *Mental Health Law for Nurses* Blackwell Science

Ellis, Norman *Employing Staff* British Medical Journal

Hoggett, Brenda *Mental Health Law* Sweet and Maxwell

Hurwitz, Brian *Clinical Guidelines and the Law* Radcliffe Medical Press (1998)

Ingman, Terence *English Legal Process* Blackstone Press

James *Introduction to English Law* Butterworths

Jones, Richard *Mental Health Act Manual* Sweet and Maxwell

Kidner, Richard *Blackstone's Statutes on Employment Law* Blackstones

Kloss, Diana *Occupational Health Law* Blackwell Science

Knight, Bernard *Legal Aspects of Medical Practice* Churchill Livingstone

Miers, David & Page, Alan *Legislation* Sweet and Maxwell

Morgan, Derek and Lee, Robert G. *Human Fertilisation and Embryology Act 1990* Blackstone Press

Selwyn's Law of Employment Butterworth

Smith and Keenan *English Law* Sweet and Maxwell

Speller's Law Relating to Hospitals (ed John Finch) Chapman and Hall Medical

Steiner, Josephine *Textbook on EC Law* Blackstone Press

Street on Torts (ed Margaret Brazier) Butterworths Tolley

Thompson, Robin & Thompson, Brian
Dismissal: A basic introduction to your legal rights
Equal Pay
Health and Safety at Work
Injuries at Work and work related illnesses
Women at work

All published by Robin Thompson and Partners and Brian Thompson and Partners London.

White, Richard, Carr, Paul & Lowe, Nigel *A Guide to the Children Act 1989* Butterworths

Health and Safety

Guidance for health care worker's protection against infection with HIV and Hepatitis The Committee of Expert Advisory Group on AIDS, HMSO (1994)

Immunisation against infectious disease Department of Health, Welsh Office and Scottish Home and Health Department, HMSO (1990)

Management of Health and Safety at Work: approved code of practice Health and Safety Commission, HMSO (1992)

Manual Handling Regulations: approved code of practice Health and Safety Commission, HMSO (1992)

Guidelines on Manual Handling in the Health Services Health and Safety Commission, HMSO (1992)

Useful Addresses

Action for Sick Children
Argyle House
300 Kingston Road
Wimbledon Chase
London SW20 8LX
Tel 0181 542 4848
Fax 0181 542 2424
e-mail action-for-sick-children-
    edu@msn.com

**Action for the Victims of Medical
    Accidents**
44 High Street
Croydon
Surrey CR0 1YB
Tel 0181 686 8333
Fax 0181 667 9065

Age Concern
Astral House
1268 London Road
London SW16 4ER
Tel 0181 679 8000
Fax 0181 765 7211
www.ace.org.uk

Alzheimer's Disease Society
Gordon House
10 Greencoat Place
London SW1P 1PH
Tel 0171 306 0606
Fax 0171 306 0808
Helpline 0845 300 0336
e-mail info@alzheimers.org.uk
www.alzheimers.org.uk

Association for Residential Care
ARC House
Marsden Street
Chesterfield
Derbyshire S40 1JY
e-mail arc@btinternet.com

**Association of Community Health
    Councils**
30 Drayton Park
London N5 1PB
Tel 0171 609 8405
Fax 0171 70 1152
e-mail achew@compuserve. com

**Association of Chartered
    Physiotherapists in Sports Medicine**
c/o 81 Heol West Plas
Coity
Bridgend
Glamorgan CF35 6BA

**Association of Paediatric Chartered
    Physiotherapists**
c/o Church Cottage
East Hagbourne
Didcot
Oxfordshire OX11 9LQ

Barnardo's
Tanners Lane
Barkingside
Ilford
Essex IG6 1QG
Tel 0181 550 8822
Fax 0181 551 6870
www.barnardos.org.uk

British Association for Service to the Elderly
The Guildford Institute
Ward Street
Guildford
Surrey GU1 4LH
Tel 01483 451036
Fax 01483 451034
e-mail base@intonet.co.uk
www.base.org.uk

British Association of Sport and Medicine
Membership Office
12 Greenside Avenue
Frodsham
Cheshire WA6 7SA
Tel and fax 01928 732961
e-mail basmoffice@compuserve.com

British Association of Social Workers
16 Kent Street
Birmingham B5 6RD
Tel 0121 622 3911
Fax 0121 622 4860
e-mail 106737.1414@compuserve.com
www.basw.demon.co.uk

British Colostomy Association
15 Station Road
Reading RG1 1LG
Tel 0118 939 1537
Fax 0118 956 9095
Freephone 0800 328 4257
e-mail sue@bcass.org.uk
www.bcass.org.uk

British Diabetic Association
10 Queen Anne Street
London W1M 0BD
Tel 0171 323 1531
Fax 0171 637 3644
e-mail bda@diabetes.org.uk
www.diabetes.org.uk

British Epilepsy Association
Anstey House
40 Hanover Square
Leeds LS3 1BE
Tel 0113 243 9393
Fax 0113 242 8804
e-mail epilepsy@bea.org.uk
www.epilepsy.org.uk

British Heart Foundation
14 Fitzhardinge Street
London W1H 4DH
Tel 0171 935 0185
Fax 0171 486 5820

British Homoeopathic Association
27a Devonshire Street
London W1N 1RJ
Tel 0171 935 2163

British Institute of Learning Disabilities (BILD)
Wolverhampton Road
Kidderminster
Worcs DY10 3PP
Tel 01562 850251
Fax 01562 851970
e-mail bild@bild.demon.co.uk
www.bild.org.uk

British Red Cross
9 Grosvenor Crescent
London SW1X 7EJ
Tel 0171 235 5454
Fax 0171 245 6315
www.redcross.org.uk

Cancer Relief Macmillan Fund
15/19 Britten Street
London SW3 3TZ
Tel 0171 351 7811
Fax 0171 376 8098
www.macmillan.org.uk

Carers National Association
20–25 Glasshouse Yard
London EC1A 4JT
Tel 0171 490 8818
Fax 0171 490 8824
Carers Line 0171 490 8898
e-mail internet@ukcarers.org.uk
www.carersuk.demon.co.jk

Centre for Policy on Ageing
25–31 Ironmonger Row
London EC1V 3QP
Tel 0171 253 1787
Fax 0171 490 4206
e-mail cpa@cpa.org.uk
www.cpa.org.uk

Chartered Society of Physiotherapy
14 Bedford Row
London WC1R 4ED
Tel 0171 306 6666
Fax 0171 306 6611

Child Accident Prevention Trust
4th Floor Clerk's Court
18–20 Farringdon Lane
London EC1R 3HA
Tel 0171 608 3828
Fax 0171 608 3674
e-mail safe@capt.demon.co.uk

Child Growth Foundation
2 Mayfield Avenue
Chiswick
London W4 1PW
Tel 0181 995 0257/0181 994 7625
Fax 0181 995 9075

Children's Legal Centre
University of Essex
Wivenhoe Park
Colchester
Essex CO4 3SQ
Tel 01206 873820
Fax 01206 874026
e-mail clc@essex.ac.uk
www2.essex.ac.uk/clc

College of Occupational Therapists
106–114 Borough High Street
London SE1 1LB
Tel 0171 357 6480
Fax 0171 450 2299
www.cot.co.uk

College of Speech and Language Therapists
7 Bath Place
Rivington Street
London EC2A 3SU
Tel 0171 613 3855
Fax 0171 613 3854
e-mail info@rcslt.org
www.rcslt.org

Council for Professions Supplementary to Medicine
Park House
184 Kennington Park Road
London SE11 4BU
Tel 0171 582 0866
Fax 0171 820 9684
www.cpsm.co.uk

Continuing Care at Home Association
54 Glasshouse Lane
Countess Wear
Exeter EX2 7BU

Counsel and Care for the Elderly
Twyman House
16 Bonny Street
London NW1 9PG
Tel 0845 300 7585

Dance UK
23 Crisp Road
London W6 9RL
Tel 0181 741 1932
Fax 0181 748 0186
e-mail danceuk@easynet.co.uk]

Data Protection Register
Wycliffe House
Water Lane
Wilmslow
Cheshire SK9 5AF

DVLA
Longview Road
Morriston
Swansea
Tel 01792 772151

Equal Opportunities Commission
Overseas House
Quay Street
Manchester M3 3HN
Tel 0161 833 9244
Fax 0161 835 1657

Family Welfare Association
501–505 Kingsland Road
Dalston
London E8 4AU
Tel 0171 254 6251
Fax 0171 249 5443

Family Welfare Association of Manchester
Gaddum House
6 Great Jackson Street
Manchester M15 4AX
Tel 0161 834 6069
Fax 0161 839 8573

Headway
(National Head Injuries Association)
7 King Edward Court
King Edward Street
Nottingham NG1 1EW
Tel 0115 924 0800
Fax 0115 924 0432
e-mail inquiries@headway.org.uk
www.headway.org.uk

Health and Safety Commission
(HSE Books)
PO Box 1999
Sudbury
Suffolk CO10 6FS
Tel 01787 881165
Fax 01787 313995
www.open.gov.uk/hse/hsehome.htm

Help the Aged
16–18 St James's Walk
Clerkenwell Green
London EC1R 0BE
Tel 0171 253 0253
Fax 0171 250 4474
e-mail info@helptheaged.org.uk
www.helptheaged.org.uk

Help the Hospices
34–44 Britannia Street
London WC1X 9JG
Tel 0171 278 5668
Fax 0171 278 1021
e-mail hth@helpthehospices.org.uk
www.helpthehospices.org.uk

Independent Healthcare Association
22 Little Russell Street
London WC1A 2HT
Tel 0171 430 0537
Fax 0171 242 2681

International Stress Management Association (UK)
Division of Psychology
South Bank University
103 Borough Road
London SE1 0AA
Tel 0700 0780 430
Fax 01992 426673
e-mail stress@isma.org.uk
www.stress.org.uk/isma

The Manipulation Association of Chartered Physiotherapists
c/o Dept of Physiotherapy
University of Hertfordshire
College Lane
Hatfield
Herts AL10 9AB

Marie Curie Memorial Foundation
(Marie Curie Cancer Care)
28 Belgrave Square
London SW1X 8QG
Tel 0171 235 3325
Fax 0171 823 2380
www.mariecurie.org.uk

Medical Devices Agency
(Adverse Incident Centre)
Hannibal House
Elephant and Castle
London SE1 6TQ
Tel 0171 972 8000
e-mail mail@medical-devices.gov.uk
www.medical-devices.gov.uk

MENCAP (see Royal Society of Mentally
  Handicapped Children and Adults)

Mental Aftercare Association
25 Bedford Square
London WC1B 3HW
Tel 0171 436 6194
Fax 0171 637 1980

Mental Health Foundation
20–21 Cornwall Terrace
London NW1 4QL
Tel 0171 535 7400
Fax 0171 535 7474
e-mail mhf@mentalhealth.org.uk
www.mentalhealth.org.uk

Migraine Action Association
178a High Road
West Byfleet
Surrey KT14 7ED
Tel 01932 353468
Fax 01932 351257
e-mail info@migraine.org.uk
www.migraine.org.uk

Migraine Trust
45 Great Ormond Street
London WC1N 3HZ
Tel 0171 831 4818
Fax 0171 831 5174

MIND
National Association for Mental Health
Granta House
15–19 Broadway
Stratford
London E15 4BQ
Tel 0181 519 2122
Fax 0181 522 1725
e-mail info@mind.org.uk

**Multiple Sclerosis Society of Great
  Britain and Northern Ireland**
25 Effie Road
London SW6 1EE
Tel 0171 736 6267
Fax 0171 736 9861
e-mail info@mssociety.org.uk
www.mssociety.org.uk

**Muscular Dystrophy Group of Great
  Britain and Northern Ireland**
7–11 Prescott Place
London SW4 6BS
Tel 0171 720 8055
Fax 0171 498 0670
e-mail muscular-
  dystrophy@gpo.sonnet.co.uk
www.sonnet.co.uk/muscular-dystrophy

**National Association for Patient
  Participation**
PO Box 999
Nuneaton
CV11 5ZD
Tel and fax 0151 630 5786

National Association for Staff Support
9 Caradon Close
Woking
Surrey GU21 3DU
Tel and fax 01483 771599
e-mail nassupport@compuserve.com

**National Association of Health
  Authorities and Trusts**
see NHS Confederation

National Autistic Society
393 City Road
London EC1V 1AG
Tel 0171 833 2299
Fax 0171 833 9666
www.oneworld.org./autism–uk

**National Council for Hospice and
  Specialist Palliative Care Services**
7th Floor, 1 Great Cumberland Place
London W1H 7AL
Tel 0171 723 1639
Fax 0171 723 5380
e-mail inquiries@hospice/spc/
  council.org.uk

National Council of Voluntary Organisations
Regent's Wharf
8 All Saints Street
London N1 9RL
Tel 0171 713 6161
Fax 0171 713 6300
e-mail ncvo@ncvo-vol.org.uk
www.ncvo-vol.org.uk

National Schizophrenia Fellowship
28 Castle Street
Kingston-upon-Thames
Surrey KT1 1SS
Tel 0181 547 3937
Fax 0181 547 3862
e-mail info@nsf.org.uk
www.nsf.org.uk

National Sports Medicine Institute
c/o The Medical College of
St Bartholomew's Hospital
Charterhouse Square
London EC1M 6BQ
Tel 0171 251 0583
Fax 0171 251 0774
e-mail library@nsmi.org.uk
www.nsmi.org.uk

NHS Confederation
Birmingham Research Park
Vincent Drive
Birmingham B15 2SQ
Tel 0121 471 4444
Fax 0121 414 1120
www.nhsconfed.net

PhysioFirst: The Organisation of Chartered Physiotherapists in Private Practice
8 Weston Chambers
Weston Road
Southend-on-Sea
Essex SS1 1AT
Tel 01702 392 124
Fax 01702 392 125
physiofirst.org.uk

Parkinson's Disease Society
215 Vauxhall Bridge Road
London SW1V 1EJ
Tel 0171 931 8080
Fax 0171 233 9908
www.shef.ac.uk/misc/groups/epda/home.html

Princess Royal Trust for Carers
142 Minories
London EC3N 1LB
Tel 0171 480 7787

Public Trust Office, Protection Division
Stewart House
24 Kingsway
London WC2B 6JX
Tel 0171 644 7000

Rainbow Trust
Claire House
Bridge Street
Leatherhead
Surrey KT22 8BZ
Tel 01372 363488
Fax 01372 363101

Rehabilitation Services and Supplies Association (RSSA)
Box 100 Greyfriars
Hill Foot Lane
Burnbridge
Harrogate HG3 1NT

Richmond Fellowship for Community Mental Health
8 Addison Road
Kensington
London W14 8DL
Tel 0171 603 6373
Fax 0171 602 8652

Registered Nursing Homes Association
Calthorpe House
Hagley Road
Edgbaston
Birmingham B16 8QY
Tel 0121 454 2511
Fax 0121 454 0932

The Relatives Association
c/o Counsel and Care (see above)

**Royal Association for Disability and
    Rehabilitation (RADAR)**
Unit 12, City Forum
250 City Road
London EC1V 8AF
Tel 0171 250 3222
Fax 0171 250 0212
www.radar.org.uk

**Royal Society for Mentally
    Handicapped Children and Adults
    (MENCAP)**
Mencap National Centre
123 Golden Lane
London EC1Y 0RT
Tel 0171 454 0454
Fax 0171 608 3254

Samaritans
10 The Grove
Slough
Berks SL1 1QP
Tel 0345 909090 (linkline)
www.samaritans.org.uk

Shaftesbury Society
16 Kingston Road
London SW19 1JZ
Tel 0181 239 5555
Fax 0181 239 5580
e-mail reception@shaftesburysoc.org.uk
www.shaftesburysoc.org.uk

Spinal Injuries Association
76 St James's Lane
London N10 3DF
Tel 0181 444 2121
Fax 0181 444 3761
e-mail sia@spinali.demon.co.uk
jgrweb.com.sia

Stroke Association
Stroke House
Whitecross Street
London EC1Y 8JJ
Tel 0171 490 7999
Fax 0171 490 2686
www.stroke.org.uk

Terrence Higgins Trust
52–54 Gray's Inn Road
London WC1X 8JU
Tel 0171 242 1010 (helpline, noon–10pm)
0171 831 0330 (admin)
0171 405 2381 (legal line, Mon & Wed
    7–9pm)
www.tht.org.uk.

Index